C0-BXP-722

A.A.O.S.:

Symposium on

The Spine

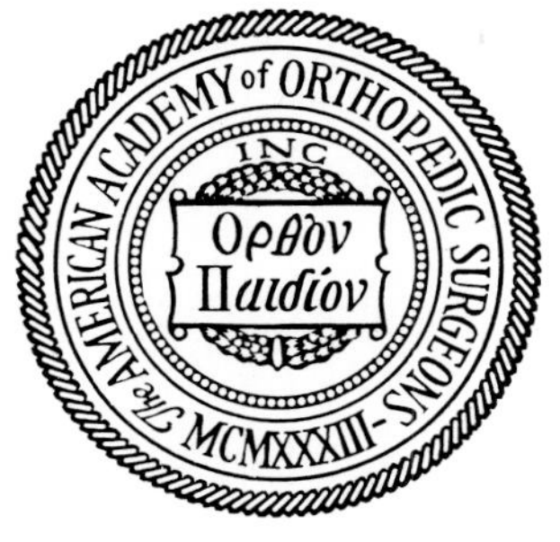

American Academy
of
Orthopaedic Surgeons

Symposium on The Spine

Cleveland, Ohio
November, 1967

With 558 illustrations

Saint Louis
The C. V. Mosby Company
1969

Printed in the United States of America

Standard Book Number 8016-0007-3

Library of Congress Catalog Card Number 74-78338

Distributed in Great Britain by Henry Kimpton, London

Contributors

Walter P. Blount, M.D.

Emeritus Professor of Orthopaedic Surgery, Marquette University School of Medicine; Consulting Staff, Milwaukee Children's Hospital and Milwaukee County Hospital; Staff, Columbia Hospital, Milwaukee, Wisconsin

Mark B. Coventry, M.D.

Professor of Orthopaedic Surgery, Mayo Graduate School of Medicine: Head of Section of Orthopaedic Surgery, Mayo Clinic, Rochester, Minnesota

Victor H. Frankel, M.D.

Associate Professor of Orthopaedic Surgery, Case Western Reserve University; Director, Biomechanics Laboratory, Division of Orthopaedic Surgery; Associate Orthopaedist, Department of Surgery, University Hospitals; Associate Orthopaedist, Rainbow Hospital; Chief, Orthopaedic Surgery, Veterans Hospital, Cleveland, Ohio

J. Neill Garber, M.D., Med. Sc.D.

Professor of Orthopaedic Surgery, Indiana University School of Medicine; Attending Orthopaedic Surgeon, Methodist and Community Hospitals, Indianapolis, Indiana

J. Leonard Goldner, M.D.

Professor and Chairman, Division of Orthopaedic Surgery, Duke University Medical Center, Durham, North Carolina

Louis A. Goldstein, M.D.

Clinical Professor of Orthopaedic Surgery, University of Rochester Medical Center; Senior Attending Orthopaedic Surgeon, Strong Memorial Hospital; Consulting Orthopaedic Surgeon, Genesee Hospital, Rochester, New York; Consulting Orthopaedic Surgeon, Veterans Hospital, Batavia, New York

Scott R. Inkley, M.D.

Associate Clinical Professor of Medicine, School of Medicine, Case Western Reserve University, Cleveland, Ohio

Stanley F. Katz, M.D.

Resident in Orthopaedic Surgery, Barnes Hospital, St. Louis, Missouri

Ian Macnab, M.B., Ch.B., F.R.C.S.(Eng.), F.R.C.S.(C)

Assistant Professor of Surgery, University of Toronto; Chief of Division of Orthopaedic Surgery, The Wellesley Hospital, Toronto, Canada

Donald E. McCollum, M.D.

Associate Professor of Orthopaedic Surgery and Chief of Orthopaedics, Affiliated Veterans Administration Hospital, Duke University Medical Center, Durham, North Carolina

John H. Moe, M.D.

Professor and Director, Department of Orthopaedic Surgery, University of Minnesota Hospitals, Minneapolis, Minnesota; Chief of Staff, Gillette State Hospital for Crippled Children, St. Paul, Minnesota

Fred C. Reynolds, M.D.

Professor of Orthopaedic Surgery, Washington University School of Medicine, St. Louis, Missouri

Albert C. Schmidt, M.D.

Professor of Orthopaedic Surgery, Marquette University School of Medicine; Attending Staff, Columbia, Lutheran, and Milwaukee Children's Hospitals; Consulting Staff, Milwaukee General Hospital, Milwaukee, Wisconsin

George E. Spencer, Jr., M.D.

Associate Professor of Orthopaedic Surgery, Case Western Reserve University School of Medicine, Cleveland, Ohio

Richard N. Stauffer, M.D.

Resident in Orthopaedic Surgery, Mayo Graduate School of Medicine, Rochester, Minnesota

James R. Urbaniak, M.D.

Resident in Orthopaedic Surgery, Duke University Medical Center, Durham, North Carolina

Leon L. Wiltse, M.D.

Assistant Clinical Professor of Orthopaedic Surgery, University of California at Irvine, College of Medicine, Long Beach, California

Foreword

This *Symposium on the Spine* has been developed from the Course on the Spine organized and presented by the Committee on Injuries, American Academy of Orthopaedic Surgeons, which was given in Cleveland in November, 1967.

Committee on Publications

Fred C. Reynolds, *Chairman*
George T. Aitken
Mark B. Coventry
Charles V. Heck

Preface

The source material for this monograph has been taken from the presentations made by the faculty of the continuing education course entitled "Current Concepts on Management of Disease and Injury Involving the Spine."

Held in Cleveland, Ohio, on November 27 to 29, 1967, it was sponsored by the Committee on Injuries, the American Academy of Orthopaedic Surgeons, and by the Department of Orthopaedic Surgery, Case Western Reserve University School of Medicine.

Over 300 practicing physicians and residents from 42 states attended the course. The following specialties were represented: orthopaedic surgery, neurosurgery, neurology, general surgery, internal medicine, physiatrics, radiology, and general practice.

The Cleveland Course Program chairman was Dr. George E. Spencer, Jr., Associate Professor of Orthopaedic Surgery, Case Western Reserve University School of Medicine. The members of his committee were Dr. William A. Mast and Dr. Robert W. Widow. The Advisory Committee included Dr. Charles S. Herndon and Dr. Frederick C. Robbins.

The Program Committee developed the curriculum, selected the faculty, and arranged the details necessary to stage this 3½-day program. Their preparation was flawless and they richly deserve the words of praise sent in by numerous members of the audience.

The faculty included most of the authorities whose contributions on the "back" have influenced current diagnostic and therapeutic trends. Their presentations were of superior quality, and their early response to the request for detailed manuscripts has made this publication possible.

The Committee on Publications of the American Academy of Orthopaedic Surgeons recognized the educational value of reproducing this material. Acting on the recommendation of the Executive Committee of the Academy, the Publications Committee assumed responsibility for attending to the details of editing and organizing the papers. Their great skill in doing so has made this publication possible.

The monograph is intended both to reinforce the knowledge gained by those who attended this course and to serve as an excellent review of "back problems" for all other interested physicians.

Committee on Injuries
Walter A. Hoyt, Jr., *Chairman*

George N. Aldredge, Jr.
Frank H. Bassett III
Rocco A. Calandruccio
Rolla D. Campbell
C. Robert Clark
Bruce F. Claussen
Charles F. Gregory
J. Paul Harvey
James A. Heckman
Richard E. King
Peter LaMotte
John D. Leidholt
Norman D. Logan
Wood W. Lovell
William R. MacAusland, Jr.
Virgil R. May, Jr.
Charles S. Neer II
Byron J. Park
Herbert E. Pedersen
Homer C. Pheasant
Charles A. Rockwood, Jr.
Augusto Sarmiento
George E. Spencer, Jr.
William S. Stryker
Robert E. Wells
Howell E. Wiggins

Contents

1. Biomechanics of the spine (Victor H. Frankel, M.D.), 1

2. Acceleration-extension injuries of the cervical spine (Ian Macnab, M.B., Ch.B.), 10

3. Fracture and fracture-dislocation of the cervical spine (J. Neill Garber, M.D., Med. Sc.D.), 18

4. Lumbosacral strain and instability (Leon L. Wiltse, M.D.), 54

5. Herniated lumbar intervertebral disc (Fred C. Reynolds, M.D., and Stanley F. Katz, M.D.), 84

6. Pathogenesis of symptoms in discogenic low back pain (Ian Macnab, M.B., Ch.B.), 97

7. Anterior disc excision and interbody spine fusion for chronic low back pain (J. Leonard Goldner, M.D., Donald E. McCollum, M.D., and James R. Urbaniak, M.D.), 111

8. The multiply operated back (Mark B. Coventry, M.D., and Richard N. Stauffer, M.D.), 132

9. Spondylolisthesis: classification and etiology (Leon L. Wiltse, M.D.), 143

10. Osteoporosis and fractures of the spine (George E. Spencer, Jr., M.D.), 168

11. Pulmonary function in scoliosis (Scott R. Inkley, M.D.), 180

12. Nonoperative treatment of scoliosis (Walter P. Blount, M.D.), 188

13. Methods and technique of evaluating idiopathic scoliosis (John H. Moe, M.D.), 196

14. Turnbuckle and Risser localizer casts in the correction of scoliosis: selection of patients and techniques (Louis A. Goldstein, M.D.), 241

15. Concave rib resection and ligament release for correction of idiopathic thoracic scoliosis (Louis A. Goldstein, M.D.), 254

16. Osteotomy of the fused scoliotic spine and use of halo traction apparatus (Albert C. Schmidt, M.D.), 265

A.A.O.S.:

Symposium on

The Spine

1. Biomechanics of the spine

Victor H. Frankel, M.D.

Emphasis has been placed on the pathomechanics of the spine as a cause of disability by man for many bipedal generations. Such terms as "backbreaking toil" are common to many languages. Osler has stated "Always listen to the patient; he is trying to tell you what is wrong." Perhaps this also applies to why it is wrong. Man has observed the effects of forces and motion on the spine and has intuitively developed a cause and effect relationship that has been established not only in the medical texts but also in our compensation and liability laws. The industrial and scientific revolution has multiplied the varieties of ways in which the spine may be injured, but it has also offered us techniques and tools for investigating the normal and pathomechanics of the spine.

It is the purpose of this paper to establish an outline or schema for the study of the biomechanics of the spine. It is hoped that this outline will serve as a focus for reading, thinking, and investigations on the subject of the mechanics of the spine. Studies of the pathomechanics of the spine have been performed for the past century and have kept pace with the introduction of pertinent engineering techniques and concepts. We change our ideas of the mechanics of the spine not because the spine has changed but because refined methods of analysis not available to our predecessors are available for our use. In the past thirty years medical-engineering teams have studied the various aspects of the mechanical problems of the spine. Exchange of ideas and laboratory personnel in a free manner has contributed greatly to the development of techniques and utilization of research data. It is my hope that this outline will allow the orthopaedist to develop an idea of the various aspects of research that must be performed and to categorize our present knowledge. This paper is then not an exhaustive review of past and current work in the field, with value judgments, but an attempt to show what must be known if one is to be knowledgeable of the biomechanics of the spine.

The spine carries loads and is subjected to forces. The forces have external effects causing accelerations, and internal effects producing states of stress and strain in the structure. The spine is flexible with motion taking place at many levels and in several different kinds of joints. Like other earthly mechanical structures, its behavior during motion and under load must follow certain well-defined laws of physics. The situation is further complicated by the fact that the biological tissues making up the spine exhibit nonlinear viscoelastic anisotropic behavior.

A study of the biomechanics of any region of the body requires development of knowledge in four areas: (1) the mechanical properties of tissues, (2) the mechanical properties of substructures, (3) motion between substructures, and (4) the effect of loading on structures.

Mechanical properties of tissues

The spine contains tissues like those found generally throughout the body; cortical and cancellous bone, ligaments, striated muscles, articular cartilage, and synovium have their counterparts in other regions of the body. Studies performed on these generally distributed tissues may be applied to such tissues as they occur in the spine.[3, 8, 29, 31]

In addition, the spine contains specialized tissue not found elsewhere in the body: the annulus fibrosus and the nucleus pulposus. Investigations of the mechanical behavior of tissue in the spine have dealt mainly with these specialized tissues.[2, 13, 17, 19, 30]

Study of the mechanical properties of tissues involves determinations of the elastic properties, failure criteria, and energy relationships. These determinations are made by loading tissues and measuring the deformations. The load-deformation data can be expressed in terms of a stress-strain curve if proper measurements are made. It is quite important to realize that the time relationships in testing are basic to the completion of meaningful experiments. The biological collagenous tissues are viscoelastic, and testing must take this into account. Two examples of the basic time-dependent behavior of spinal component tissue are illustrated in Fig. 1-1. Reproduced are stress-strain curves for cortical bone and ligamentum nuchae. Note that the stress-strain relationships are very dependent on the rate of elongation. A test in which the strain rate or the load rate is not indicated is of very little use, as the data cannot be reproduced. In addition, a loading or strain rate may be chosen that is not meaningful in the physiological sense. The stress-strain curve will also be different, according to the type of forcing condition. Either the strain rate or the load rate can be varied. However, it is necessary to specify which has been used, as different stress-strain curves will be generated.

The stress-strain curves may also indicate the energy that is stored during loading and released during unloading. Any net loss in energy during the loading and unloading cycle can be determined and a hysteresis loop constructed. If loading is carried to failure, the energy required to cause failure can be assessed by measuring the area under the stress-strain curve. This again demonstrates the importance of specifying the strain rate in a test; the energy required for failure of the specimen depends upon the strain rate, as can be seen in Fig. 1-1. From this data it is evident that bone or other collagenous tissue does not have a simple

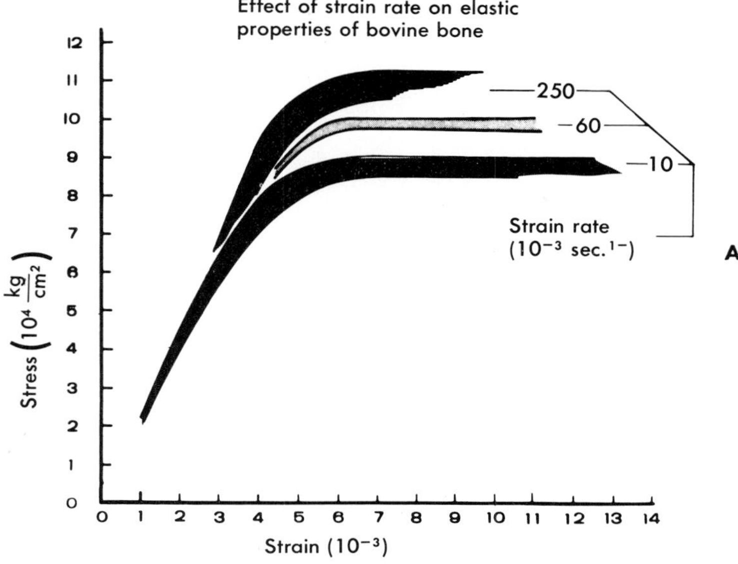

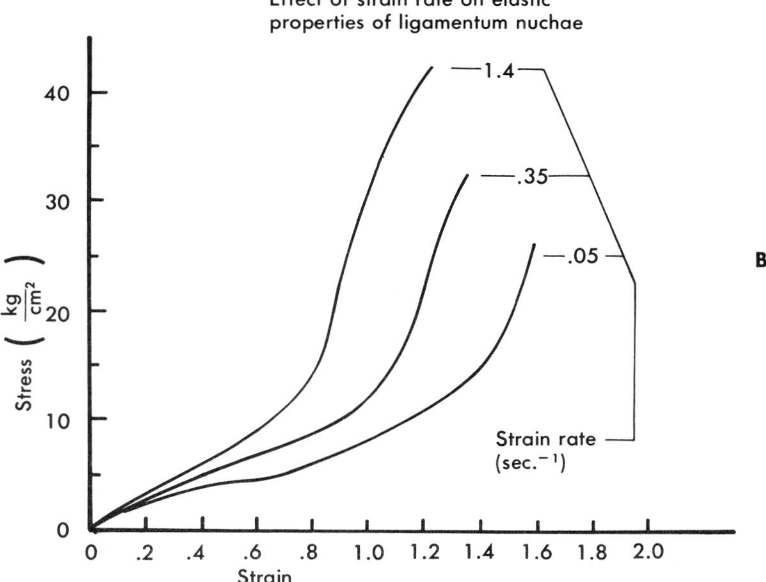

Fig. 1-1. Stress-strain curves for ox ligamentum nuchae tissue, **B,** and cortical bone, **A,** three strain rates. The stress, strain, and energy absorption at failure depended upon the strain rate. (**A** from Burstein, A. H., and Frankel, V. H.: The design of orthopaedic implants and prostheses,* New York, 1967, American Society of Mechanical Engineers.)

*This study was supported by grants from the John A. Hartford Foundation and the Social and Rehabilitation Service, Department of Health, Education, and Welfare.

"strength" measured as ultimate stress, strain, or energy absorption at failure but that the "strength" depends upon the loading or strain rate. In addition, the studies shown in Fig. 1-1 were performed with a simple one-dimensional strain. To completely determine the mechanical properties of the tissues multidimensional loading must be utilized at various strain rates. Of course careful control of the testing environment and specimen preparation is necessary.

From the stress-strain curve it is possible to determine the elastic limits for tension in bone and ligaments. An approximately straight line in the stress-strain curve for bone in Fig. 1-1 is the linear elastic portion of the curve. The slope of this line represents the modulus of elasticity, which is a measure of stiffness of the specimen. If the load is carried beyond the straight-line portion of the curve, a permanent deformation will be present when the bone is unloaded. Specimens of ox cortical bone also exhibit a plastic region before failure, in which the bone has continued to elongate without a progressive increase in stress.

Studies on the specific vertebral tissues ligamentum annulus and intervertebral discs have been performed for many years. Galante[13] has demonstrated the viscoelastic properties of the ligamentum annulus. He noted the presence of a hysteresis loop in loading cycles. The tensile properties were found to be dependent upon the location and orientation of the specimen. The average elongation and energy dissipation at failure decreased with age up to 30 years of age and were thereafter constant.

Nachemson[22-24] demonstrated the presence of hydrostatic pressure in normal disc tissue. In degenerated disc tissue this phenomenon was lost. Much work remains to be performed in establishing the mechanical properties of the tissues acting upon the spine in the normal state before one can assess the changes wrought by age, disease, or treatment on the tissues themselves.

Mechanical properties of substructures

The substructure that concerns us in the spine is the "motor unit" of Schmorl and Junghans.[28] This consists of two articulating vertebrae. It is useful to further subdivide this for study into the body-disc-body segment and the posterior elements and associated joints. Again, we find the kind of structures generally distributed throughout the skeleton and other structures specific to the spine. Study of the mechanical properties of the substructures involves placing the structure under load and observing the deformations.[9, 17, 20] In addition, measurements of the amount and distribution of tissue must be made. It is desirable to assess the stiffness, strength, and failure criteria of the substructure.[26] It is necessary to take into account the viscoelastic properties of the tissues, which have been determined according to the previous section, in choosing the loading or strain rates. Meaningful loading techniques must be selected. It must be learned which of the possible loading configurations—tension, compression, bending, torsion, or shear—is applicable. Intervertebral discs with attached bone have been tested in compression, and load-deformation data reported. Farfan[10] has tested the discs in torsion, with the production of lifelike annular ruptures. He demonstrated permanent deformation of the disc, following torsion of more than 3 to 6 degrees, and an abrupt failure as torsion was continued. Torsion was utilized as a loading configuration in order to elucidate the mechanical reasons for the incidence of clinical disc pathology associated with asymmetrical facet orientation.[11]

As the stiffness and strength of the structure depend not only upon the amount of material present but also on its distribution, it is necessary to measure the area moment of inertia (I) and the polar moment of inertia (J) for the various bending and torsion axes utilized. The stiffness in tension or compression will depend upon the modulus of elasticity (E) and the area. The stiffness in bending will be equal to the product (E • I). In torsion, the stiffness will depend upon the shear modulus (G) and is expressed as J • G.

Load strength of the structure in tension and compression is expressed as σ, the normal stress at failure measured as pounds per square inch. The strength of the structure in bending is given by the formula $\frac{I}{Y}\ \sigma_{max}$ in which I is the area moment of inertia, Y is the distance to the outermost fiber, and σ_{max} is the maximum normal stress. For torsion the strength is expressed by the formula $\frac{JT_{max}}{R_{max}}$ in which J is the polar moment of inertia, R_{max} is the maximum radius to the outermost fiber, and T_{max} is the maximum shear stress. Small changes in the distribution of material in the structure may have profound effects on the strength.

It is necessary to assess the methods of failure of the substructure. A failure may be one of three types: plastic failure, in which the material "flows" before rupturing; brittle failure, in which the material has no plastic area; and fatigue failure, in which failure occurs at loads that when applied only a few times do not produce failure. The mode of failure can be determined from load-deflection or torque-deflection curves in a manner similar to that shown in Fig. 1-1 for stress-strain curves. The rate and method of loading are important parameters.

From the above discussion it should be evident that studies of the mechanical properties of the substructures involve careful control of the same parameters as in the study of tissues. In addition, the geometry of the structure must be considered.

Relative motion between osseous substructures

This portion of a study of the biomechanics of the spine utilizes the tools of kinematics. The necessary measurements in any kinematic study are basically simple. They are measurements of the linear and angular displacements of one body in reference to another. In addition, it is necessary to record the time during which each increment of the motion took place. From this data the velocity and accelerations can be calculated and plotted. Data for the spine have been gathered, utilizing bone pins and various forms of roentgenography.[15]

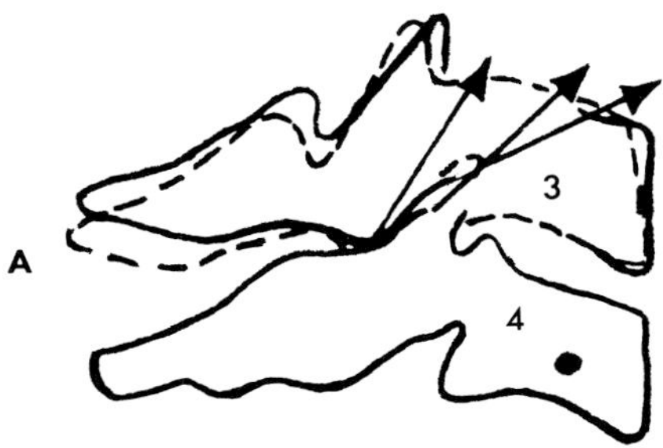

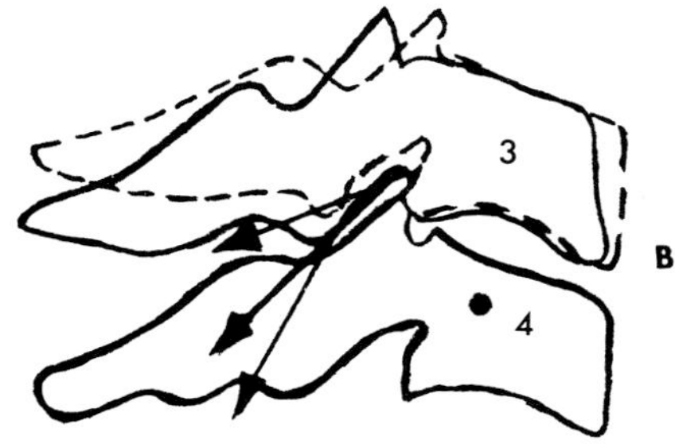

Fig. 1-2. Instant center study of C3-C4 motion in normal 19-year-old female. **A,** The instant center for motion from extension (dotted outline) to neutral (solid line) is indicated and lies on the body of C4. The velocity directions at the contact surfaces of the facet joints are tangent to the surface of the facet as indicated by the arrows. **B,** The same normal function when C3 moves from flexion (dotted line) to neutral (solid line). The arrows indicate that the velocity direction is tangent to the surface.

An important phase of the kinematic description is the location of the point about which the bodies are rotating at any particular instant. This point is termed the instant center if it has been determined from velocity data and the centroid if it has been derived from displacement data. The centroid for each of various spinal areas has been recorded by a number of authors, for both normal and abnormal discs.[14, 16, 18, 25, 27] As the segment goes from flexion to extension, the centroid may change its relative anatomical relationship. In Fig. 1-2 the centroid for the C3-C4 level in a normal 19-year-old girl is reproduced. Note how the centroid changes as the spinal segment goes from flexion to extension. If one considers the full implications of the instant center, it is evident that at any one moment all structures are rotating around the center. The velocity of any point in the structure can be determined by connecting that point to the instant center and dropping a perpendicular to it. This is analogous to twirling a ball on a string. At any instant when the string is cut the ball will follow a tangent to the circle about which it is rotating, and the velocity direction will be perpendicular to the particular radius at the instant of release. In going back to the vertebrae in Fig. 1-2 it is now evident that the centroid or instant center is a powerful tool in determining the behavior of tissues at any location in the structure. If one considers the facet joints, it is evident that a point in the joint will be moving in a direction perpendicular to a line joining that point and the instant center. The surfaces will then be sliding over each other in the complete range of motion from flexion to extension in the normal joint.

In Fig. 1-3 the instant center for an abnormal disc level has been determined. All parts of the vertebrae are forced to rotate about this center as the bones go from flexion to extension. When the facets are considered, it is seen that the velocity at the joint surface is such as to force segments of the joint together in extension and also in flexion. This perhaps accounts for the painful and limited

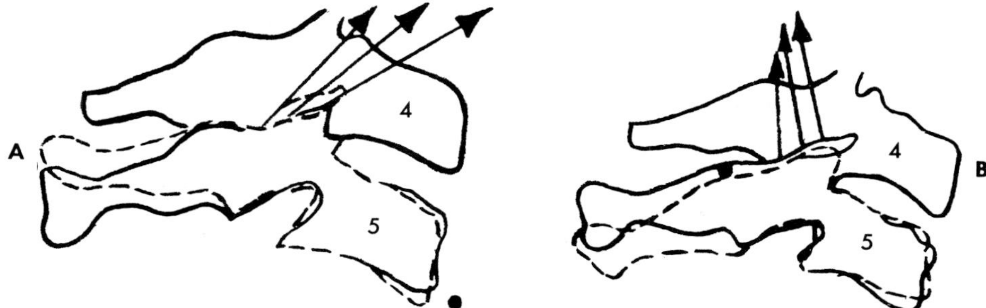

Fig. 1-3. Instant center study of motion between C4 and C5 in patient with neck pain following acceleration injury. **A,** In moving from neutral (solid line) to extension (dotted line) the instant center lies anterior to the load of C5. The velocity directions at the facet joint surface are maldirected and tend to force the joint surfaces into slight compression. **B,** In moving from neutral (solid line) to flexion (dotted line) the bodies move around an instant center that lies on the spinous process of C5. The velocity directions at the joint surface tend to severely compress the joint.

neck extension in the patient. Pennel and Kohn[25] have correlated abnormally placed instant centers in the lumbar spine with clinical disc disease.

Functional loading of structures

The loads that are applied to the structures of the spine are derived from two sources. These loads may be induced by motion or they may be necessary to produce the motion. Loads induced by motion may arise from external effects or from the elastic restraints in the spine. An example of a load arising from motion due to external effects would be the loading which results from a fall on the buttocks. Because of the motion and contact with an external object a force is produced in the spine.

Loads arising from elastic restraints are common and can be illustrated by considering the spinal segment shown in Fig. 1-2. As stated above, during an instant of motion all parts of the vertebra are rotating about the instant center. If one considers the anterior longitudinal ligament and the adjacent ligamentum annulus, it becomes evident that these are under tension as the spine goes into extension. The tensile force in the ligaments must be opposed by a compressive force in the disc for equilibrium. Even during passive motions in the spine forces will be exerted on the discs and other structures, due to tensile forces arising as the ligaments are stretched to allow the desired motion.

Loads are also present because they are necessary to produce the force needed for the motion.[5] These loads arise from three sources: external loads, muscles, and joint reaction. The external loads in the case of the spine are present as a result of a burden being lifted or carried. In this case, the functional loading due to an external load may be quite difficult to calculate. It is now well known that portions of the load being lifted by the arms may be transmitted to the pelvis not only by the spine but also by a hydrodynamic system developed in the abdominal viscera contained in a column by a firm anterior abdominal wall.[1, 4, 6, 7, 12, 21] In studying the effects of an external load on the spine it is necessary to adhere to the principles of engineering as expressed in the development of a free body of the area being considered. In the construction of a diagram all forces and moments that act on the plane under consideration must be represented if equilibrium is to be achieved. If this is done properly and data can be obtained for such forces as those found in the abdominal cavity, the effect of external forces on various portions of the spine can be calculated.

Forces are developed as a result of the muscle activity necessary to produce a given motion. Studies of the forces acting on the head of the femur, which have now been confirmed experimentally, revealed that a large portion of the total force acting over a joint is developed by muscle forces. In the case of a person standing on one leg, the muscle force necessary to balance the pelvis is approximately two times body weight. If this force is added to the force of the superincumbent weight, a total force acting on the hip joint will reach levels of nearly three times body weight. Similar calculations can be performed for loading at any spinal segment. As there is a large muscle bulk spanning most of the spine, it is not surprising that a sudden tetanic contraction such as is produced during electroshock therapy may produce a fracture of a vertebral body.

Forces are also developed during motion because of joint reactions. Muscles are able to move segments of the body because they develop a force couple. The force acting across a joint to produce the other half of the force couple is very close in magnitude to the muscle force acting over the joint. From the above discussion it is evident that calculating the effect of a load held in the outstretched hands on the L5-S1 spinal segment is complex. It requires not only knowledge of the geometry of the parts but also information as to what muscle forces are acting and the forces arising from stretching of ligaments.

In studying a diseased spine that is undergoing changes thought to be due to altered mechanics it is necessary to carefully consider the four listed areas of investigation in order to assign the lesion to its proper category as a basis for preventative methods and rational treatment.

References

1. Bartelink, D. L.: The role of the abdominal pressure in relieving the pressure on the lumbar intervertebral discs, J. Bone Joint Surg. **39-B:**718, 1957.
2. Brown, T., Hansen, R. J., and Yorra, A. J.: Some mechanical tests on the lumbosacral spine with particular reference to the intervertebral discs; a preliminary report, J. Bone Joint Surg. **39-A:**1135, 1957.
3. Burstein, A. H., and Frankel, V. H.: The viscoelastic properties of some biological materials, Ann. N. Y. Acad. Sci. **146:**158, 1968.
4. Davis, P. R.: Variations of the human intra-abdominal pressure during weight-lifting in different postures, J. Anat. **90:**601, 1956.
5. Davis, P. R., Troup, J. D. G., and Burnard, J. H.: Movements of the thoracic and lumbar spine when lifting: a chrono-cyclophotographic study, J. Anat. **99:**13, 1965.
6. Eie, N.: Load capacity of the low back, J. Oslo City Hosp. **16:**73, 1966.

7. Eie, N., and Wehn, P.: Measurements of the intra-abdominal pressure in relation to weight bearing of the lumbosacral spine, J. Oslo City Hosp. **12:**205, 1962.
8. Evans, F. G.: Bibliography on the physical properties of the skeletal system, Highway Safety Research Institute, University of Michigan, Ann Arbor, Report Bio-1.
9. Evans, F. G., and Lissner, H. R.: Biomechanical studies on the lumbar spine and pelvis, J. Bone Joint Surg. **41-A:**278, 1959.
10. Farfan, H.: Mechanical failure of the lumbar intervertebral joints, St. Mary's Hosp. (Montreal) Med. Bull. **9:**142, 1967.
11. Farfan, H. F., and Sullivan, J. D.: The relation of facet orientation to intervertebral disc failure, Canad. J. Surg. **10:**179, 1967.
12. Floyd, W. F., and Silver, P. H. S.: The function of the erectores spinae muscles in certain movements and postures in man, J. Physiol. (London) **129:**184, 1955.
13. Galante, J. O.: Tensile properties of the human lumbar annulus fibrosus, Acta Orthop. Scand., supp. 100, 1967.
14. Granturco, C.: A roentgen analysis of the motion of the lower lumbar vertebrae in normal individuals and in patients with low back pain, Amer. J. Roentgen. **52:**261, 1944.
15. Gregersen, G. G., and Lucas, D. B.: An in vivo study of the axial rotation of the human thoracolumbar spine, J. Bone Joint Surg. **49-A:**247, 1967.
16. Harris, R. I., and Macnab, I.: Structural changes in the lumbar intervertebral discs, their relationship to low back pain and sciatica, J. Bone Joint Surg. **36-B:**304, 1954.
17. Hirsch, C.: The reaction of intervertebral discs to compression forces, J. Bone Joint Surg. **37-A:**1188, 1955.
18. Hoover, N. W.: Methods of lumbar fusion; instructional courses, J. Bone Joint Surg. **50-A:**204, 1968.
19. Horton, W. G.: Further observations in the elastic mechanism of the intervertebral disc, J. Bone Joint Surg. **40-B:** 552, 1958.
20. Ingelmark, B. E., and Ekholm, R.: Über die Kompressibilität der Intervertebralscheiben. Eine experimentelle Untersuchung über die Intervertebralscheibe zwischen dem dritten und vierten Lendenwirbel beim Menschen, Acta Soc. Med. Upsal. **57:**202, 1952.
21. Morris, J. M., Lucas, D. B., and Bresler, B.: Role of the trunk in stability of the spine, J. Bone Joint Surg. **43-A:**327, 1961.
22. Nachemson, A.: Lumbar intradiscal pressure; experimental studies on post-mortem material, Acta Orthop. Scand., supp. 43, 1960.
23. Nachemson, A.: The influence of spinal movements on the lumbar intradiscal pressure and on the tensile stresses in the annulus fibrosus, Acta Orthop. Scand. **33:**183, 1963.
24. Nachemson, A.: The load of lumbar discs in different positions of the body, Clin. Orthop. **45:**197, 1966.
25. Pennel, G., and Kohn, G.: Point-of-motion studies of the lumbar spine, Toronto, 1966, presented at 1966 Ontario Rehabilitation Meeting.
26. Perey, O.: Fracture of the vertebral end-plate in the lumbar spine; an experimental biochemical investigation, Acta Orthop. Scand. supp. 25, 1957.
27. Rolander, S. D.: Motion of the lumbar spine with special reference to the stabilizing effect of posterior fusion; an experimental study on autopsy specimens, Acta Orthop. Scand., supp. 90, 1966.
28. Schmorl, G., and Junghans, H. In Wilk, S. P., and Join, L. S.: The human spine in health and disease, New York, 1959, Grune & Stratton, Inc.
29. Sedlin, E. D.: A rheologic model for cortical bone; a study of the physical properties of human femoral samples, Acta Orthop. Scand., supp. 83, 1965.
30. Virgin, W. J.: Experimental investigations into the physical properties of the intervertebral disc, J. Bone Joint Surg. **33-B:**607, 1951.
31. Weaver, J. K., and Chalmers, J.: Cancellous bone: its strength and changes with aging and an evaluation of some methods for measuring its mineral content. I. Age changes in cancellous bone, J. Bone Joint Surg. **48-A:**289, 1966.

2. Acceleration-extension injuries of the cervical spine

Ian Macnab, M.B., Ch.B.

Everyone is well acquainted with the common story associated with whiplash injuries. Despite the history of pain in the neck, pain between the shoulder blades, pain in the back of the head, pain down the arm, dysphagia, tinnitus, vertigo, and intermittent blurring of vision, there is remarkably little to find on examination. The usual x-ray films do not commonly show any gross abnormalities, even though there may be an alteration in the normal cervical curve. Despite the frustratingly negative examination, the patient's aches and pains fail to respond to the brownian movements of routine medical therapy. As the months roll by, it becomes increasingly apparent that the patient is grossly emotionally disturbed.

There is general agreement on the type of symptoms to be expected, but widely divergent views are held on the significance of these symptoms. These divergent viewpoints, rigidly held and hotly contested, are firmly based—on impressions only. In an endeavor to make these impressions more factually significant, the progress of 575 patients has been carefully followed. Many physicians believe that the "whiplash syndrome" is demonstrated only by a group of hysterical, neurotic, if not frankly dishonest, people. However, there are certain disturbing features apparent from an analysis of the case histories available that make it difficult to accept the belief that litigation neurosis is the sole explanation of the long drawn out disability in every instance.

Some patients had other, associated injuries. In addition to injuring their necks, they sprained their ankles or broke their wrists. Normal painless function returned to their ankles and wrists in the expected period of time. These patients did not keep on complaining for month after month about their painful ankles or about their painful wrists—but their necks still hurt. It is difficult to understand why litigation neurosis in these instances should be confined to the neck. If litigation neurosis was the sole cause for their continuation of symptoms, it is difficult to explain why these patients did not continue to have neurotic pain in their wrists or show litigation neurosis about their ankle disabilities.

Table 2-1. Side collisions

Number of collisions	44
Number of occupants	69
Number of occupants seeking medical advice	52
For neck pain only	2
For neck pain and other injuries	5
For other injuries only	45

When forward flexion of the neck is produced by acceleration or deceleration, the head stops moving when the chin touches the chest. Similarly, in lateral flexion, movement in a normal cervical spine stops when the ear hits the shoulder. In both these modalities of cervical movement, the range of the motion occurring is within physiological limits; in normal necks, even at the extreme of movement, no strain is applied to the intervertebral joints. In extension injuries of the neck, however, there is no block to movement until the occiput hits the chest wall, and this is far beyond the physiologically permitted limit.

In the series of rear-end collisions analyzed, there were 5 patients who at the moment of impact were facing the back of the car. As the result of the impact they experienced an uncontrolled flexion of the neck, but none complained of neck pain. Of the 69 patients who were passengers in vehicles involved in side collisions that resulted, one presumes, in lateral flexion movement applied to the neck, only 7 suffered neck pain (Table 2-1) and in only 2 did significant disability persist for more than two months. If neck pain following acceleration injuries is purely neurotic in origin, it is difficult to understand why patients commonly get neurotic if the head is thrown backward and rarely get neurotic if they are jolted forward or sideways. Such findings suggest that the persistence of pain following forced extension of the neck is related in some way to the fact that the neck can, and may, move beyond physiologically permitted limits.

The physiologically permitted range of extension is much less when the neck is rotated. Normally, at the limit of extension the occipitomental line is about 20 or 30 degrees above the horizontal when the chin is pointing straight forward. If the neck is rotated through 45 degrees, the amount of extension permitted is only about half this amount. Because the permitted physiological range of extension is very short when the neck is slightly rotated, the posterior joints can soon be pushed beyond their physiological range and injury result from an extension strain.

An interesting observation on the significance of litigation neurosis comes from a follow-up of these patients after settlement of court action (Table 2-2). There were 266 patients in whom all the legal problems had been settled two or more years before the follow-up. As in any review of this type, it was impossible to get all these patients back for study. Only 145 patients were examined personally; of these, 121 were continuing to have symptoms. It is obvious that in a follow-up such as this, where attendance for review may seem pointless, time-consuming, and

Table 2-2. Analysis of results—two years after settlement of court action

Total suitable for review	266
Number of patients reviewed	145
Number of patients with symptoms	121
Persistence of symptoms two years after settlement	
121 out of 266	45%

difficult, the patients most likely to attend are those with continuing symptoms. To avoid bias of this type, it is necessary that we regard all patients who did not come back as being completely cured. On this basis then, it can be said that out of 266 patients, 121 continued to have some measure of symptoms. In other words, satisfactory conclusion of settlement or court action failed to relieve symptoms in 45% of the group studied—a group that is not, of course, representative of every whiplash injury. It is a special group, consisting of patients referred for specialist opinion because of severity of symptoms or because of undue persistence of symptoms. It represents, therefore, the more severe disabilities, whether they be physiogenic or psychogenically induced.

These results at first sight may appear to be grossly at variance with Gotten's often quoted review. Gotten[1] in 1956 published a survey of 100 cases of whiplash injury reviewed after settlement of legal action. It was stated in this review that 88% had "largely recovered"; 12% were still significantly disabled. Reading his report the other way round, one can say that out of 100 patients reviewed, many had some sort of symptoms; and even after the passage of several years 12%, a significant number, were seriously disabled and 3% were still losing time from work.

In order to assess the injury sustained by patients subjected to acceleration forces of this type, it is necessary that we should understand more of the pathological changes that can take place. Therefore, it was decided to try reproducing the injury experimentally by subjecting animals to an extension strain of the neck produced by sudden acceleration.[2] Because of the difficulties of obtaining a standard force, it was decided to use the force of gravity. Anesthetized animals were strapped to a steel platform attached to two vertical guide rails, and the platform was dropped over a distance varying from 2 to 40 feet. On striking the bottom of the runway, the animal's head and neck were suddenly extended over the edge of the platform, producing an acceleration strain as in rear-end collisions. The degree of force applied to the neck could be varied by altering the height of the drop.

It is realized, of course, that this apparatus does not accurately reproduce the forces involved in rear-end collisions, but the method was used to determine whether recognizable acceleration injuries did indeed occur.

By altering the height of the drop, various lesions were produced. Muscle injuries were noted, varying in severity from minor tears of the sternomastoid to

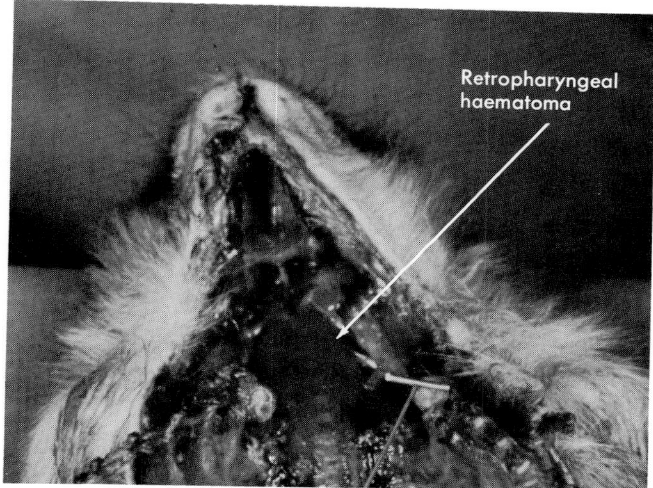

Fig. 2-1. Gross hematoma in relation to the anterior aspect of the cervical vertebrae in a monkey due to tearing of the longissimus colli.

more serious tears of the longissimus colli (Fig. 2-1). These muscle injuries are of significance when assessing clinical symptoms described by patients. Spasm of the sternomastoid, particularly if unilateral, can interfere with the neck-righting reflex and produce the veering and weaving type of dizziness or unsteadiness that many of the patients complain of. Any tear of the longissimus colli, no matter how small, was associated experimentally with a retropharyngeal hematoma. Hemorrhages were also seen in the muscle coats of the esophagus. Esophageal damage and retropharyngeal hematomas could account for the early dysphagia that is occasionally a complaint made by victims of acceleration-extension injuries of the neck. Damage to the longissimus colli can be associated with damage to the cervical sympathetic plexus and this might explain the Horner syndrome, the intermittent blurring of vision, and some instances of vertigo seen clinically.

The vertebral artery is vulnerable to extension strains of the neck. It is readily stretched as it passes from the second to the first cervical vertebra (Fig. 2-2). When there are marked degenerative changes in the mid cervical spine, this part of the spine does not move well; the full brunt of an extension strain is felt, therefore, by the upper cervical segments, particularly C1 and C2. Excessive extension between the atlas and the axis may lead to a significant stretching of the vertebral artery. This older group of patients frequently also have concomitant atherosclerotic changes involving the vertebral artery, and it is in this group that the various types of vertebral artery syndrome are to be recognized.

One of the most interesting lesions was a tearing of the anterior longitudinal ligament and separation of the disc from the associated vertebra (Fig. 2-3). This lesion never occurred without damage to the anterior cervical muscles. The disc in-

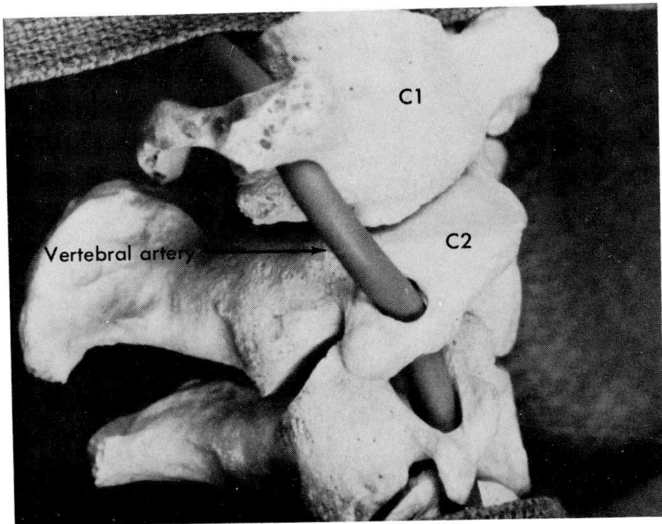

Fig. 2-2. The vertebral artery courses posteriorly from the vertebral artery foramen of Cl to the vertebral artery foramen of the atlas. Extension of the atlas in relation to the axis may put a significant stretch on the vertebral artery.

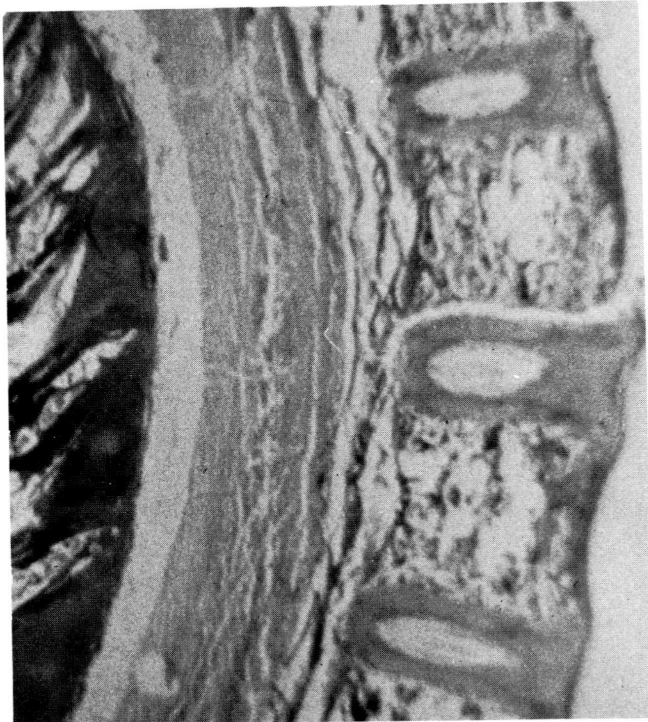

Fig. 2-3. Section of cervical spine of a monkey subjected to an acceleration-extension injury. Note how the disc has been separated from the vertebral body above.

jury in the monkeys could not be detected on x-ray examination, even after the passage of several months.

It is always difficult and at times dangerous to translate the findings of experimental investigation into the sphere of clinical experience. However, I would like to suggest that these experiments show that recognizable lesions can be produced. They indicate that the lesions can vary: some may be very minor injuries, such as tear of the muscle fibers; others may constitute serious lesions, such as separation of the disc or damage to the posterior joints. It is reasonable to presume that the same variation is seen clinically, with the majority of patients sustaining minor injuries only, but with some having a lesion of more serious significance. In considering the clinical syndrome presented, we have to accept the fact that a vast majority of patients show a marked emotional overlay.

When a patient breaks his neck, even though the injury may involve litigation, a functional overlay is not common. Similarly, when patients break their wrists or sprain their ankles, even if this lesion is associated with an acceleration-extension injury of the neck, normal painless function usually returns to the ankles and wrists in the expected period of time without any functional overlay. Surely these observations suggest that broken necks are treated adequately, sprained ankles are treated adequately, broken wrists are treated adequately; and surely these findings suggest that, by failure to treat the whiplash injury adequately, the physician himself may be responsible for producing some of the so-called litigation neurosis.

If the physician in his treatment is to avoid an iatrogenic neurosis, then the following points bear consideration. When first seen, if it appears that the patient may have sustained significant injury, as evidenced by the nature of the impact, by marked spasm of the sternomastoid, or by complaints suggestive of damage to the anterior soft tissues of the neck, then the neck should be splinted. If the neck needs splinting at all, then it needs splinting well. The best way to do this is to apply at least three soft cervical ruffs. The only way to rest the neck completely is to remove the weight of the head, and the only way this can be achieved is to confine the patient to bed. If, in twelve or twenty-four hours, the patient is relatively symptom-free, he can get up. Otherwise he should stay in bed for a week. Traction may be given at this stage if it relieves pain. If a patient is asked to stay in bed for a week, it is essential that he be given some form of sedation. Without this, and in view of the fact that he feels relatively well, he is unlikely to carry out this form of therapy, because it seems unreasonable. These patients' only symptom is pain. The need for rest in bed must be explained to them; otherwise, they will not cooperate. At the end of a week the majority should be able to go to work. They should be given instructions on how to avoid extension strains of the neck in the activities of daily living and, most important of all, they must be told the difference between hurting themselves and harming themselves. They must be told that many things they do during the day may hurt them and they should be informed of the fact that flare-up of pain does not necessarily signify increasing damage to the neck. They should be told that if they restrict their activities because of fear of harm, they are mistaken. Many patients, fearful of harming themselves, restrict their activities unnecessarily in the honest but mistaken belief that this was their physician's advice. Their problems are compounded of apprehension and misapprehension, and the physician must deal firmly with both.

The patient should not be given unnecessary and expensive medication. As the cost of "frantic" medication rises, so does the cost of injury and each failure of the "Try this, try that" school of therapeutics engraves more deeply on the patient's mind the seriousness of his injury. Mild analgesia to take the edge off his discomforts and mild sedation to take the edge off his anxieties are all that is required. The nature and the purpose of the drugs must be explained to the patient. It is dishonest, and bad medicine, to give the patient a tranquilizer in a sly manner, pretending it is something to take his neck spasms away. If he is disabled by a psychogenic magnification of his symptoms, he must be told so and must be told that he is being given sedation to treat this aspect of his problem.

Physiotherapy, if ordered, must be along rational lines. Heat in all its modalities, massage, and traction may make the patient feel easier temporarily but do nothing to speed the resolution of the underlying lesion. If attendance at a physiotherapy department makes the patient take time off from work, it is probably harmful in that it further impresses him with the severity of the lesion. Traction can be used at home, but should be prescribed only if the patient gets relief of pain while traction is actually being applied and for some time afterward. Traction is not curative; its function is solely to make the patient more comfortable and to cut down on the use of analgesics. The patients must be told this. If a patient does not feel comfortable in a soft homemade ruff type collar, then there is no point in ordering any other kind. If he does indeed feel better in a collar and can work more efficiently while wearing it, then there is no psychologically sound reason for withholding it. If the patient's symptoms are severe enough to warrant putting him to bed for a week, then he will probably have daily discomfort for six weeks. If at the end of six weeks the patient is still conscious of some measure of discomfort all day long, then he may well have intermittent discomfort for a further six months or a year. The patient must be told the expected duration of symptoms. There is nothing more demoralizing than expecting a cure day by day from some new pill or from some new apparatus at the physiotherapy department. Unless the physician honestly believes that his patient will get better in a week or ten days as the result of the treatment he is giving, he must tell the patient what to expect. However, the patient must be told at the same time that the lesion in the neck alone and the discomfort derived from it are not adequate reason to withdraw completely from the activities of daily living.

These patients must be watched carefully. There is no doubt that they do have for some time daily discomfort of varying severity. There is also no doubt that the persisting ache, resulting in interference with daily activities and coupled with doubts as to the future, may trigger a latent depression; it may initiate an anxiety neurosis or may precipitate a conversion hysteria. When the physician feels that the patient is becoming more disabled by the functional overlay than by the pain itself, then the patient must be told honestly that opinion. This should be recognized early and a second opinion be sought early.

In teaching patients to live within the limits of minor discomforts, the attitude of the physician is of paramount importance. He must accept the possibility of injury and investigate its probability in each patient. He must not be perfunctory in treatment; yet he must never overtreat the patient. His treatment should not interfere with the patient's daily routine. Only a few—a very few—come to surgery, and in teaching the rest of his patients to accept and live within the limits of minor discomforts, the physician must be honest: honest about the treatment he is giving, honest about the patient's physical and mental well-being, and honest about the prognosis. Above all, he must take care not to fan the flames of hostility that these patients so commonly exhibit, and thereby initiate, aggravate, or perpetuate a financially motivated exaggeration of symptoms.

References

1. Gotten, N.: Survey of 100 cases of whiplash injury after settlement of litigation, J.A.M.A. **162:**865, 1956.
2. Macnab, I.: Acceleration injuries of the cervical spine, J. Bone Joint Surg. **46-A:**1797, 1964.

3. Fracture and fracture-dislocation of the cervical spine

J. Neill Garber, M.D., Med. Sc.D.

The diagnosis "broken neck" often has a terrifying impact upon the patient and his family, implying that he has received an injury which is almost incompatible with continued existence and from which there is little chance of recovery if he does survive.

Fractures and dislocations of the cervical spine are not uncommon. The majority are caused by vehicular accidents; others result from diving into shallow water, contact sports, and falling.

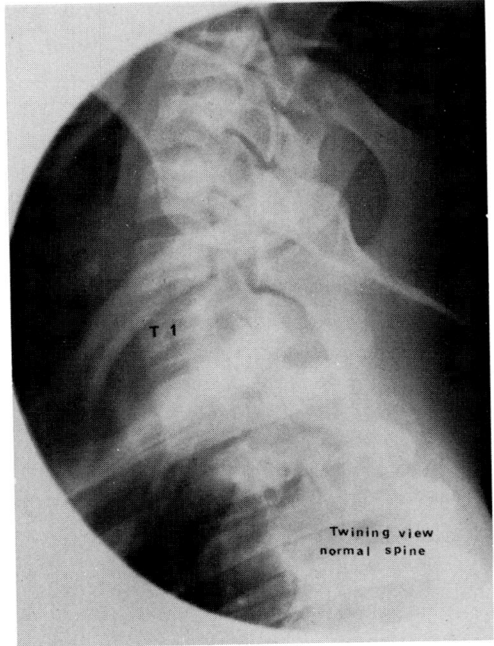

Fig. 3-1. Twining view for visualization of cervicodorsal junction.

Many traumatic and many congenital lesions of the neck are not complicated by seriously disabling or permanent neurological changes.

The purpose of this presentation is to discuss some of the typical lesions at various levels in the cervical spine that ordinarily are not accompanied by disabling neurological involvement and to consider the indications for conservative and surgical treatment.

It is true that some of these patients may have profound motor and sensory changes in one or more of the extremities immediately after an injury. The physician must be precise to differentiate between paresis and paralysis when he first examines the patient, and he should note carefully the degree of sensory and motor impairment. A flicker of toe motion or the presence of some sensation in the extremities affords a better prognosis because cord conduction has not been completely interrupted.

An accurate evaluation of the true extent of cord damage is very difficult, if not impossible, to make within the first few hours after injury. It is not uncommon to see profound paresis clear rapidly with rest and skull traction.

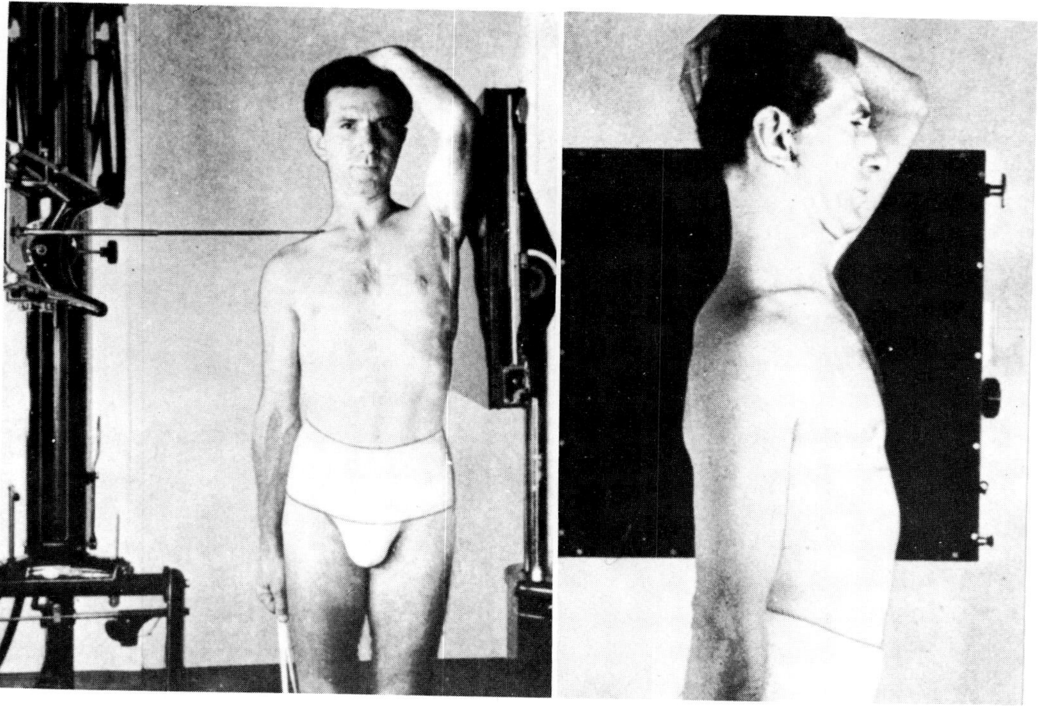

Fig. 3-2 **Fig. 3-3**

Fig. 3-2. Position for Twining view—frontal. (From Merrill, V.: Atlas of roentgenographic positions, vol. 1, ed. 3, St. Louis, 1967, The C. V. Mosby Co.)
Fig. 3-3. Position for Twining view—side. (From Merrill, V.: Atlas of roentgenographic positions, vol. 1, ed. 3, St. Louis, 1967, The C. V. Mosby Co.)

Complete loss of sensory and motor function frequently indicates transection of the cord with a permanent fixed disability. Laminectomy, often performed to make certain that everything possible is being done to give the patient a chance for recovery, does not alter the course of such a case.

Every patient who has had a head injury should be carefully examined for injury to the neck as well. Roentgenographic studies should include the entire cervical spine and the cervicodorsal junction. Routine studies may show only the fifth or sixth vertebra distally, especially if the patient has a short, fat neck. Fractures and dislocations at C6, C7, and T1 may be overlooked if the physician does not insist upon special views for this region of the spine.

Roentgenographic visualization of the cervicodorsal junction by the Twining view is illustrated in Fig. 3-1. The patient may stand against the upright cassette or lie upon the table in a similar position.[2] (See Figs. 3-2 and 3-3.)

Fractures of the atlas—Jefferson's fracture

Sir Geoffrey Jefferson[1] presented his theory of the mechanism of fracture of the atlas in a paper published in 1920. This injury is caused by a fall on the

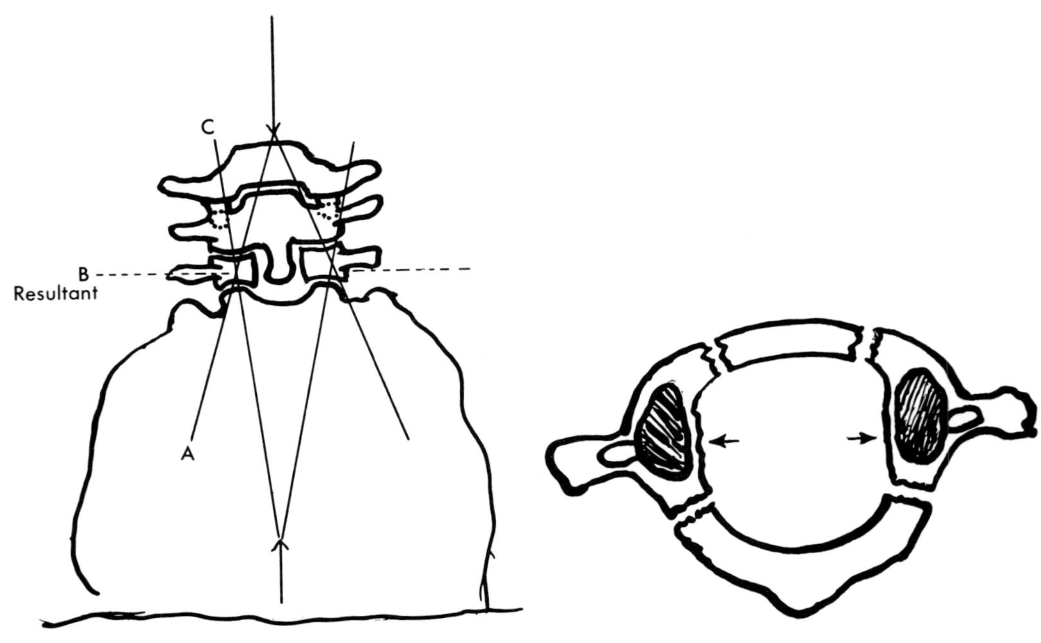

Fig. 3-4

Fig. 3-5

Fig. 3-4. Mechanism of fracture of the atlas vertebra. (Modified from Jefferson, G.: Brit. J. Surg. **7**:407, 1920.)

Fig. 3-5. Resultant of forces fractures the ring of the atlas. (Modified from Jefferson, G.: Brit. J. Surg. **7**:407, 1920.)

head or by a severe blow on top of the head. (See Fig. 3-4.) The resultant of the opposing forces is exerted laterally on the ring of the atlas and usually causes fractures at the thinnest and weakest point of the ring where the posterior arch joins the lateral masses (Fig. 3-5). Cord injury is not common in those who survive the isolated fracture. Passageway for the cord through the atlas is large. When fracture occurs, the fragments spread outward to enlarge the circumference of the atlas.

A middle-aged lady, E. R., came in for examination because of neck pain that followed an auto collision occurring seven months before. She had been thrown so violently upward by the impact that she was knocked unconscious when her head hit the roof of the car. A defect in the posterior arch of the atlas near its junction with the lateral masses seen in lateral roentgenograms is probably an old fracture. (See Figs. 3-6 and 3-7.)

Fracture in the posterior arch of the atlas may also be caused by extreme hyperextension of the neck. L. M. (Fig. 3-8) had fractures of C1 and C2. Force acting first on the face has pushed the head back, apparently fracturing C1 by compressing it between the occiput and C2. The pedicles of C2 were also fractured.

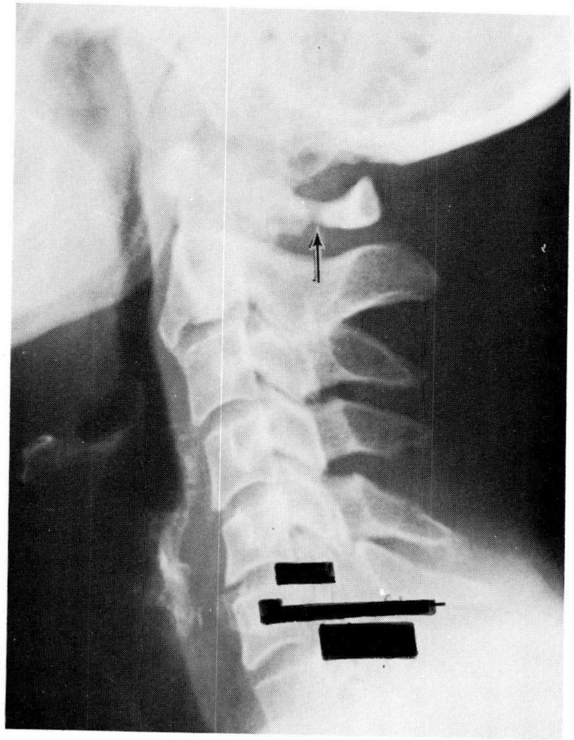

Fig. 3-6. E. R. This defect (arrow) may be an old fracture in the posterior arch of the atlas. Seven months after injury. (From Garber, J. N.: J. Bone Joint Surg. **46-A:**1782, 1964.)

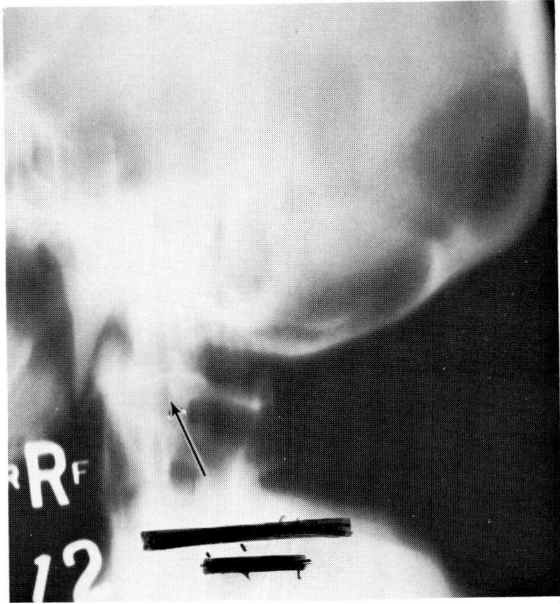

Fig. 3-7. E. R. Tomogram—seven months after injury.

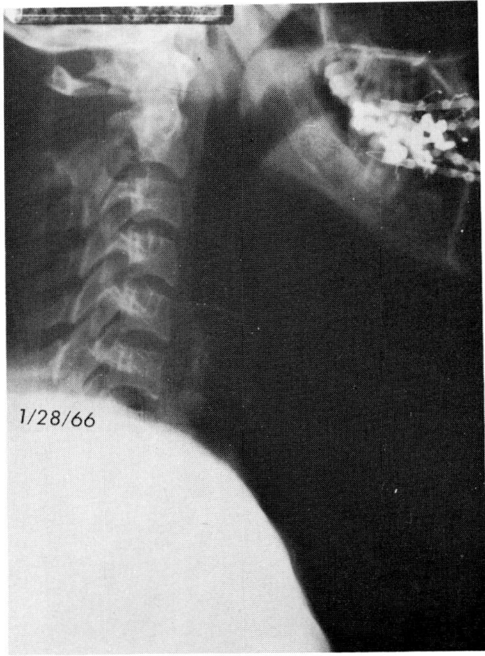

Fig. 3-8. L. M. Fractures are present in the posterior segments of the atlas and the axis. (Courtesy Dr. Robert Brueckmann, Indianapolis.)

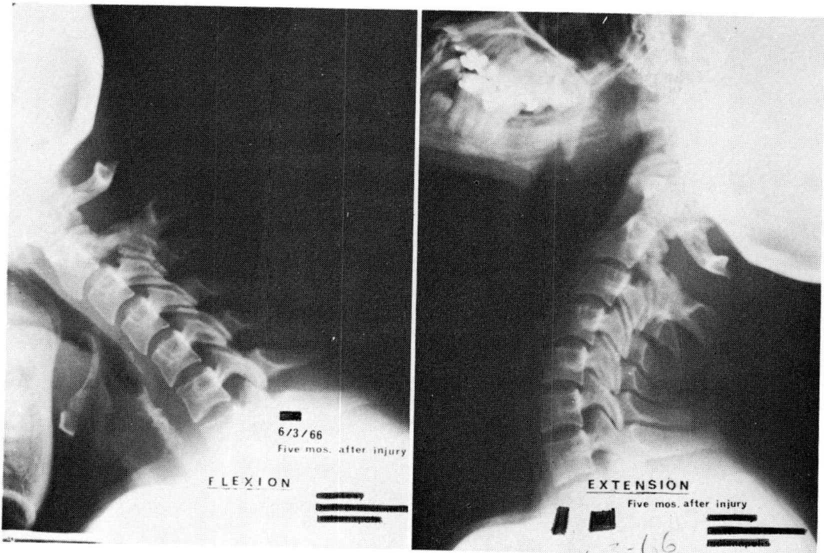

Fig. 3-9. L. M. Five months after injury. (Courtesy Dr. Robert Brueckmann, Indianapolis.)

There were no neurological complications. Progress was satisfactory with an initial period of six weeks in skull traction followed by brace support. The fractures healed in stable position as demonstrated in flexion and extension studies made five months after injury (Fig. 3-9).

Although this case has been included here under fractures of the atlas, it probably belongs under the classification of traumatic spondylolisthesis of the axis to be discussed later.

This double fracture involving the first two vertebrae may even be a separate entity. I have observed 2 other such cases, and Dr. Robert Brashear has reported 1 in his series of 16 cases of fractures of the neural arch of the axis (A.O.A. program—May, 1966).

Patients with this injury do well on conservative treatment. Laminectomy is not indicated unless there are in-driven fragments of bone.

Fractures of the axis

Fracture of odontoid process

Fracture of the odontoid process occurs near its base at the junction with the body of the axis. The history of injury, such as a fall, followed by neck stiffness and soreness, is the common picture. Neurological signs are infrequent.

Roentgenograms should include the open-mouth anteroposterior view of the cervical spine along with the usual lateral projection. A cartilage plate at the base of the odontoid may persist until early adulthood and should not be mistaken for a fracture line.

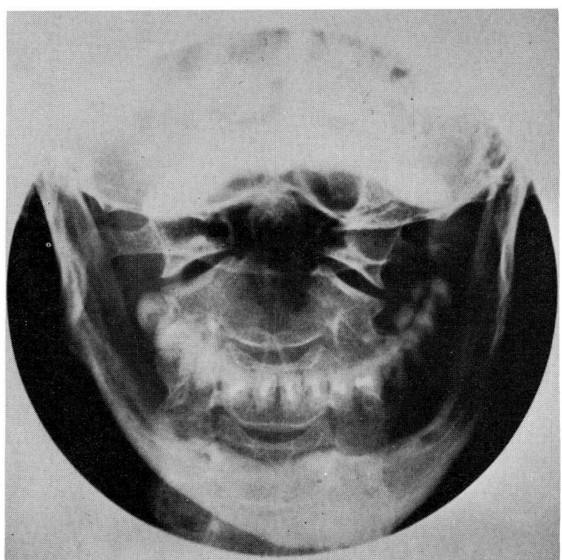

Fig. 3-10. O. H. There is a fracture line near the base of the odontoid. (From Garber, J. N.: J. Bone Joint Surg. **46-A:**1782, 1964.)

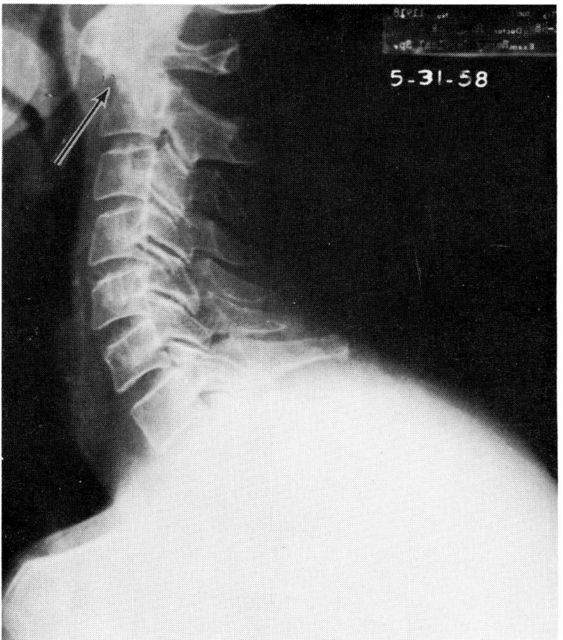

Fig. 3-11. O. H. There is anterior displacement of the atlas due to fracture of the odontoid. (From Garber, J. N.: J. Bone Joint Surg. **46-A:**1782, 1964.)

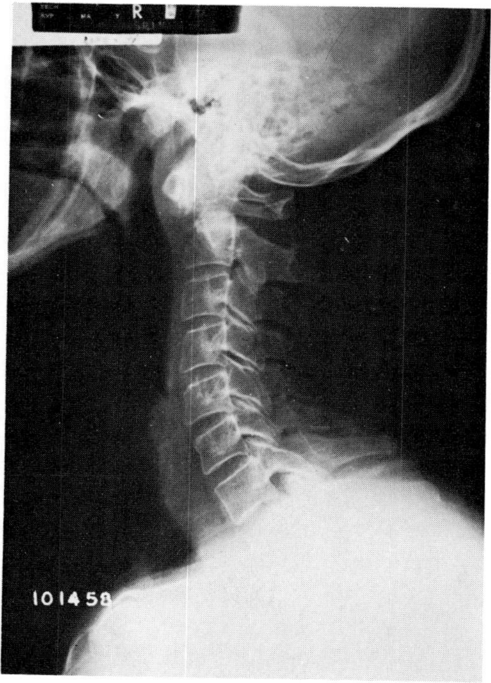

Fig. 3-12. O. H. Neutral position—five months after injury.

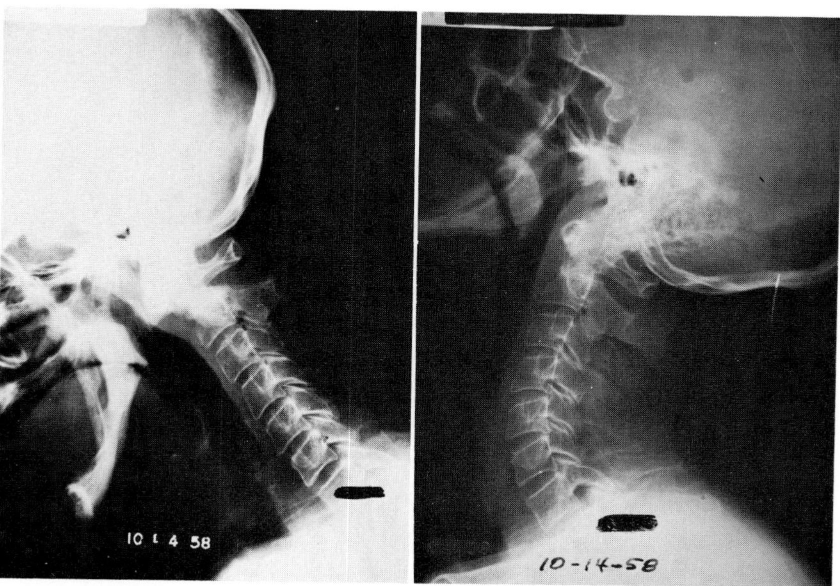

Fig. 3-13. O. H. Flexion and extension—five months after injury.

An elderly man, O. H., fell down a flight of steps at home in May, 1958. There is, in the open-mouth view, an irregular fracture line across the base of the odontoid (Fig. 3-10). The odontoid fragment and the atlas are displaced anteriorly in the lateral roentgenogram. (See Fig. 3-11.) After five months of conservative treatment with traction and brace the fracture has healed in a stable position (Figs. 3-12 and 3-13).

These fractures heal by fibrous or bone union and, in the usual case, conservative treatment with traction followed by a Minerva jacket or a brace suffices.

Traumatic spondylolisthesis of the axis

In 1958 I reported 8 cases of fractures through the pedicles of the axis with forward displacement of the body of the vertebra (Combined Meeting of the Orthopaedic Associations of the English Speaking World, Washington, D. C., May, 1958). This number of identical lesions and several more of the same type that have been reported since then—8 by Schneider and co-workers[3] in 1965, 16 by Dr. Robert Brashear in 1966 (A.O.A. program), and additional cases by Dr. Thomas Delorme and Dr. Herbert Pedersen in 1967 (A.O.A. program)—are sufficient to classify this injury as a definite entity.

All of the fractures in my series occurred in auto accidents and probably were caused by hyperextension of the neck. Neurological complications were either nonexistent or were of a minor degree and cleared with rest and traction.

A 21-year-old girl, E. F., was thrown from her car in an auto collision in June, 1965. In the lateral roentgenogram made at the time of injury there are fractures through the pedicles of the axis with minimal anterior displacement of the vertebral body (Fig. 3-14). This patient had moderate weakness of the right arm, which cleared rapidly with rest and skull traction.

The spinal canal, normally of ample size for the cord at this level, is made even larger by the anterior displacement of the vertebral body.

Seven months later, after treatment with traction and a brace, lateral studies in flexion and extension revealed complete healing of the fractures (Figs. 3-15 and 3-16).

Traction has little reducing effect upon the displaced body of the vertebrae because the body has been virtually disconnected from the posterior part of the segment.

Conservative treatment is adequate when the fragments of the pedicles are not widely separated.

Cases in which there is much wider separation of the fragments should probably have fusion of the first three vertebrae. An example of this is demonstrated in the lateral roentgenograms of J. B., one made after skull traction had been applied for a few days after she was injured in an auto accident. No improvement in the anterior displacement of the body or in the approximation of the pedicle fragments followed the application of skull traction as seen in the roentgenogram on the left; the one on the right was taken after surgical fusion. (See Fig. 3-17.)

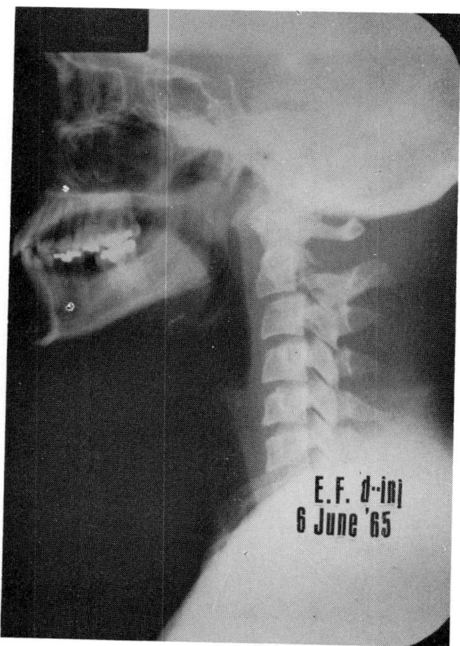

Fig. 3-14. E. F. There are fractures through the pedicles of the axis vertebra—"traumatic spondylolisthesis"—day of injury.

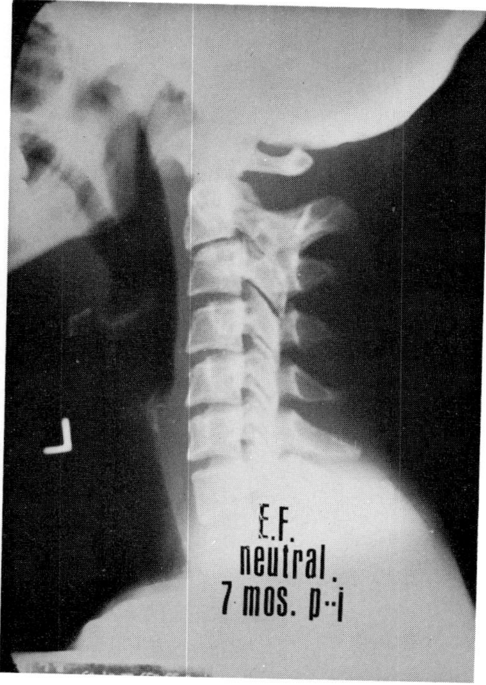

Fig. 3-15. E. F. Lateral view in neutral position—seven months after injury.

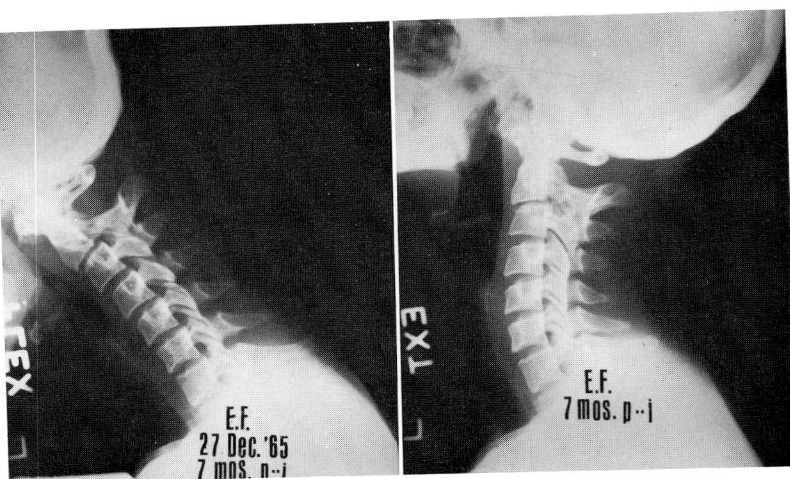

Fig. 3-16. E. F. The fractures have healed and the spine is stable after conservative treatment—seven months after injury.

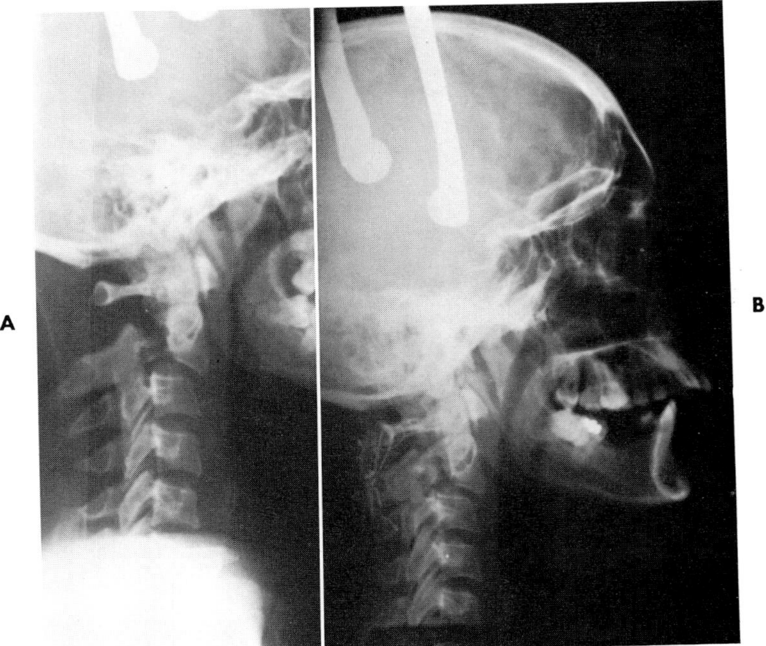

Fig. 3-17. J. B. **A,** Skull traction has not altered the position of the body of the axis. **B,** Roentgenogram made a few days after spine fusion. (From Garber, J. N.: J. Bone Joint Surg. **46-A:**1782, 1964.)

Dislocation without fracture

It is believed by some authors that dislocation in the cervical spine cannot occur without fracture. Possibly this is true, but occasionally dislocations are seen in which a fracture cannot be demonstrated.

Dislocations occur most commonly at the level from C3 to C7. These are unstable lesions in that they may be easily reduced by traction or manipulation, and, at the end of a reasonable period of immobilization, they recur. A dislocation easily reduced will just as easily recur unless fusion is done.

There is a dislocation of C4 on C5 in the roentgenogram of a young lady, M. J. L., made five days after an injury in July, 1954 (Fig. 3-18). Head sling traction was applied on admission to the hospital. The dislocation was still present just before manipulation under anesthesia (Fig. 3-19).

The dislocation was corrected by gentle manipulation, as indicated in this lateral projection (Fig. 3-20). Upon removal of the Minerva jacket after three months of immobilization, the dislocation was still reduced (Fig. 3-21).

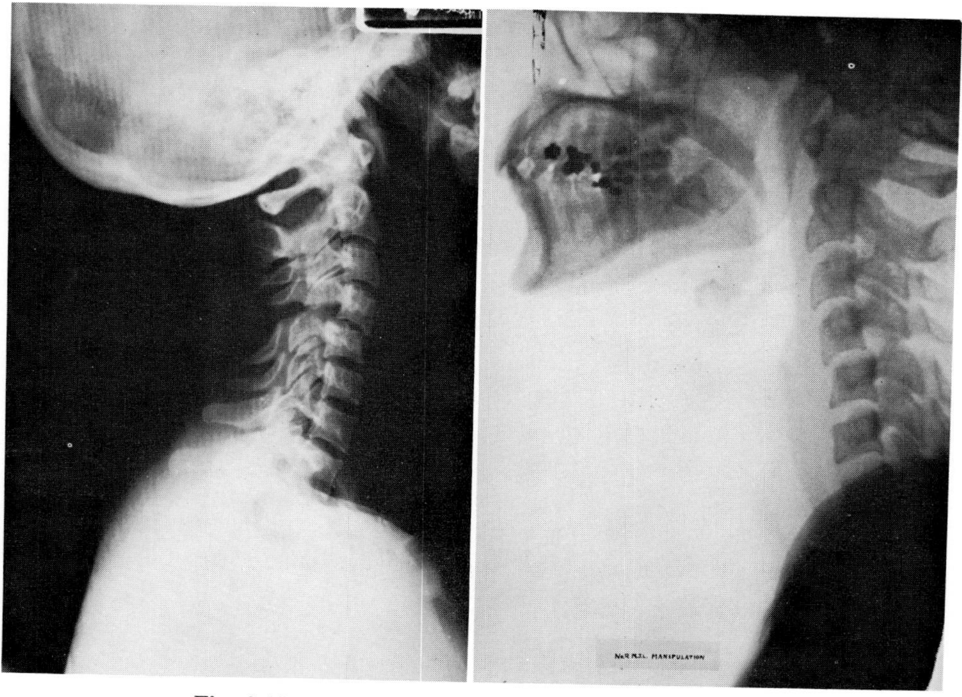

Fig. 3-18

Fig. 3-19

Fig. 3-18. M. J. L. Lateral roentgenogram taken July 28, 1954, one week after injury, shows anterior dislocation of C4 on C5.

Fig. 3-19. M. J. L. Lateral roentgenogram taken in surgery prior to manipulative reduction and the application of a Minerva jacket, August 4, 1954. (Polaroid film.)

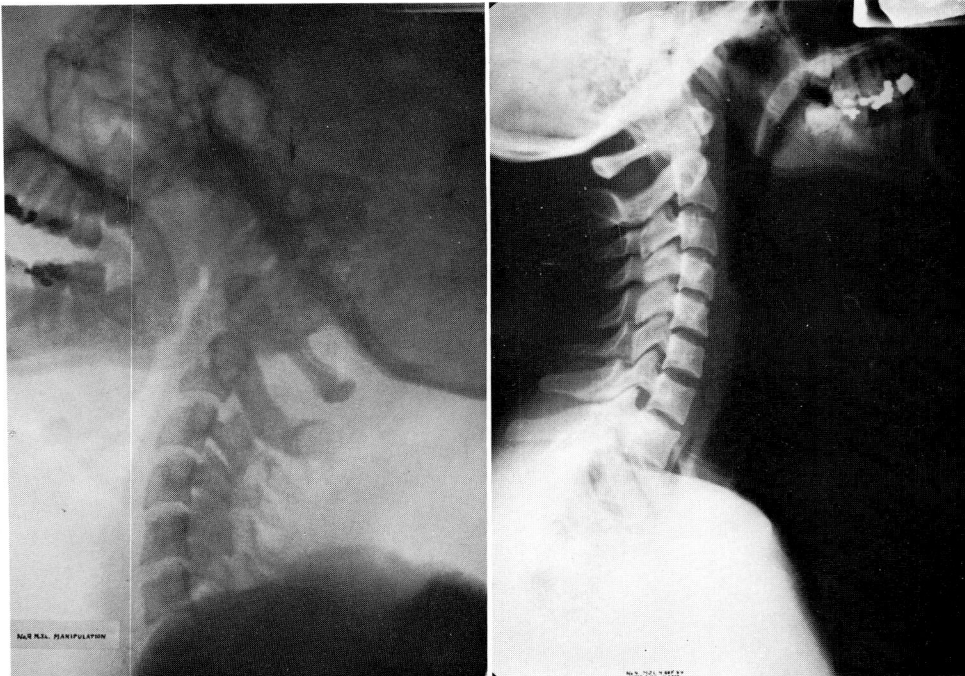

Fig. 3-20 Fig. 3-21

Fig. 3-20. M. J. L. Reduction of the dislocation of C4 on C5 has been obtained by manipulation. (Polaroid film.)
Fig. 3-21. M. J. L. Three months after reduction of the dislocation. The Minerva jacket was removed and a felt collar was applied at this time (Nov. 4, 1954).

The patient wore a felt collar for one month after the jacket was removed. A roentgenogram at that time, four months after the injury, indicated that the dislocation had recurred (Fig. 3-22). Skull traction was applied on her readmission to the hospital and fusion was done. Fusion appears to be satisfactory and position acceptable in roentgenograms taken thirteen months after the operation (Fig. 3-23).

It is obvious then that stability in the cervical spine depends upon articular capsules, ligaments, and muscles—and not upon the anatomical design of intervertebral bone and joint structure.

Cock-up dislocation

This lesion is probably caused by a blow on the head that flexes the neck. It usually occurs at the C6-C7 level. There is point-to-point contact of the articular processes (Fig. 3-24). Patients in my series have had minimal neurological changes.

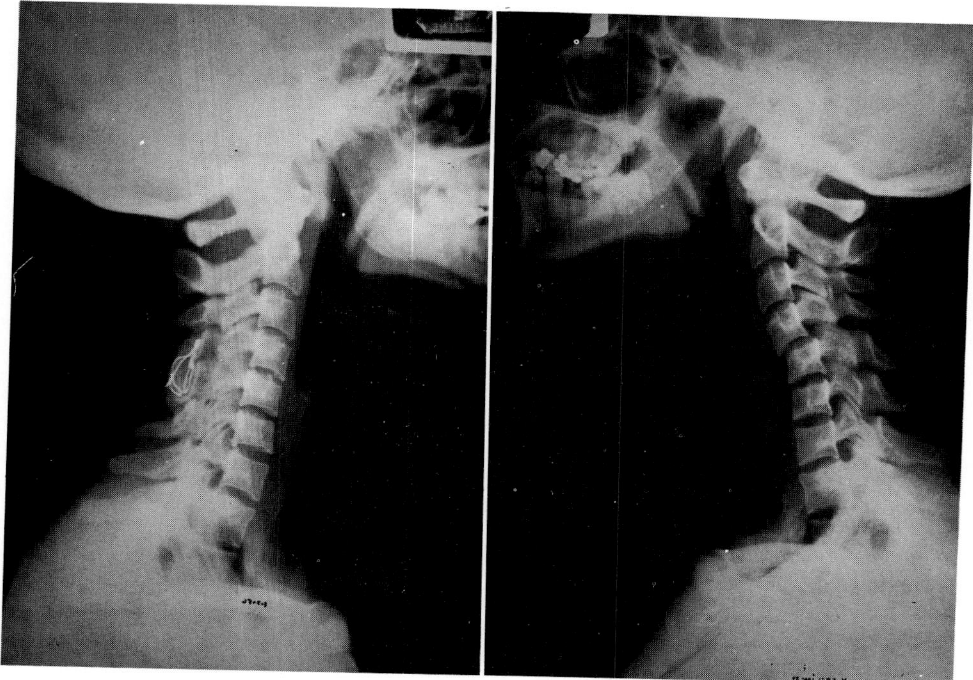

Fig. 3-22

Fig. 3-23

Fig. 3-22. M. J. L. The dislocation has recurred (Dec. 1, 1954) one month after the Minerva jacket was removed.
Fig. 3-23. M. J. L. Thirteen months after fusion of C4 and C5 (Jan. 7, 1956).

One might speculate that if the force exerted had been greater the inferior articular processes would have been pushed on over the processes below to cause severe cord damage or death.

This young girl, N. C., did not come in for examination until eleven months after she fell from a hay wagon, striking her head on the ground. At the time she did not feel that she had been severely injured and, after a few days' rest, resumed her work on the farm.

As time went on she developed neck stiffness and pain down both arms to the elbows with aggravation by strenuous activity. Her head was thrust forward.

A lateral roentgenogram reveals the cock-up point-to-point dislocation of C6 on C7 and calcification beneath the anterior spinal ligament (Fig. 3-25).

Reduction was initiated by skull traction and completed at the time of the fusion operation. Six months after operation the calcification anteriorly, which might once have been considered evidence of spontaneous fusion, has disappeared. The clasp on the necklace is not part of the fixation apparatus. (See Fig. 3-26.)

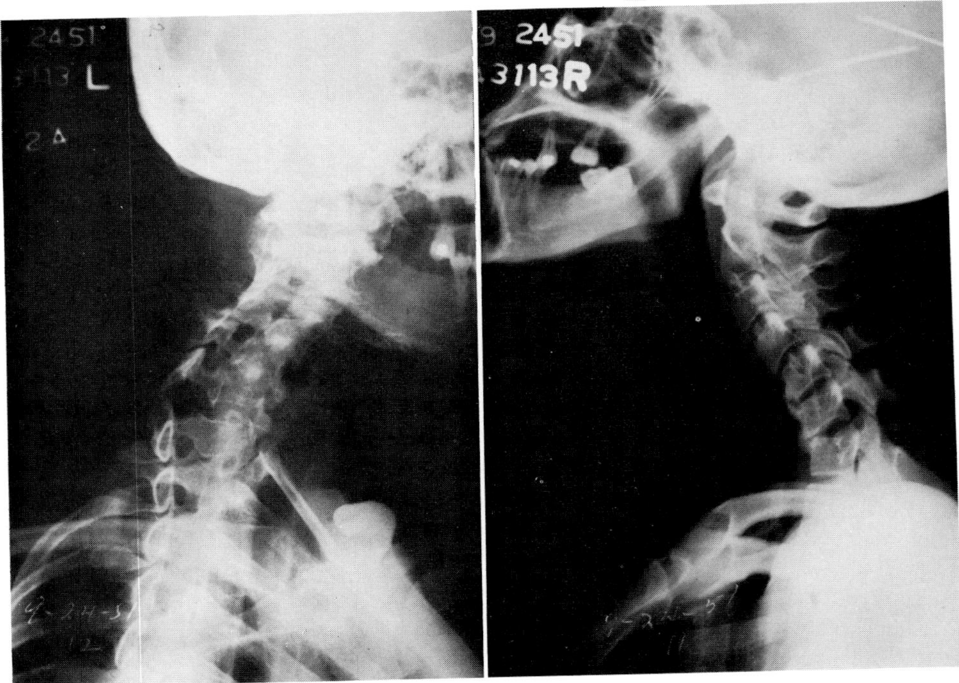

Fig. 3-24 Fig. 3-25

Fig. 3-24. N. C. There is point-to-point contact of the articular processes of C6 and C7.
Fig. 3-25. N. C. Cock-up dislocation of C6 on C7 eleven months after injury (Sept. 24, 1951). There is narrowing of the anterior third of the disc space between the two vertebrae, and calcification is present beneath the anterior spinal ligament connecting C5, C6, and C7.

Single and multiple fractures of the vertebral bodies

Compression or vertical fractures involving one or more vertebrae between C2 and T1 have a higher incidence of severe and permanent cord damage. Neurological complications may be acute and profound at the time of injury, or they may appear months later and become progressively more severe due to a slowly increasing kyphotic deformity of the neck.

It is highly probable that wide displacement of the bodies, or fragments of them, also occurs with these single and multiple compression lesions at the moment of injury. Such a dislocation may reduce spontaneously or it may be lessened during transportation of the victim to the hospital. This may explain those situations in which there is marked cord involvement, yet the bone injury in the roentgenogram is of only moderate severity.

A diving accident caused a bursting type fracture of C5 in an 18-year-old boy, F. H. He had extensive quadriparesis that improved with skull traction. Fusion from C4 to C6 was done. (See Fig. 3-27.) It was felt that the positive stability

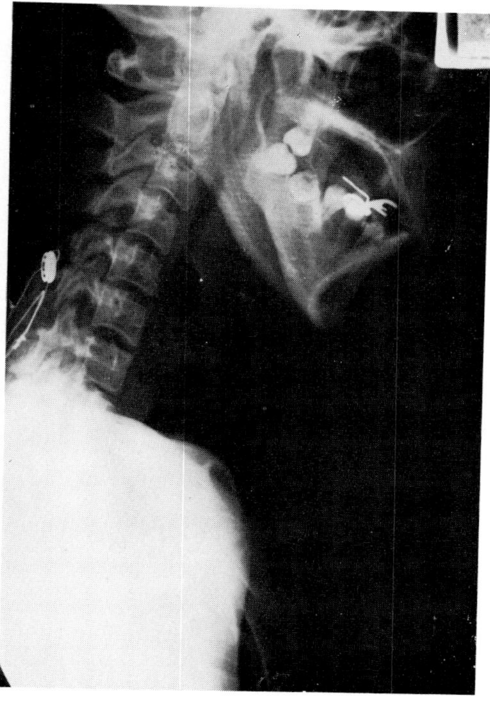

Fig. 3-26. N. C. Six months after fusion operation. Calcification under anterior spinal ligament has disappeared. (The oval metallic shadow is that of a necklace clasp.)

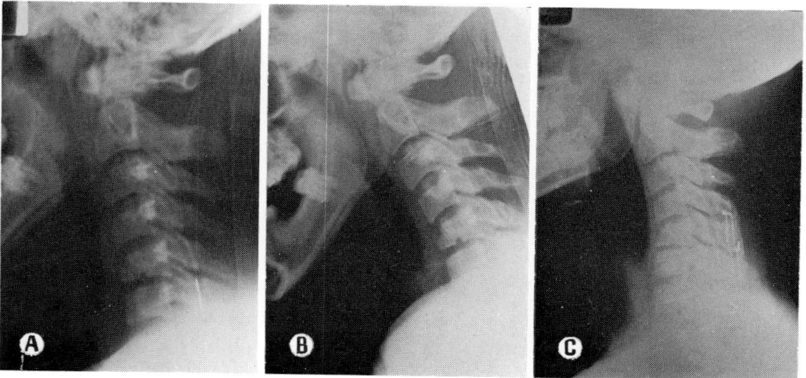

Fig. 3-27. B, A bursting fracture of C5 at the time of accident. **A,** Improvement after skull traction. **C,** The position four months after fusion.

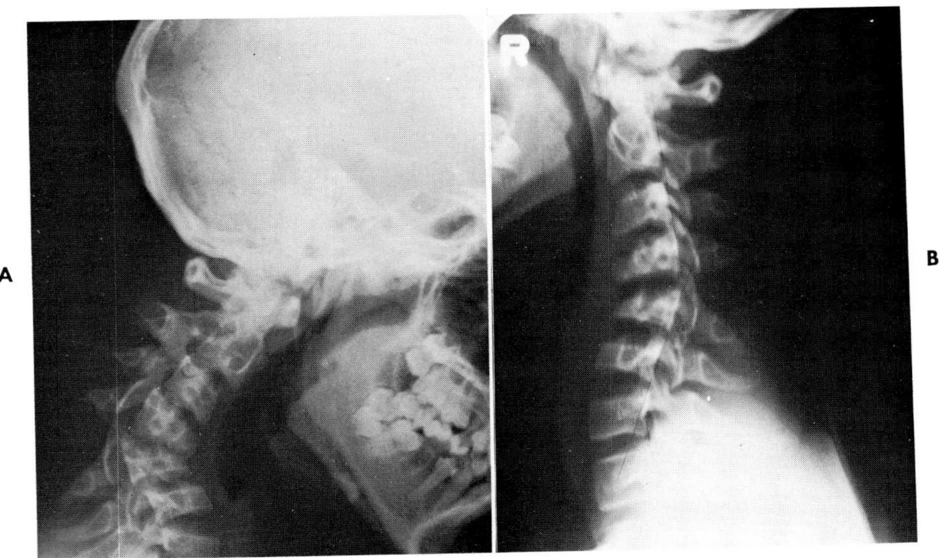

Fig. 3-28. G. G. **A,** Lateral roentgenogram made on hospital admission eight months after injury. **B,** Improvement in alignment after application of skull traction.

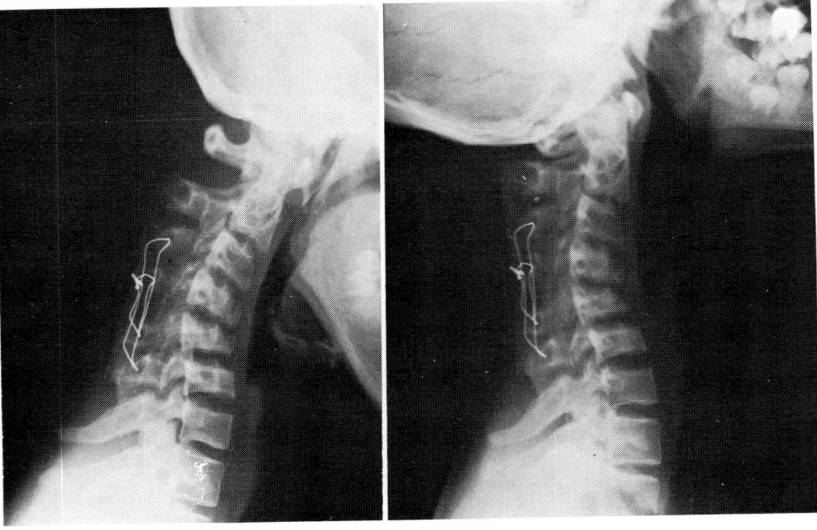

Fig. 3-29. G. G. Lateral roentgenograms in flexion and extension made almost six months after fusion.

provided by fusion was necessary because of the extensive damage to the single vertebral body.

There is a vertical fracture of the body of C5 with posterior displacement of fragments shown in roentgenogram *B* of Fig. 3-27. *A* in this illustration indicates improvement after skull traction, and the roentgenogram *C* on the right was made four months after operation.

Another young man, G. G., on regaining consciousness four days after an auto accident in 1954, was found to have a left hemiparesis as a result of multiple fractures in the cervical spine. Original treatment with skull traction for seven weeks followed by a Forrester brace relieved most of the motor weakness within three months.

He was admitted to the Indiana University Hospitals in March, 1955, eight months following the accident. He complained of a gradually increasing deformity of the neck and exhibited symptoms of an upper motor neuron type. The multiple fractures present in the roentgenogram taken at this later hospital admission are seen in Fig. 3-28.

The neck has straightened after the reapplication of skull tongs and fusion, illustrating again that even months after injury some lesions can be improved by traction and stabilization (Fig. 3-29).

Injuries to the arthritic spine

Mention should be made of pathological changes with or without injury, which are sometimes seen in the arthritic spine.

W. B., a 55-year-old man, has had extensive rheumatoid arthritis for seven years. He has had no severe injury at any time; but during this period, as a sequela of the disease or of the treatment or both, there has been a dissolution of the transverse ligament of the atlas, permitting progressive dislocation of this vertebra over the axis below. There is beginning displacement of the atlas in roentgenograms made in 1961; progressive forward displacement has occurred over the four years to 1965. (See Figs. 3-30 and 3-31.) The swan-neck appearance in the lateral projection is typical of long-standing atlantoaxial displacement (Fig. 3-32).

Another man, H. H., with Marie-Strümpell ankylosing arthritis of long duration reversed the usual rear-end collision story and, instead, hit a car in front of him. His "brittle neck" broke at the level receiving the maximum force—the C6 body. (See Fig. 3-33.) Neurological changes that were minimal in severity immediately after the injury disappeared with conservative therapy.

Such cases should, in my opinion, be managed with great care and with emphasis on conservatism. Sudden drastic changes in alignment, which could be made by strong traction or manipulation, might produce profound and even total cord damage. Furthermore, for other reasons an individual with this type of problem is often not the most desirable candidate for surgery.

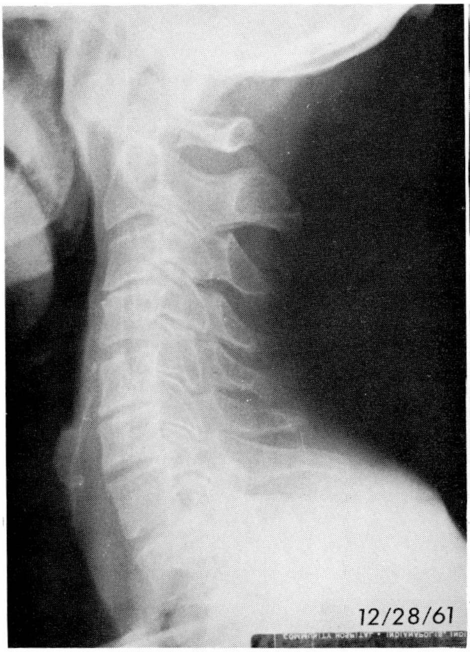

Fig. 3-30 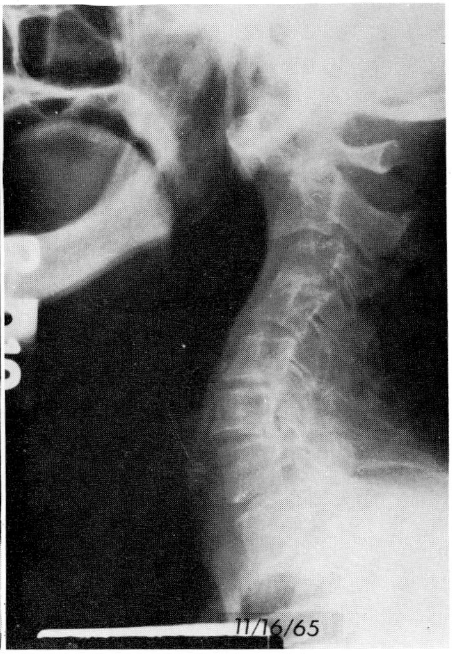 **Fig. 3-31**

Fig. 3-30. W. B. Marie-Strümpell's ankylosing spondylitis of seven years' duration in 1961. **Fig. 3-31.** W. B. Four years later in 1965.

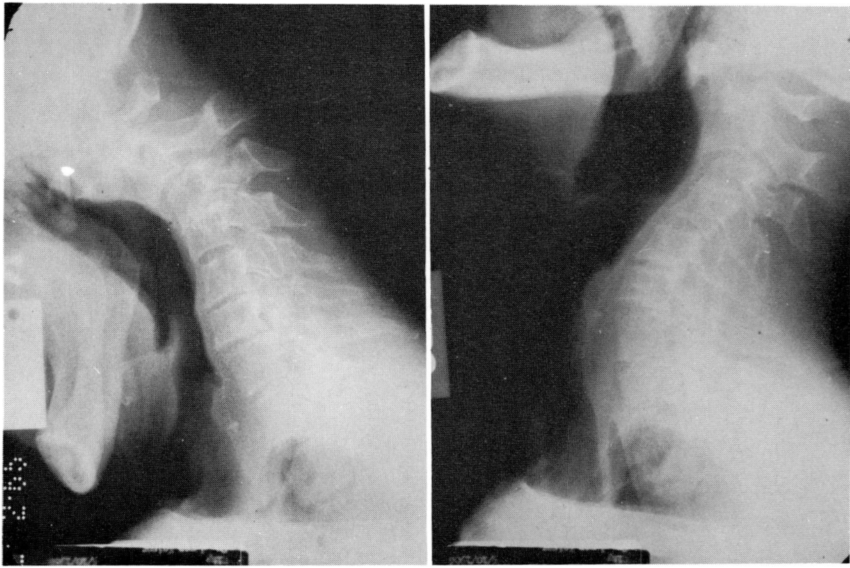

Fig. 3-32. W. B. Flexion and extension—1965.

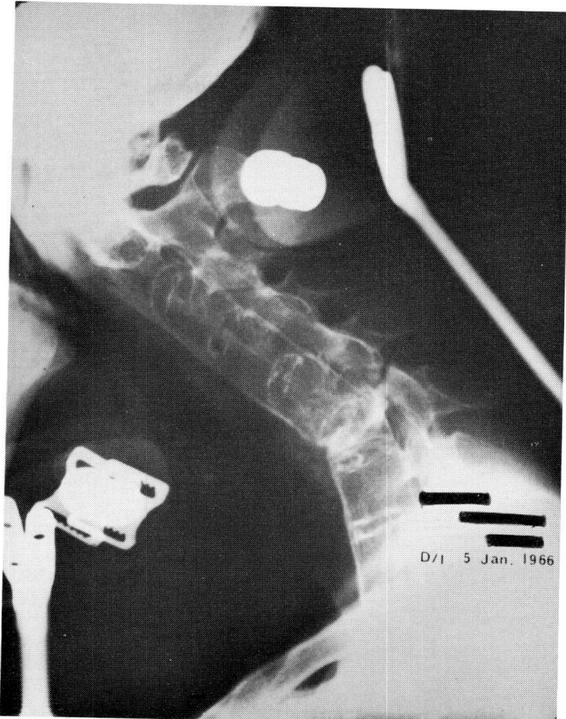

Fig. 3-33. H. H. Fracture of ankylosed spine after "reversed" rear-end collision. (Courtesy Dr. Henry Tanner, Indianapolis.)

Congenital anomalies of the atlas and axis

Congenital defects in the cervical spine must be considered together with traumatic lesions. Frequently the congenital anomalies are first discovered when roentgenograms are made because of neck injury.

Atlas

Two female patients, one 24 years of age and the other 45 years old, developed neck pain after rear-end auto collisions. These people had had no neck complaint prior to the accidents, and they had no neurological changes afterward.

There is complete absence of the posterior arch of the atlas in the younger woman, D. O. (Fig. 3-34). There appears to be a calcified mass posteriorly in the soft tissue (Fig. 3-35). The neck is stable in flexion and extension (Fig. 3-36).

In the second, M. O., there is failure of development of the posterior arch of the atlas adjacent to the lateral masses (Fig. 3-37). There is no abnormal excursion of the atlas in flexion and extension (Fig. 3-38).

H. A., a 17-year-old girl, had a mild neck strain from a rear-end collision in April, 1966. Bilateral defects are seen in the posterior arch of the atlas in a

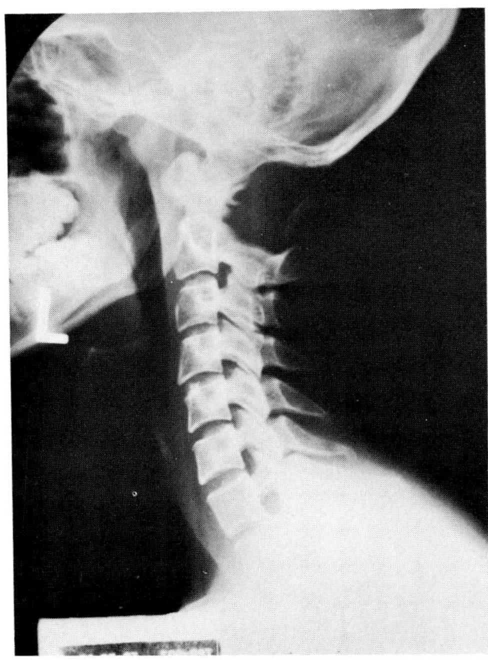

Fig. 3-34. D. O. Absence of posterior arch of the atlas. (Courtesy Dr. Thomas A. Brady, Indianapolis.)

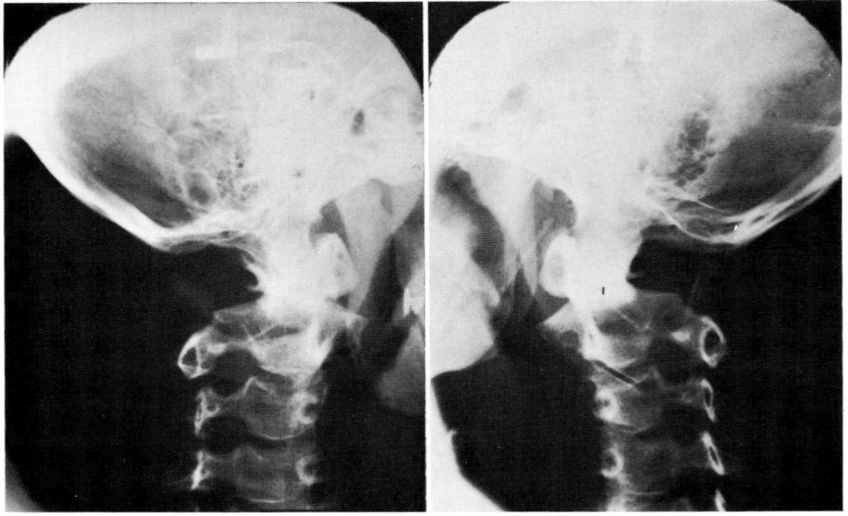

Fig. 3-35. D. O. Absence of posterior arch of the atlas. Oblique views.

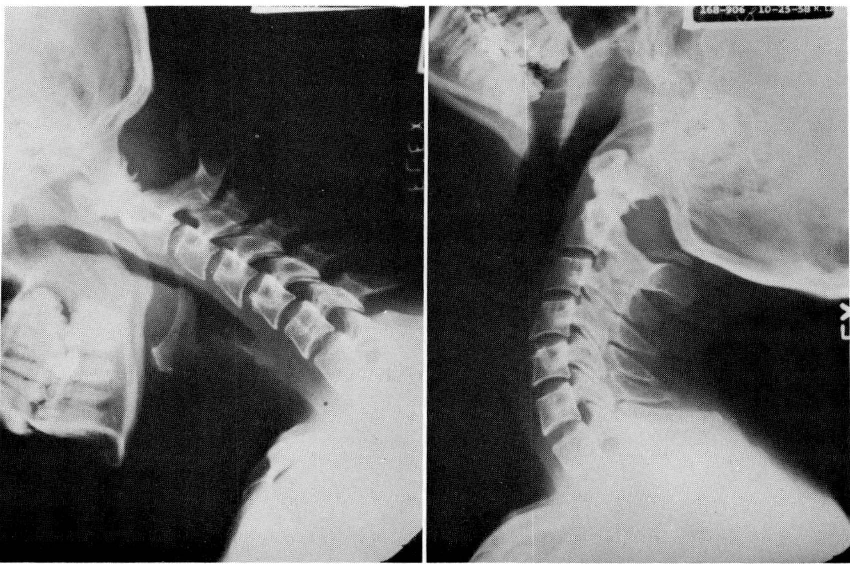

Fig. 3-36. D. O. Flexion and extension. (From Garber, J. N.: J. Bone Joint Surg. **46-A:**1782, 1964.)

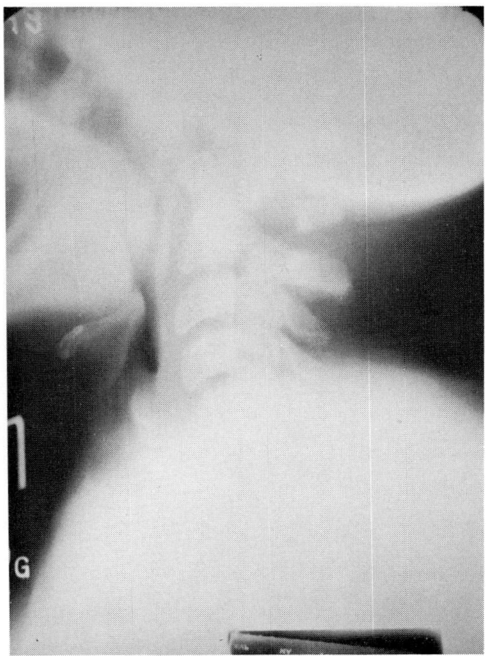

Fig. 3-37. M. O. Failure of development of posterior arch of the atlas. (Courtesy Dr. Raymond O. Pierce, Indianapolis.)

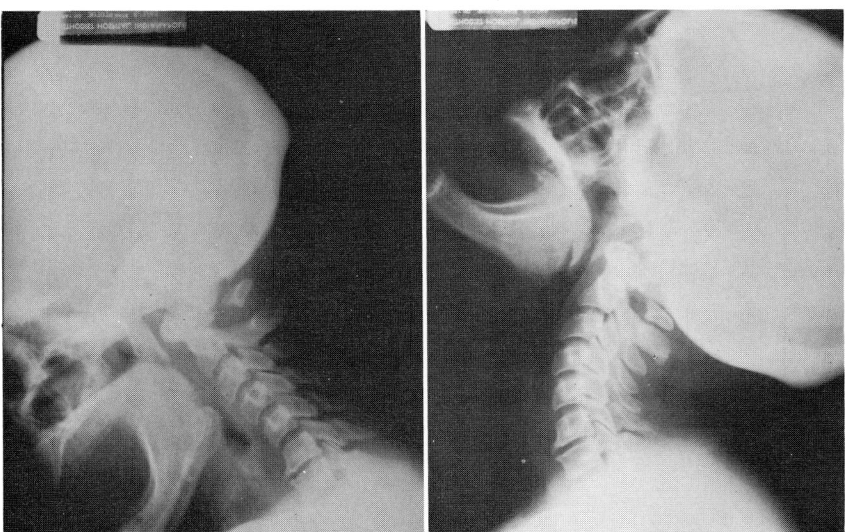

Fig. 3-38. M. O. Flexion and extension. (From Garber, J. N.: J. Bone Joint Surg. **46-A:**1782, 1964.)

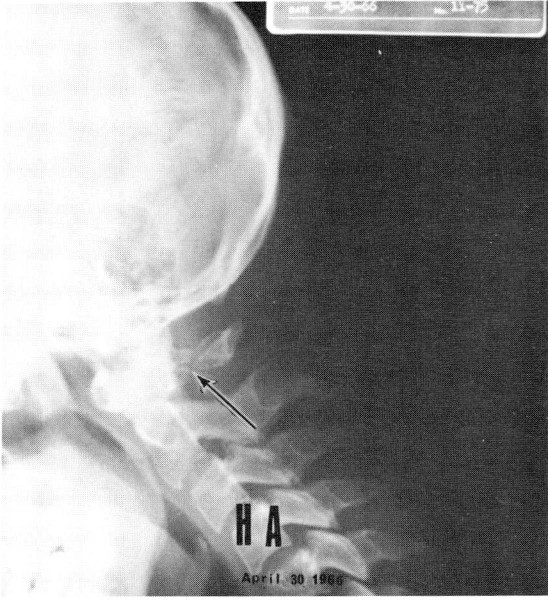

Fig. 3-39. H. A. A fresh fracture (at arrow) in 1966? (Courtesy Dr. Robert M. Palmer, Indianapolis.)

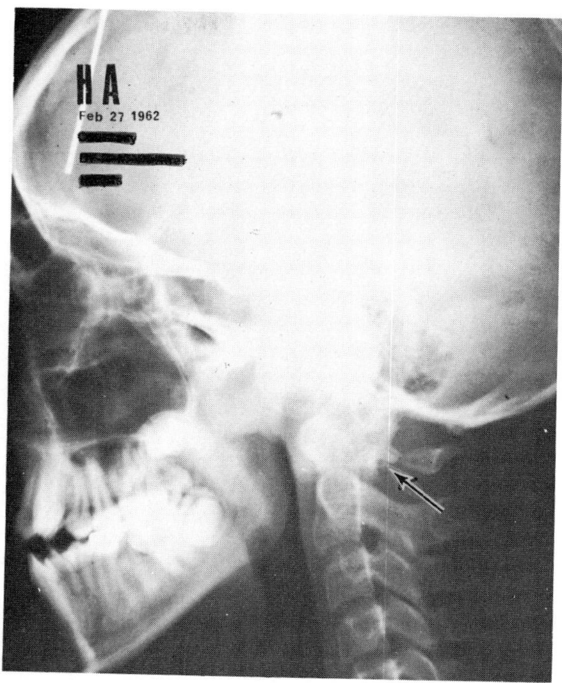

Fig. 3-40. H. A. The defect (arrow) in the posterior arch of the atlas was present in this roentgenogram made for dental purposes in 1962.

lateral roentgenogram (Fig. 3-39) taken at that time. Does the arrow indicate a fresh fracture?

Fortunately, a roentgenogram of the skull had been made for dental purposes four years before. The defects in the atlas were present then and are congenital in origin. (See Fig. 3-40.)

These congenital anomalies undoubtedly would not have been found had it not been for the accidents. Once the true nature of the lesions was apparent here, the further study by roentgenograms in flexion and extension was most important to demonstrate that neither the congenital anomalies nor the injuries had any effect upon the stability of the spine.

F. S. was examined within a few hours after an auto accident because of pain and stiffness in her neck (Fig. 3-41).

The bone "fragment" below the anterior arch of the atlas in the lateral roentgenogram was at first thought to be fractured from the arch. On closer examination, this so-called fragment is found to have smooth margins with a thin rim of cortical density, suggesting that it is an intercalary bone of developmental origin rather than a fragment from the atlas. (See Fig. 3-42.)

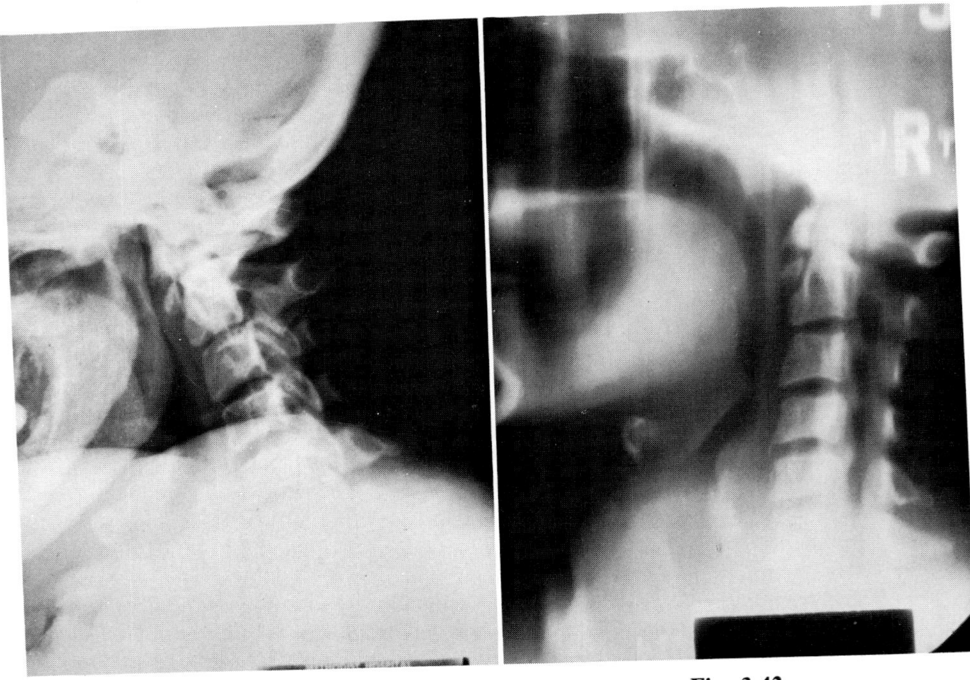

Fig. 3-41

Fig. 3-42

Fig. 3-41. F. S. Lateral roentgenogram showing questionable fracture of the atlas. (Courtesy Dr. Raymond O. Pierce, Indianapolis.)
Fig. 3-42. F. S. Lateral tomogram.

Furthermore, if this were a fracture the resulting hemorrhage would have widened the cervicolaryngeal space, a space between the posterior wall of the larynx and the upper corner of the third cervical vertebra, which does not exceed 5 mm. in the normal neck.

Here we find that this space is not widened, which gives added evidence against the diagnosis of acute fracture (Fig. 3-43). An intercalary bone at this level is a rare finding; these bones are occasionally seen lower, at the C5-C6 level.

Recognition of such defects as congenital rather than traumatic lesions becomes of greater importance as the number of neck injury cases increases.

Axis

Partial or total absence of the odontoid process allows an abnormal range of excursion of the atlas over the axis. Fortunately, a wide range of motion can occur at this level in the cervical spine without causing severe damage to the cord because of ample space in the spinal canal.

Vague neck discomfort and headache may be the only complaint. Other

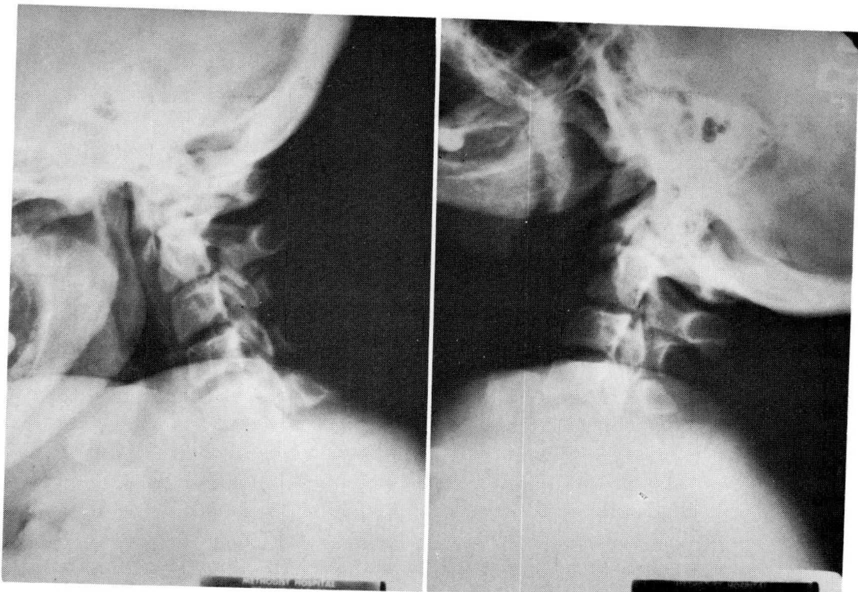

Fig. 3-43. F. S. Flexion and extension.

patients may have attacks of transitory quadriparesis following injury from a relatively minor force such as the Nelson hold in wrestling or a moderately severe bump on the head.

One patient in my series who has a rudimentary odontoid process developed progressive hemiparesis.

Trauma to the head and neck has precipitated the symptoms in almost all of the patients. The severity of the symptoms, particularly when quadriparesis occurs, is out of proportion to the relatively moderate force of the trauma. The normal neck would be expected to withstand such force without difficulty.

In the lateral roentgenogram of the *normal* cervical spine the only bone structure that lies in front of a line projected along the anterior margins of the cervical vertebrae is the profile of the anterior ring of the atlas (Fig. 3-44).

Absence of the odontoid process is seen in this roentgenogram of a 35-year-old man, D. S., who had repeated attacks of quadriparesis after blows of moderate severity on the back of the head (Fig. 3-45). On one occasion generalized weakness caused him to fall to the floor when he raised his head too soon under a low bridge while wheeling a hand truck. There is wide excursion of the atlas on the axis as the neck is flexed and extended (Fig. 3-46).

A 13-year-old boy, J. S., was examined because of a congenital abnormality of the odontoid process.

At the age of 2 years he fell out of his crib. Following this injury he had stiffness of the neck and held his head in a cocked position. An x-ray examination

Text continued on p. 48.

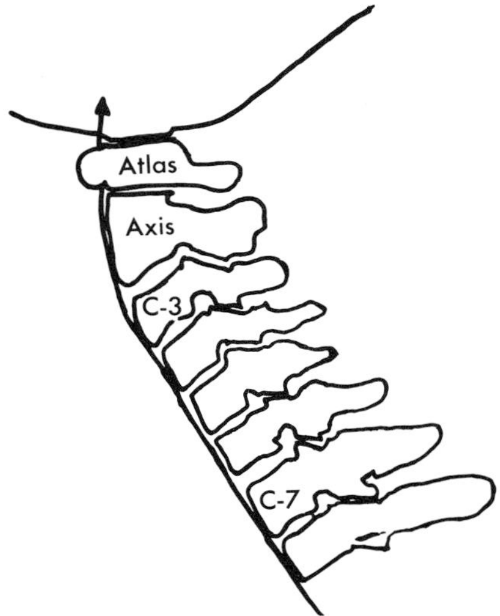

Fig. 3-44. Anterior projected line in the normal cervical spine. In the lateral roentgenogram of the normal cervical spine the only bone structure that lies in front of a line projected along the anterior margins of the cervical vertebrae is the profile of the anterior ring of the atlas.

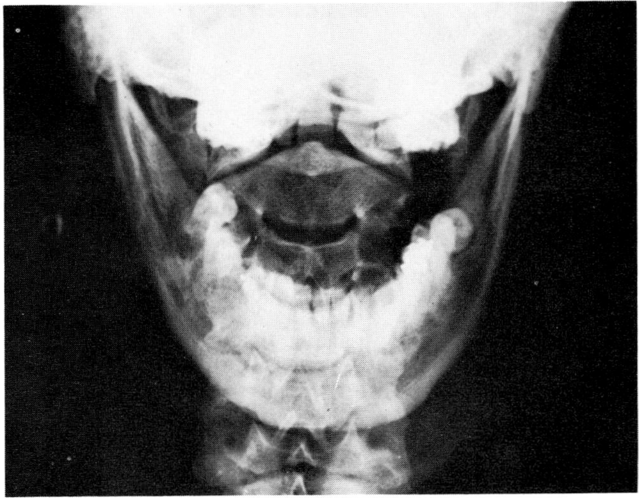

Fig. 3-45. D. S. A rudimentary odontoid process. (From Garber, J. N.: J. Bone Joint Surg. **46-A:**1782, 1964.)

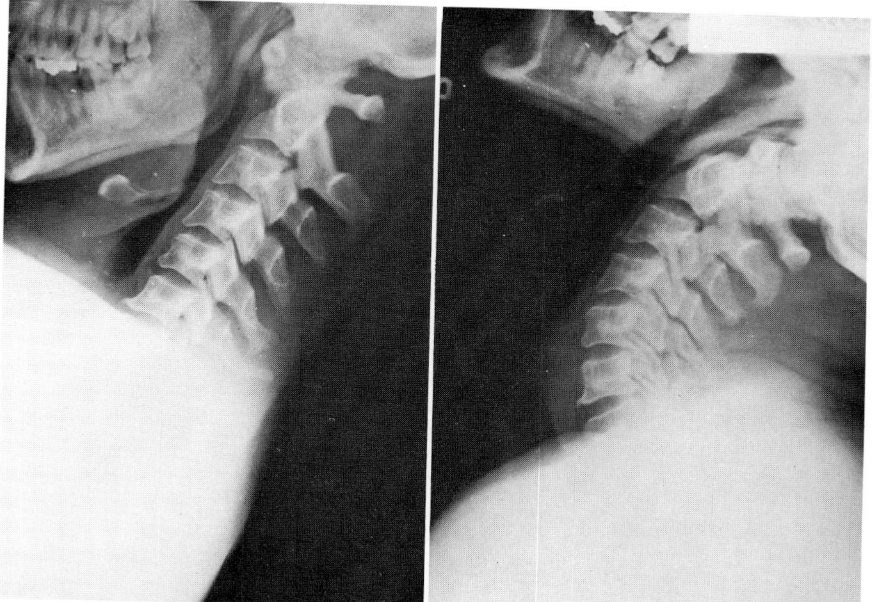

Fig. 3-46. D. S. There is wide excursion of the atlas over the axis in flexion and extension. (From Garber, J. N.: J. Bone Joint Surg. **46-A:**1782, 1964.)

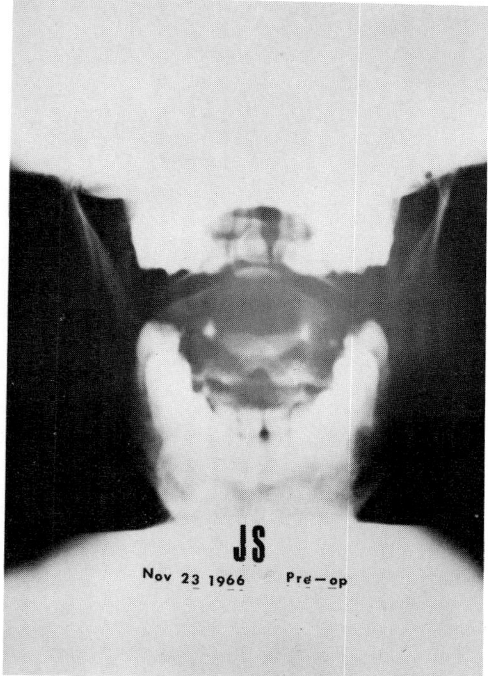

Fig. 3-47. J. S., age 13. Open-mouth anteroposterior view shows a rudimentary odontoid process with an os odontoideum or an ununited fracture of the odontoid from an old injury—probably the former.

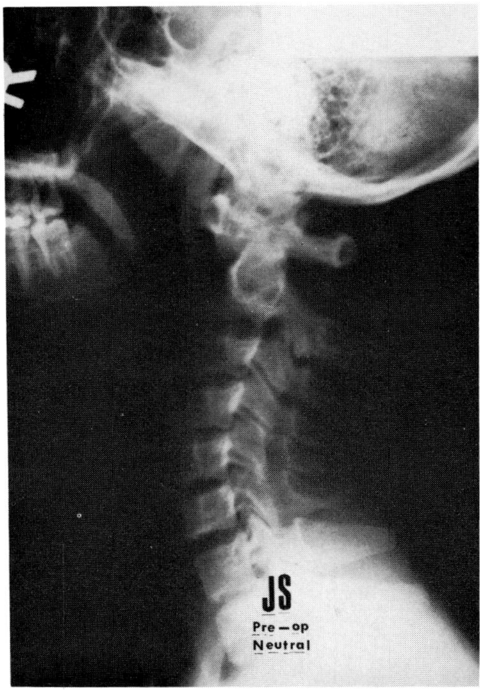

Fig. 3-48. J. S. Even though the head is in a neutral position the atlas is displaced forward on the axis.

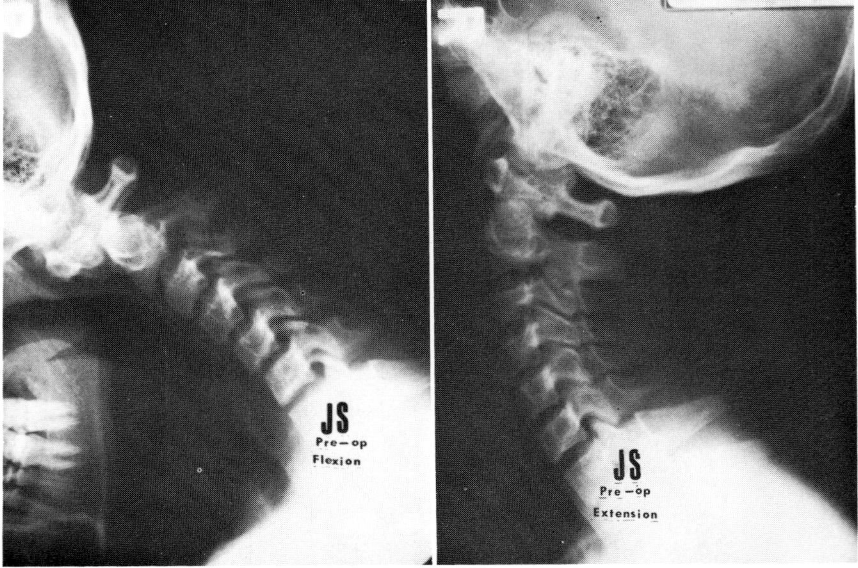

Fig. 3-49. J. S. Lateral roentgenograms in flexion and extension (November, 1966).

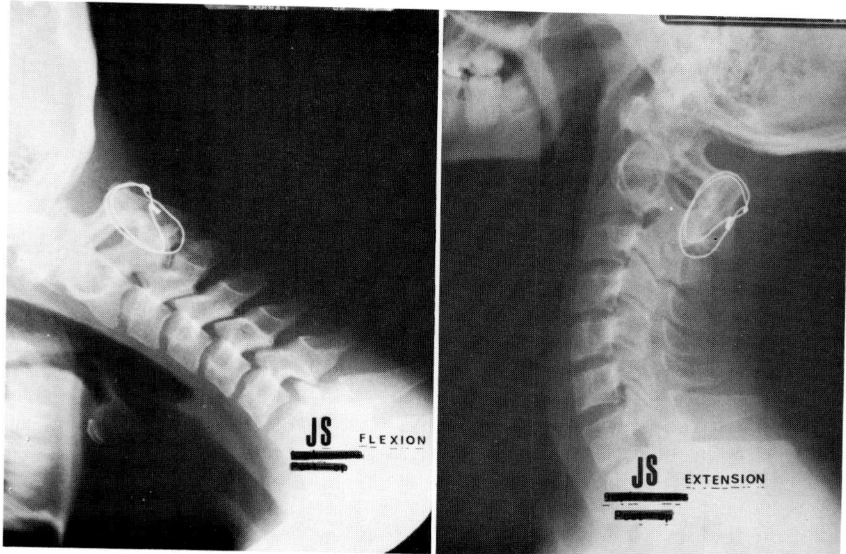

Fig. 3-50. J. S. Lateral roentgenograms made nine months after the fusion operation.

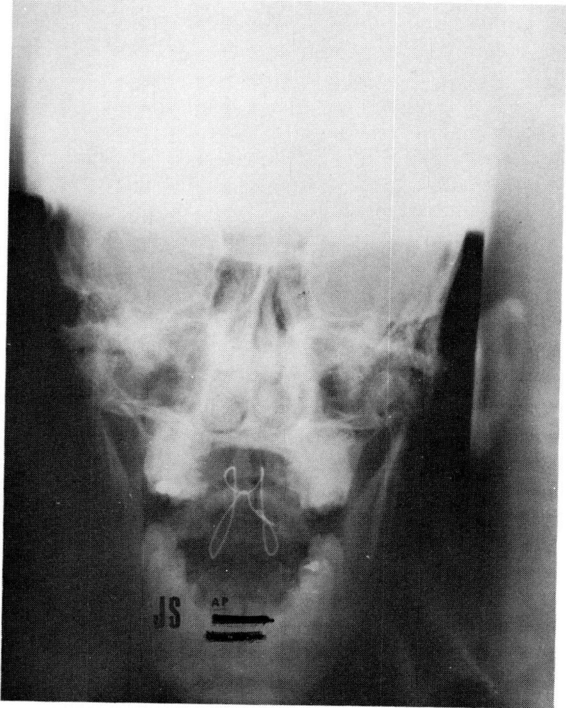

Fig. 3-51. J. S. An anteroposterior roentgenogram taken after the fusion operation shows the course of the wire holding the block graft.

then is said to have shown some abnormality of the odontoid process, either of a congenital nature or due to trauma of the fall. His symptoms disappeared after he wore a collar for several weeks.

Through the ensuing years he played basketball and football in grade school without difficulty until he was kicked in the side of the head during a football game in November, 1966. Pain and stiffness in the neck with limited head motion followed this injury. There was no nerve involvement and after three weeks of conservative treatment all symptoms subsided.

In the open-mouth anteroposterior roentgenogram there is either a rudimentary odontoid with an os odontoideum or a nonunion of an old fracture (Fig. 3-47).

There is forward displacement of the atlas in the neutral position (Fig. 3-48) and on flexion of the neck. Only when the neck is fully extended does the atlas come back to its normal relationship with the axis. (See Fig. 3-49.)

This fine, well-adjusted lad, 13 years old and 6 feet 3 inches in height, is intensely interested in athletics and, as you may well imagine, is the apple of the eyes of his coaches.

With this in mind and considering his probable anticipated life-span of sixty active years, I felt that his C1-C2 level should be stabilized. The fusion was done on Feb. 2, 1967.

Satisfactory stability is evident nine months after operation, in roentgenograms made in flexion and extension (Fig. 3-50). The anteroposterior roentgenogram illustrates the course of the wire holding the block graft (Fig. 3-51).

Stabilization of the upper cervical spine by fusion of the first two or three vertebrae relieves the symptoms in these patients. Some patients may be reluctant to undergo surgery of this magnitude, particularly if their symptoms are not severe and are not present all of the time. These people should be warned to avoid any situations in which there might be a blow to the head, and probably they should be advised to wear a protective collar while riding in a car.

Fusion is definitely indicated for those patients who have transitory or progressive neurological symptoms.

Treatment of injuries of the cervical spine

Immobilization of the head by whatever means are available, for transportation from the scene of the accident, and then the application of traction, first through a head sling and later by skull tongs if needed, are of paramount importance in the early treatment of neck injuries.

I have used the posterior fusion procedure when surgical stabilization was indicated. For this, the patient is placed prone with the head supported on the cerebellar rest. Traction with 5 to 10 pounds of weight is maintained throughout the procedure and continued afterward. (See Fig. 3-52.)

Diagrams in Fig. 3-53 illustrate the technique of the Gallie fusion of the first two cervical vertebrae as it was reintroduced by Dr. J. William Fielding a few years ago (A.A.O.S. audiovisual program—January, 1966).

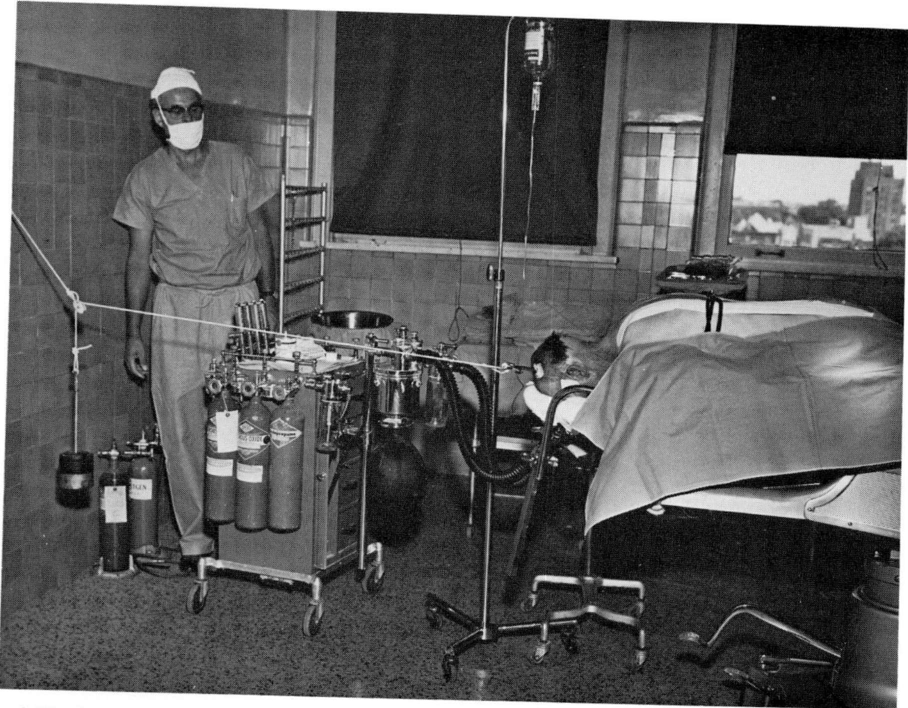

Fig. 3-52. Position of patient on the operating table for posterior fusion. The head is supported on a cerebellar rest.

I have changed this slightly by putting two drill holes instead of notches near the upper corners of the iliac block graft to prevent the wires' sliding together at the top. Two ends of the wire loop are passed through these holes and then beneath the posterior arch of the atlas and the laminae of the axis.

One end of the wire goes through the loop and, as the block is brought down in place, the ends of the wire are twisted as illustrated. Notches at the two lower corners of the graft keep the wires apart here. A much larger notch cut in the center of the lower part of the graft lets it slip down onto the lamina of the axis around its spinous process. (See Fig. 3-53.)

The technique of the classic posterior fusion from C2 downward is shown in the diagrams in Fig. 3-54. Laminae are denuded of cortical bone with a rongeur. One should never pound with a mallet on the cervical spine. Some surgeons believe that denuding the laminae is not necessary; they place strips of iliac graft over the laminae which are stripped only of soft tissue.

Years before we had the Stryker frame and the circle bed I used this type of bed arrangement for patients with neck injuries (Fig. 3-55). A long, firm bed board is placed beneath the mattress and the patient is reversed in bed with his

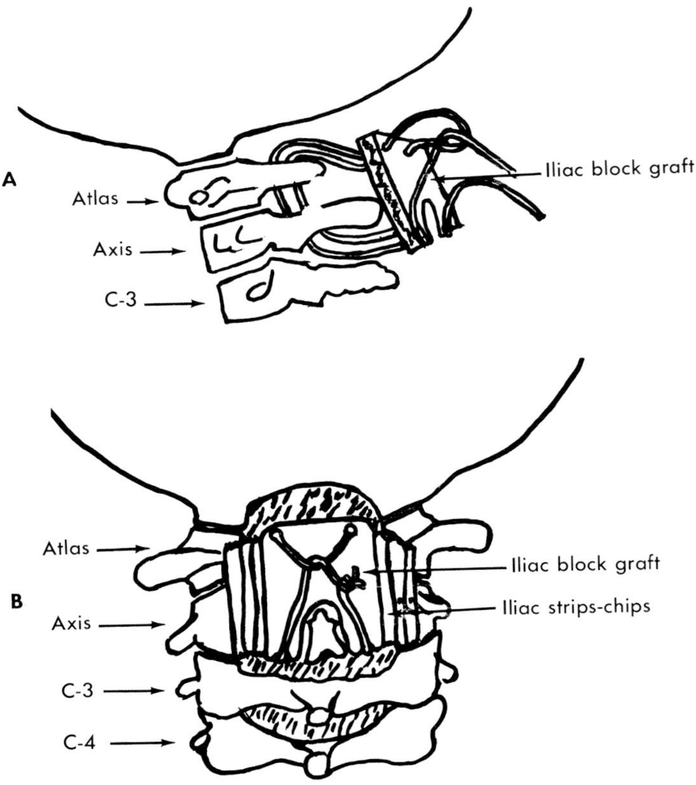

Fig. 3-53. Diagrams of the Gallie technique to fuse the atlas and the axis vertebrae. **A,** Lateral view. **B,** Posterior view. (After Dr. J. William Fielding.)

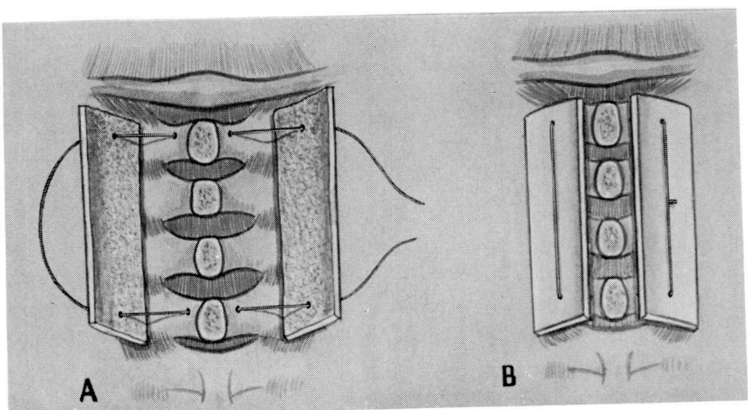

Fig. 3-54. Diagrams illustrating the technique of wiring iliac shingle grafts in place if two spinous processes are to be wired together, as in fusion for a dislocation. **A,** The processes are first wired together. **B,** Then the grafts are wired in place over them as shown here. (From Garber, J. N.: J. Bone Joint Surg. **46-A:** 1782, 1964.)

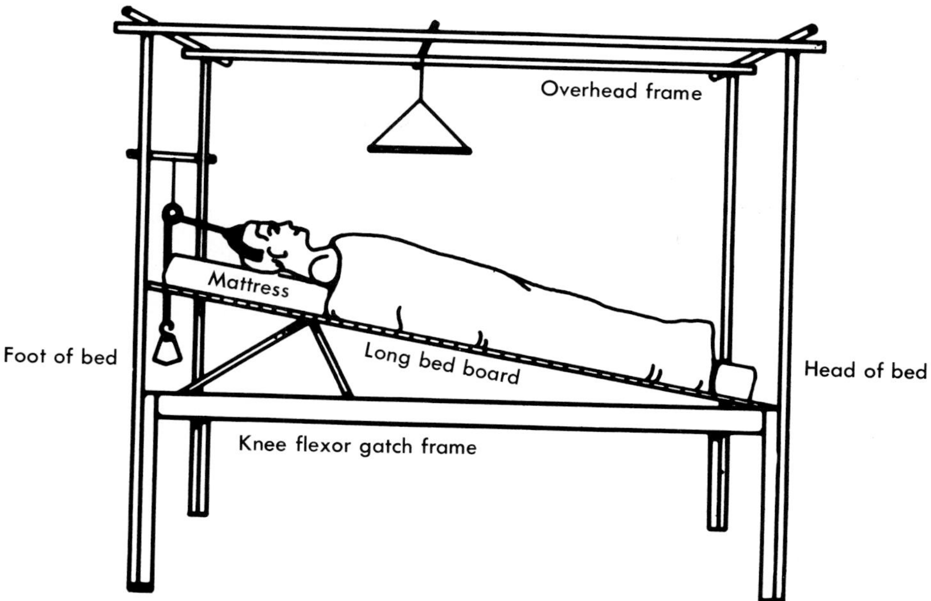

Fig. 3-55. A bed arrangement that may be used in the care of neck injuries.

head at the foot. As the knee flexion part of the Gatch frame is raised, the patient is brought up to any desired level of an inclined plane. This provides countertraction to any weight used through the head tongs or sling. The desired axis of pull can easily be maintained by adjusting the height of the crossbar of the overhead frame that carries the pulley.

There are certain advantages. The patient feels more secure on a bed of normal width than on the narrow frame. He can lie on three surfaces instead of two—both sides and his back. Care of the patient is fairly simple, and the bed will not fall apart to dump him on the floor, as frames have been known to do.

When the patient is turned to either side, sufficient pillow support is added to keep the head from tilting downward to the surface of the mattress.

Traction is continued for a period of four to six weeks after surgery. A Minerva jacket or a brace is then applied for four to five months.

During the past few years I have used a special brace in preference to the Minerva jacket. It is similar to the one used by Dr. Robert Bailey of Ann Arbor, Michigan, for the postoperative treatment of his cervical fusions. (See Figs. 3-56 and 3-57.)

It is impossible to immobilize the cervical spine completely with a plaster jacket or a brace. The jacket is usually applied with the patient supine. When he stands, the fit of the jacket changes. If a headband is included, it may cause the jacket to push down on the neck when the patient is in the upright position.

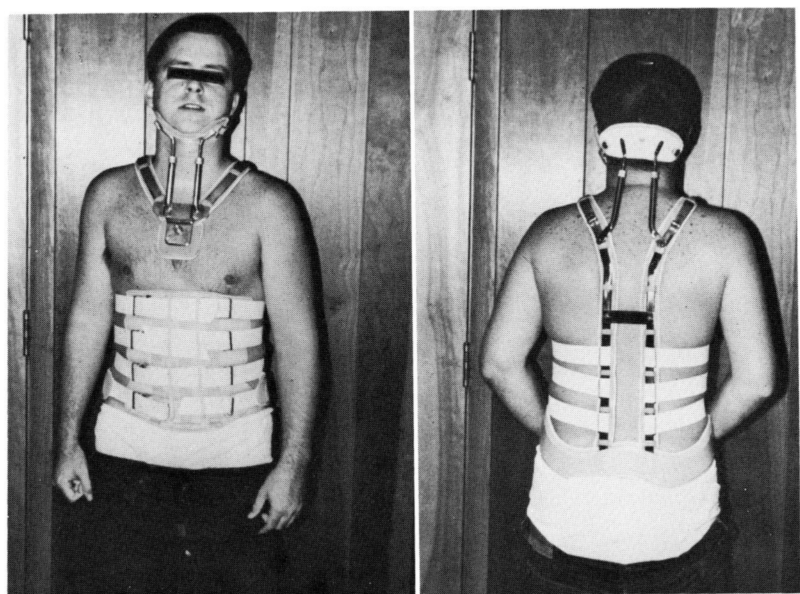

Fig. 3-56. Cervical spine brace—front and rear. (Courtesy Dr. William Irvine, Indianapolis.)

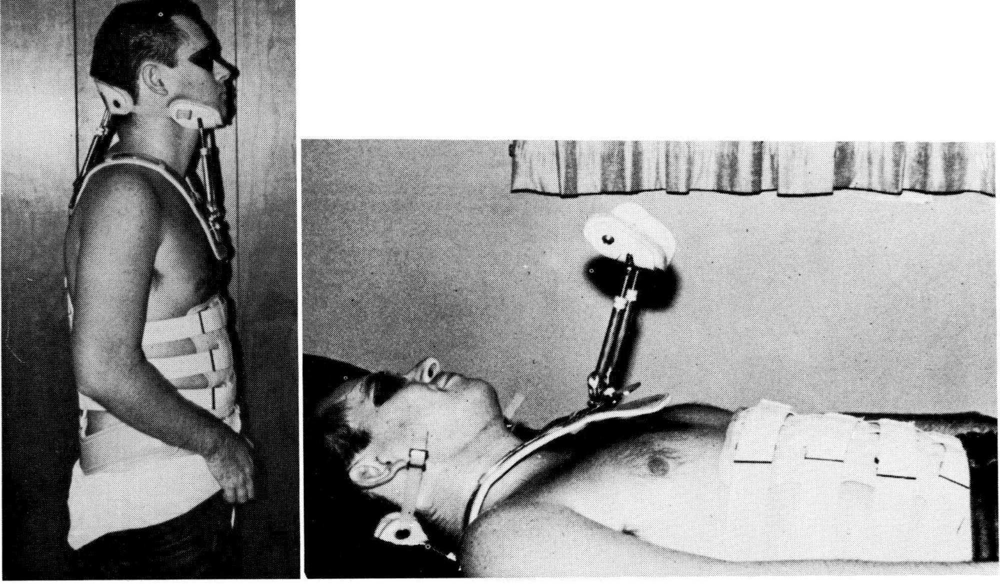

Fig. 3-57. Cervical spine brace. Patient standing and supine.

Some comment should be made about anterior cervical fusion. This is a procedure that has great merit in suitable hands and in a suitable environment. In certain cases where wide laminectomy has been done it is the only way in which the neck can be stabilized.

Conclusions

The more frequently encountered derangements of the cervical spine have been discussed here.

An attempt has been made to show that certain of these conditions will respond adequately to conservative measures, while in others stabilization by spine fusion should be done.

Fractures and dislocations of the cervical spine are common injuries and in many instances the individual so injured can be returned to a comfortable, productive existence with little disability.

References

1. Jefferson, G.: Fractures of the atlas vertebra, Brit. J. Surg. **7:**407, 1920.
2. Merrill, V.: Atlas of roentgenographic positions, vol. 1, ed. 3, St. Louis, 1967, The C. V. Mosby Co.
3. Schneider, R. C., Livingston, K. E., Cave, A. J. E., and Hamilton, G.: "Hangman's fracture" of the cervical spine, J. Neurosurg. **22:**141, 1965.

4. Lumbosacral strain and instability

Leon L. Wiltse, M.D.

In this chapter I will consider lumbosacral strain and instability as a general heading for the discussion of low back pain arising from the structural elements of the low back. These structural elements are the nucleus pulposus, the annulus fibrosus, the intervertebral joints with their synovial and cartilaginous tissues, the muscular and ligamentous structures, and the vertebrae themselves. Suggestions for conservative management of low back pain will be given. The surgical treatment will be discussed in a different chapter. The terms lumbar insufficiency, lumbago, and sciatica will be used to describe the various manifestations of lumbosacral pain.

The term *lumbar insufficiency* will be used to designate fatigue or pain in the small of the back, of more or less intermittent character. It is usually associated with bending over and picking things up; it is not completely disabling and it goes away as soon as the activity that precipitated it is stopped.

Lumbago is used to define pain in the low back which is of more severe nature, which does not go away on cessation of the activity that precipitated it, and which may be totally disabling.

Sciatica is used to define pain which starts in the low back and goes down one or both legs.

These three conditions often occur in the same individual but at different times. Often lumbar insufficiency comes on first and may be present for a period of years. This condition may be all that the patient ever has. However, lumbar insufficiency may later become lumbago, which is more or less constant and disabling. We have all seen many cases of patients who, having had backache suggestive of lumbar insufficiency for a number of years, may, following an episode of lifting or trauma, develop lumbago and, later, sciatica.

The relationship of these conditions can be explained in this way: During the period when only lumbar insufficiency is present, disc degeneration is starting. There are radial tears in the annulus fibrosus, and by microscopic examination one might find definite changes from normalcy. However, by ordinary roentgenogram or even myelogram no changes would be noted. Changes might be noted by discogram at this stage. During the period of lumbago, the same situation is present but further advanced. The third stage, that of sciatica, usually is considered to result from compromise of the nerve root near its exit. This stage often begins about ten years after the first signs of lumbar insufficiency. Of course, all variations may occur. The person may never have more than lumbar insufficiency, or occasionally his first trouble is sciatica. The sciatica may be true dermatomal radiation that follows a dermatomal pattern and results in sensory and reflex change or it may be sclerotomal in nature, following sclerotomal patterns and not producing signs of neurological deficit.

Etiological discussion of the cause of low back pain has been virtually dominated for the past thirty years by the intervertebral disc. However, there certainly are other structures in the low back that can cause pain. The capsular and ligamentous innervations of the intervertebral joints are the same as for any synovial joint and are far richer in sensory nerve endings than is the border of the annulus; therefore, they should be more sensitive to painful stimuli and give rise to symptoms readily. The interspinous and supraspinous ligaments certainly are injured occasionally, and in some patients we see that there is abnormal separation of the spinous processes on flexion, indicating injury to the supraspinous and interspinous ligaments. Drag on the ligaments in cases of primary instability may be a cause of pain. The muscles themselves may become inflamed and painful and, of course, the nerve tissues of the cauda equina, as in true polyneuritis or arachnoiditis, may be the site of pain independent of the structural elements of the low back.

Degenerative arthritic changes of the intervertebral joints are present in many persons and probably in all persons eventually. These changes generally appear somewhat later than does disc degeneration. The synovial joints of the upper lumbar area will show arthritic changes earlier than will those of the lower lumbar area,[10] but the upper lumbar spine is less often the site of severe pain. While many spines develop rather severe arthritic changes as evidenced on roentgenogram, without symptoms, there is a correlation between evidence of degenerative arthritic changes in the synovial joints of the spine and clinical symptoms, although it is not a very striking correlation.[11]

In discussing lumbosacral strain and instability, a few general observations should be made. Some of these have been accepted as true for many years, but others may elicit some argument.

Low back pain affects persons of all ages but is most common in those between 25 and 50. The most common age of onset of low back pain in the male is about 28 to 29, and that for sciatica, 35 to 36; sciatica is seldom seen before age 25 and the incidence peaks at 35 to 37.[9] The onset is usually somewhat later in the female. Attacks of lumbago are shorter in young persons and last longer as age increases. The ectomorph, the mesomorph, and the endomorph are affected by low back pain with about the same frequency. However, real obesity does increase the incidence of low back trouble.

The vast majority of attacks, at least 95%, will subside spontaneously whether treatment is given or not.

Frequency of back trouble

There are no accurate studies as to the frequency of significant low back trouble in the United States. However, Hirsch and Schajowicz[10] conducted a study in Sweden from which they concluded that 65% of the Swedish population at one time or another had had significant back trouble. There is always the problem of deciding just how much back trouble is significant. For the purpose of this chapter we will consider that an attack is significant if it causes one to lose time from work or causes him to consult a doctor.

Disc degeneration

Disc degeneration should be interpreted as a more or less normal physiological process which begins at about the age of 20 and continues throughout life. Chemically,[24] it is a process associated with (1) gradual reduction of chondroitin sulfate without coincident change in the keratosulfate fraction of the mucopolysaccharides, (2) the appearance of a β protein in increasing quantity, and (3) increased fibrillation and precipitation of collagens. The net effects on the disc include (1) loss of its gel properties, (2) thinning, and (3) defective function as an elastic body, becoming incapable of normal absorption and redistribution of stresses. It affects the sedentary worker as frequently as it does the heavy laborer.[11] However, the sedentary worker is much better able to adapt to a certain amount of back trouble than is the heavy laborer. Therefore, the sedentary worker who has symptoms of lumbar insufficiency may be able to adjust his work in such a way that he can live comfortably. In contrast, the heavy worker, if he continues in his job, would have considerable discomfort and would probably begin having real lumbago to the point where he would have to quit work or change jobs.

There is a definite correlation between the incidence of repeated attacks of back trouble and heavy work. In other words, a person who has had an attack of back trouble and who has to continue doing heavy work is much more prone to further trouble than is the sedentary worker. Among heavy laborers, according to Hult,[11, 12] injuries account for the onset of back trouble about 20% of the time. In the laborer, heavy lifting without any definite injury is associated with the onset of back trouble about 40% of the time, thus making a total of 60%, in the male, which might be considered compensable in an industrial situation.[11] No such figure is available for the female.

Very heavy work does speed up the process of disc degeneration. However, it must be emphasized that disc degeneration may develop and even attain advanced stages without ever giving rise to pain, in either the very sedentary worker or the heavy laborer. Roentgenographic signs of osteophytes and disc degeneration become increasingly common with increasing age. Friberg and Hirsch,[7] through comparative pathological and roentgenographic investigations, and Lindblom,[16] through discography, proved that advanced disc degeneration with gross radial ruptures may be present even though ordinary roentgenograms reveal no pathological signs.

There is definitely a greater incidence of symptomatic low back trouble in the presence of roentgenographic evidence of degenerated and narrowed discs than there is in more normal spines, although not as striking as one might expect. By the time one sees evidence of degeneration on the roentgenogram, months or years have gone by since the onset of disc degeneration. In his office any orthopaedist will daily come across cases showing noticeable degenerative changes up and down the spine in the form of markedly narrowed disc spaces and severe osteophyte formation; yet these patients may never have had any pain in the back. However, such a spine is more prone to injury, and if the person is placed on a job where he has to do a lot of heavy lifting,[11] he is more likely to develop significant back trouble. Yet, we have seen men in their 60's and 70's doing heavy lifting, whose spines show advanced degeneration and who will admit to no symptoms. These changes do ordinarily cause lowered resistance to strains of various types, and a person engaged in heavy and back-straining work will more frequently develop back symptoms than will a person doing lighter tasks.

Among those with back trouble, the incidence of incapacity for work rises with rising age. Employees engaged in heavy work are ten years older from the point of view of the incidence of lumbago than those engaged in light work.[12] As stated above, symptoms in the younger worker are frequently relatively mild and transient but become more severe and persistent with increasing age, resulting in a higher incidence of incapacity for work. A comparison between men engaged in light and those in heavy work will show that both mild accidents and heavy lifting are much more common causative factors in the onset of back symptoms in the group engaged in heavy work.[11]

In California at least, when a man hurts his back in the performance of his job, even though the work is heavy, it is the duty of the attending physician to get him back to his previous job. If he cannot be returned to his previous state of health, he is entitled to a certain amount of compensation, especially if he has to take work that pays less money than did his previous job. There can be little doubt that, once a man really injures his back, it will never return completely to its previous state. He may get back to his job and may not develop further symptoms even with heavy work; thus he will feel that he has made a complete recovery. But once a disc prolapse has occurred, some measure of defectiveness in function remains and a predisposition to recurrence is present. With the passage of time, however, the chance of recurrence at that level becomes less. It has been my opinion for years that we must develop better opportunities for a change to lighter work for the man who has had back injury and is showing signs of disc degeneration and yet must continue to work. We must develop methods of placing him in an occupation that he can perform even with his somewhat poor back. To send him back to his heavy work is to invite further trouble. In this state, disabilities of the low back account for the largest amount of insurance payments of any industrial condition. There is no question but that the reasonably well motivated person who becomes incapacitated for heavy work because of his back could, in all probability, perform a lighter job perfectly well, indefinitely. In the present state of our medical knowledge we are unable to prevent the occurrence of disc degeneration and the resultant changes, but we can control the job a man must do. We must accept the fact that many a person has such changes and consequently has a back in which certain types of heavy work involve real risk that his back trouble will be so intensified that he will become incapacitated for all work for

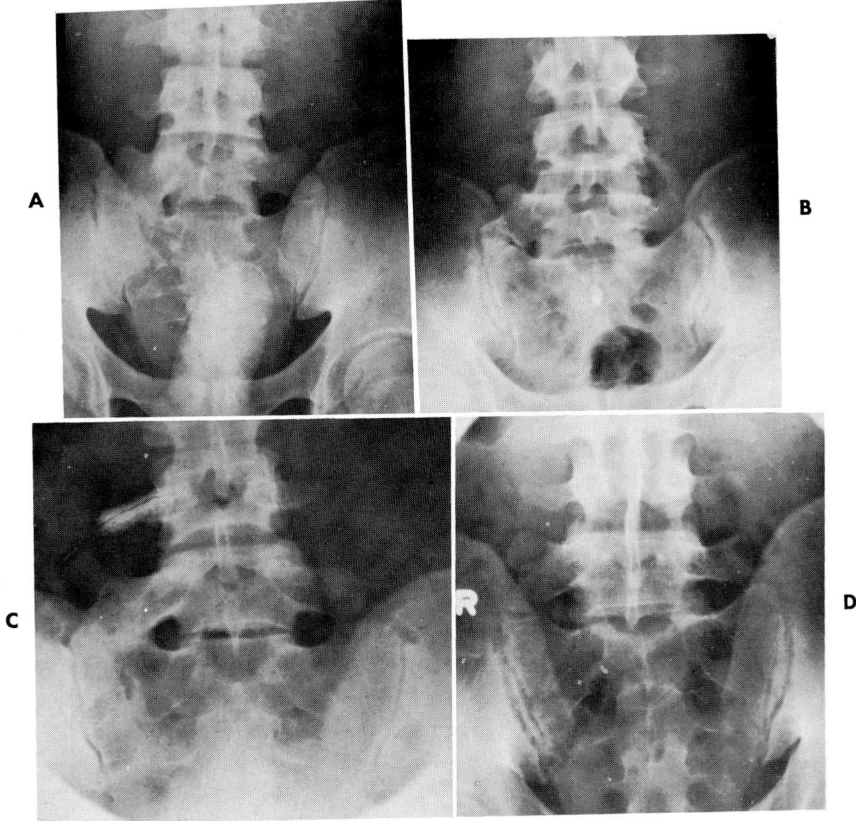

Fig. 4-1. A, On the reader's left the transverse process of L5 is solidly fused to the sacrum. There is no reason to believe that this situation would predispose to back trouble. **B,** Here we see some evidence of a pseudarthrosis on the left between the transverse process of L5 and the ala of the sacrum. **C,** There is a definite pseudarthrosis between the transverse process of L5 and the ala of the sacrum. This type of situation, theoretically, would increase the incidence of low back pain, but there are no statistics from studies of living human beings to prove this increase. **D,** This view is similar to **C,** but here the transverse process of L5 is less firmly attached to the ala of the sacrum than in **C.**

months or years. As long as such work must be carried out, it is only reasonable to require that those who are forced to perform it should be protected as much as possible.

• • •

The question of just what part some of the roentgenological variations we so commonly see in our routine back x-ray films may play in the production of symptoms has been the subject of extensive study and even more speculation.

Sacralization, lumbarization, and tropism

Sacralization of L5 or lumbarization of S1 probably has no effect on the incidence of low back pain. Hult concluded that there was absolutely no correlation in a rather large sample of industrial workers and forest workers that he studied. Recent studies by Dr. H. F. Farfan on mechanical failure of the intervertebral joints, reported in a paper read at the meeting of the Canadian Orthopaedic Association, June 18 to 23, 1967, in Montreal are of interest. It is Farfan's contention that while complete sacralization or lumbarization has nothing to do with

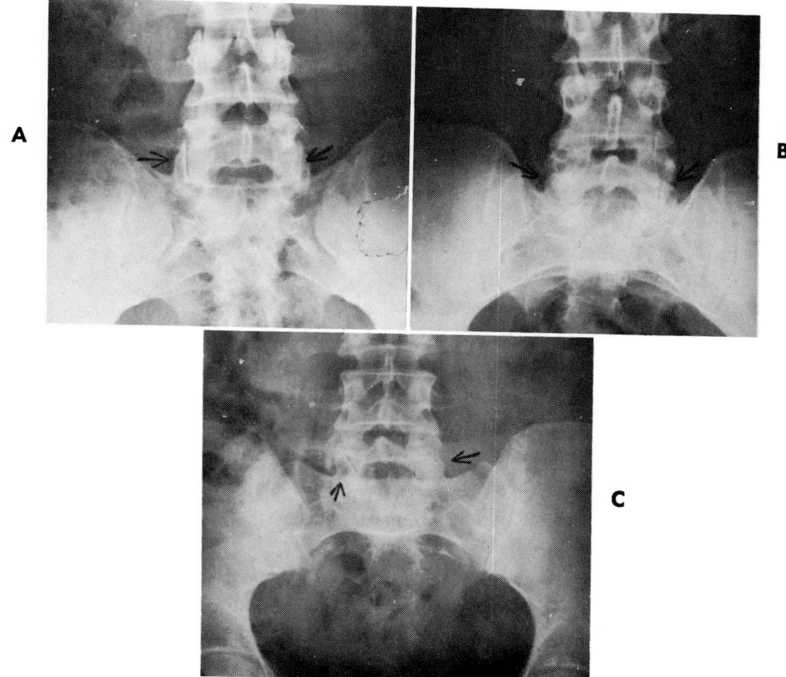

Fig. 4-2. A, In this anteroposterior roentgenogram, the facets between L5 and S1 are in a parasagittal direction. This should be an ideal situation. **B** and **C,** In each of these roentgenograms the facets between L5 and S1 are asymmetrical. On one side the facet is in a parasagittal direction and on the other it is more coronally placed. According to Farfan, this would increase the incidence of back pain.

increased incidence of rupture of the annulus fibrosus, asymmetry does. Where one transverse process is free and the other is partially tied to the sacrum (Fig. 4-1), abnormal torsional stresses are created, which do increase the incidence of rupture of the annulus. Farfan believes that the same thing is true in tropism (Fig. 4-2) where, because of the difference of angle of the two facets, one side holds better than the other and thus abnormal rotary motions are permitted. It is his contention that there is a very definitely increased incidence of disc rupture and thus disc symptoms in the presence of tropism. He also says that one reason discs rupture more frequently in the lower lumbar area than they do in the upper lumbar area is that in the upper lumbar area the facets are more sagittally placed and thus tend to prevent rotation. In the lower lumbar area they are more transversely placed. Rotary motions, he says, are much more prone to produce ruptures than are the anterior-posterior motions of flexion and extension.

Farfan and Sullivan[4] found in clinical studies a high correlation between asymmetrical orientation of the facet joints and the segment of disc pathology. In only 2 of the 78 patients whose findings were analyzed was this not true. Furthermore, the same high correlation was seen between the side of the disc prolapse and the side of the more obliquely oriented facet. The more obliquely oriented a facet is, the less mechanically suited it is to resist rotation. When one facet is rotated against its fellow, the joint is forced apart on that side. This "cam" effect of the facet and rotation toward the side of the oblique facet combine to produce maximal strain at the posterolateral angle of the annulus fibrosus, which is the point where the rupture usually occurs.

I have had a feeling, based on a simple observation and a bit of deductive reasoning, that if there is an asymmetrical lowest lumbar vertebra where the enlarged transverse process is tied loosely to the sacrum on one side but is completely free on the other, the free side is more prone to be the side of rupture of the annulus. Farfan's studies tend to bear this out.

The vacuum phenomenon

Appearance of the vacuum phenomenon on roentgenogram is definite evidence of advanced disc degeneration.[13] There is the same correlation between this appearance and symptoms in the low back as there is for the appearance of any advanced disc degeneration in the spine and symptoms in the low back.

Lumbar lordosis

In clinical studies that have been conducted, lumbar lordosis shows no correlation with low back pain.[11, 12] In Splittoff's[29] study there was actually a decrease in the angle of inclination of the superior sacral segment in his patients with back pain, but this could be explained on the basis of the fact that persons with low back pain often automatically flatten their backs because this is the most comfortable position.

We have all been taught that lumbar lordosis beyond 70 degrees certainly increases the incidence of back trouble.[5] However, these are usually theoretical conclusions and not based on clinical studies. We also know by simple observation of patients that if the person with back symptoms will flex his pelvis and thus eliminate some of his lordosis, his back pain may be relieved. It is when one starts his study from random samples of people without any selection as to whether or not they have back trouble that the rather surprising observation is made that there is no correlation between lordosis and low back pain.

Lumbosacral tilt

Orthopaedists have always felt that lumbosacral tilt is a factor in the production of low back pain; when we see a patient with severe lumbosacral tilt, we are inclined to ascribe his low back pain (which is the reason we saw him in the first

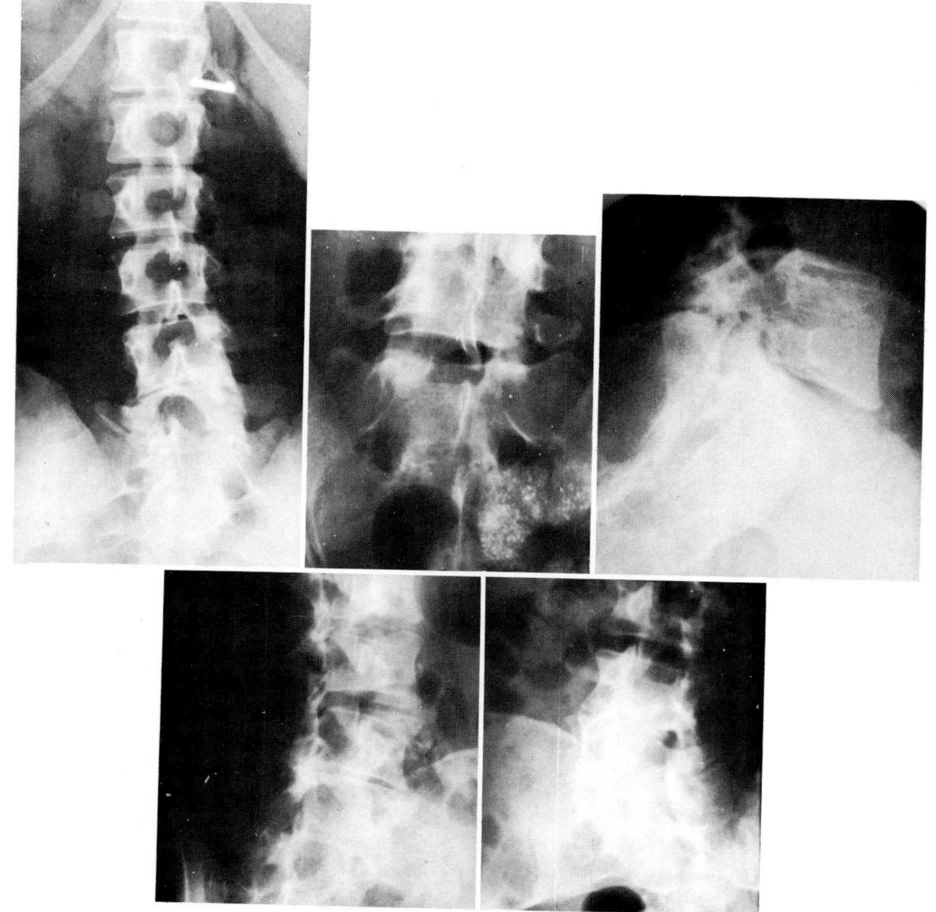

Fig. 4-3. We have always considered this situation as productive of back pain. Theoretically it should be, but statistically there is no proof that it is.

place) to this abnormal and unstable condition at the lumbosacral joint. To my knowledge there are no population studies to either confirm or refute this notion, but certainly from the theoretical point of view a situation such as is shown in Fig. 4-3 should be productive of low back pain.

Differences in the level of the sacrum between the ilia

It will be noted that in some patients the sacrum sits high in the pelvis between the ilia, and in others deep down between (Fig. 4-4). This condition is just a normal variation and of no consequence from the standpoint of producing symptoms.

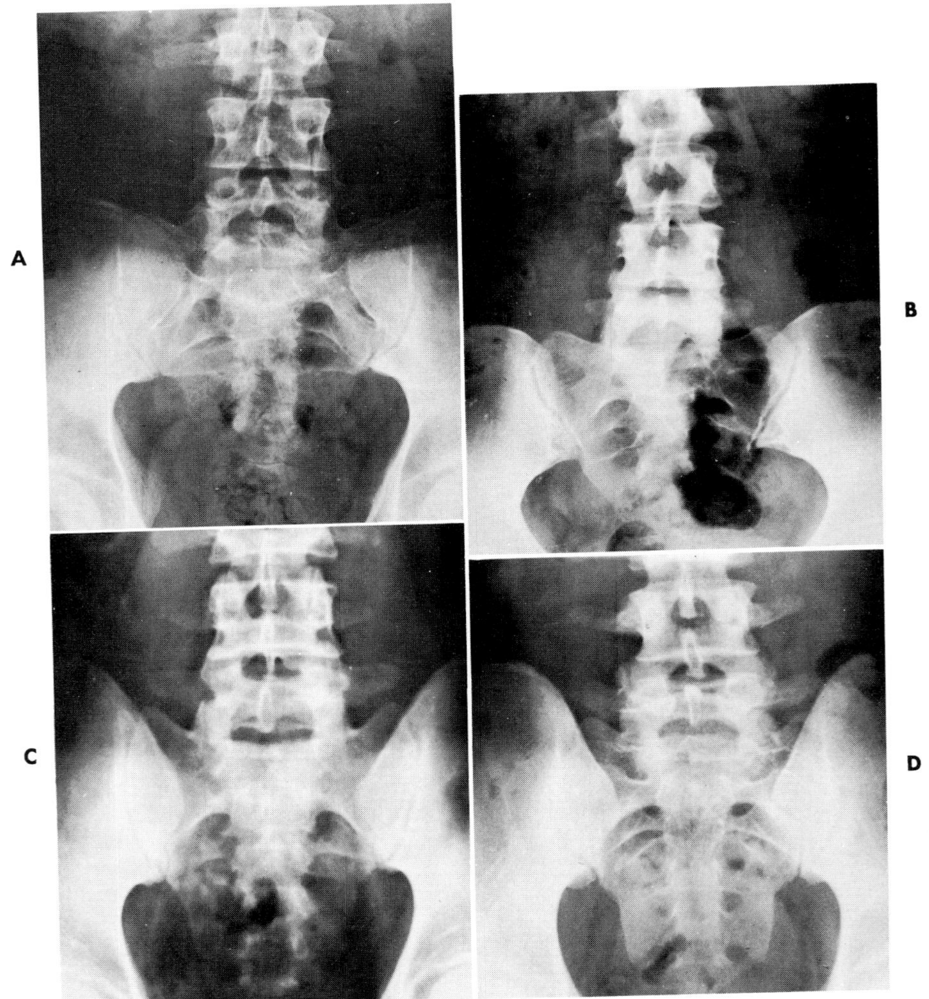

Fig. 4-4. A, Note that the top of the sacrum is level with the tops of the ilia. This is not an illusion. **B** to **D,** These show examples where the sacrum sits more deeply between the ilia. There is no known clinical significance to this phenomenon.

Defects in the pars interarticularis

Spondylolisthesis and spondylolysis do definitely increase the incidence of back pain. Hult,[11, 12] in one significant group of patients, found the percentage of low back trouble in the entire number of subjects to be 59.9%. However, those with spondylolisthesis had an incidence of 84.0%. Disc degeneration likewise was increased in the presence of spondylolisthesis (Fig. 4-5). Macnab[16a] has found that in the younger groups, up to age 25, the presence of spondylolisthesis has very definitely increased the incidence of back trouble. After that age, the difference was less remarkable. It has been generally thought but there is no statistical proof that the presence of a unilateral pars defect would increase the incidence of back trouble. Even though the vertebra is a brittle ring, there may be some spring in the bone with a unilateral pars defect, which could account for a buildup of fibrocartilaginous material at the point of defect. The unilateral defect would also place abnormal torsional stresses on the disc and perhaps increase the incidence of herniation.

Thoracic spine

In regard to the thoracic spine, the following generalizations can be made.

Scoliosis

Thoracolumbar scoliosis does not increase the incidence of low back pain or sciatica.

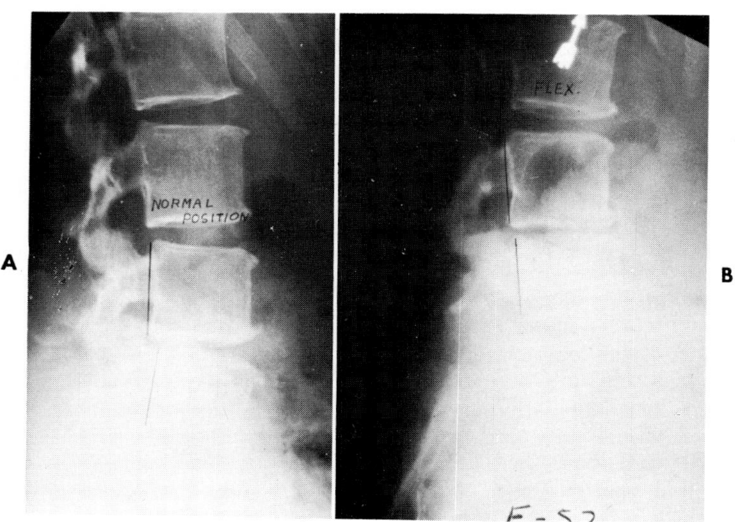

Fig. 4-5. Severe disc degeneration definitely does increase the incidence of back symptoms. **A,** Note that in the normal position there is definite retro-spondylolisthesis. **B,** On flexion, the posterior slip disappears. This is evidence of rather severe disc degeneration.

Ruptured disc in the thoracic spine

Although disc degeneration is demonstrated roentgenologically in the thoracic spine as often as in the cervical and lumbar spine areas, the incidence of symptoms such as backache that can be referred to the thoracic spine is less than 5%. This finding may be due to the fact that the anatomical conditions promoting intervertebral disc protrusion giving rise to symptoms are not present in the thoracic spine. This lack of symptoms is due not only to the stability of the thoracic spine but also to the fact that rupture of the annulus occurs most frequently on the concave side of the curve of the spine and, of course, this is in front in the thoracic spine. According to Farfan's[4] studies, there is another reason for this situation: because of the way the facets are set, coupled with the more oval shape of the bodies of the thoracic vertebrae, the point of the annulus most likely to rupture is located anteriorly in an area that will cause no trouble.

Kyphosis

Kyphosis of the thoracic spine does not increase the incidence of low back pain. Seventy-six percent of thoracic kyphosis is due to Scheuermann changes in the vertebrae.[11, 12] Both kyphosis and Scheuermann changes are found twice as often in children who had done heavy work very early in life. Kyphosis of the thoracic and thoracolumbar spine is of cosmetic importance only.

Primary instability

Anterior-posterior slip on backward and forward bending as seen on roentgenogram does herald the onset of disc degeneration.[19] It is an earlier sign than is narrowing or osteophyte formation, but slip on bending is not always present when there is roentgenographic evidence of disc degeneration, nor is it always present when there are symptoms. If one has a patient with back pain (Fig. 4-6) and takes flexion and extension roentgenograms according to the technique of Knutsson and does see the backward and forward slipping with parallelism, he has presumptive evidence that the level showing the slip is the point that is producing the pain.[14] However, according to Mensor and Duvall,[17] if one performs this test on a random sampling of patients, about 15% of the patients having symptoms will show this backward and forward slip, but 8% will also show this sign without having any symptoms. Therefore, primary instability, although it is a sign of disc degeneration, does not necessarily mean that a person is having pain; but spines with primary instability are statistically a little more likely to be symptomatic than those without it.

Other conditions found on physical examination

Restriction of motion of the spine

There is a definite statistical relationship between restriction of motion of the spine and back pain. We constantly see persons who have never had back trouble who nevertheless have rather severe restriction of back motion, but persons with

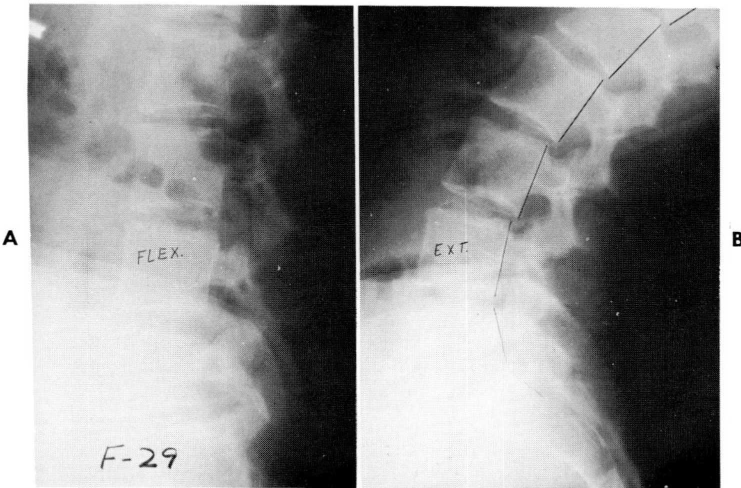

Fig. 4-6. A, In flexion the posterior borders of the vertebral bodies are even. **B,** Note the posterior slip of each vertebral body: L3 on L4, L2 on L3, etc. This slip is normal, as evidenced by the lack of parallelism and the fact that the slip is not localized to one vertebral body.

back pain are more likely to have restriction of motion than are those without it. One must be careful in measuring back motion, however, to be sure that he is measuring the actual motion in the lumbar spine and not motion in the hips. The American Orthopaedic Association has published *A Manual of Orthopaedic Surgery,* which gives an excellent method of measuring motion in the spine.

Tenderness over the tips of the spinous processes

There is a definite correlation between pain on pressure over the lumbar spinous processes and back pain.[11, 12]

Sciatic tension tests and neurological deficit

There is a very high correlation between a history of low back pain and sciatica and positive sciatic tension tests. The same is true for neurological deficit.

Differences in leg length

Differences in leg length, even up to 1½ inches, do not increase the incidence of low back symptoms.[11] Beyond this point there may be correlation. It is well known that correcting leg length discrepancy often relieves back pain in the person who already has back pain; thus, changing the statics of the spine may relieve symptoms that are already present. (See Fig. 4-7.)

Postural foot deformities

There is no correlation betwen flat feet and back trouble. It is a well-known fact that some patients' backaches are remarkably relieved by arch supports. These

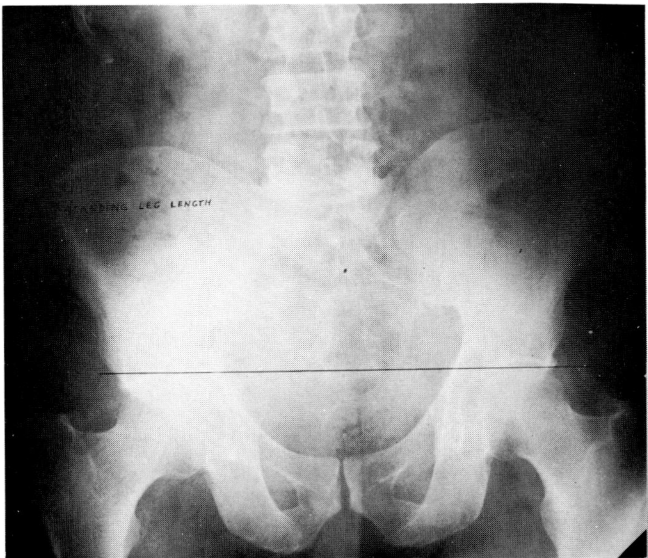

Fig. 4-7. During the past ten years we have measured leg length by having the patient stand in stockinged feet in front of a level cassette while a pelvic roentgenogram was being taken. By measuring from the top of the head of the femur to the lower edge of the film, one can get a measurement of leg length differences that is accurate to about 3/16 of an inch. The technologist must be sure that the patient stands level, with both knees in the same degree of extension. Such conditions as flatfoot on one side or old fracture of the calcaneus will cause a difference in leg length that will not be picked up by other methods of leg length measurement. This method of leg length measurement, however, will not be accurate in cases of contracture of the tensor fascia lata.

do alter the statics in the spine and may actually cause a person to walk with a little less lumbar lordosis, thus relieving his pain either temporarily or permanently, but in large population studies the presence of flat or pronated feet does not increase the incidence of low back trouble beyond that of the population as a whole.[11, 12]

Heredity

Heredity is thought to play a part in disc degeneration[10] and since there is a definite relationship between roentgenographic evidence of disc degeneration and low back pain, we may postulate that it also plays a part in the incidence of low back trouble. Although I know of no studies in the human being to definitely establish the hereditary nature of disc degeneration, most of us have observed families in which several members have had disc operations, and it is a common observation among veterinarians that some breeds of dogs, such as the dachshund and Pekinese, are affected by disc degeneration and disc herniation more than other breeds. This predisposition is not related to the length of the spine nor its mobility but has been shown by Hansen[8] to be directly related to the predisposition of these breeds to degeneration of the disc. In prolapse-prone breeds, the gelatinous nucleus prematurely disappears at the age of 3 or 4 months and at 1 year is a fibrocartilaginous mass, thus paralleling the changes that have been observed in man.

Personality types

Many authors have suggested that there is a personality type which is prone to discogenic disease. It has been said that the tense, emotionally high-strung person is more likely to develop trouble. In 1955, Scott[27] reported that voles, which are a type of field mouse, when subjected to emotional stress with the attendant increase in adrenocortical activity, were found to have a greater volume of the nucleus pulposus than that of control animals. It has also been postulated that abnormal imbibition of water into the disc may predispose to herniation. This observation would support the possibility of a relationship between the emotional makeup of an individual and disc degeneration and perhaps rupture. Admittedly, it is only a "straw in the wind."

Cervical symptoms

There is a definite statistical correlation between cervical pain and the lumbosciatic syndrome.[12] Both clinical signs and roentgenological findings indicate that the genesis is associated with degenerative changes in the intervertebral discs. Most of us have noted in our patients a relationship between cervical symptoms and lumbar symptoms. One prominent orthopaedist of my acquaintance has stated facetiously that any time a patient is being operated on for a cervical disc if one will look at the patient's back he will find a ten-year-old laminectomy scar in the lumbar area, implying that lumbar disc pain and cervical disc pain occur in the same patient and that the low back is about ten years ahead of the neck in its degenerative process.

Causes of sciatica

The question arises as to just what does cause pain in sciatica. This has been the subject of a lot of investigation. Compression and irritation of a spinal nerve in the intervertebral foramina by a bulging or ruptured disc have been chiefly incriminated. However, compression alone can hardly be the whole answer. When pressure is exerted on a nerve, the first fibers to be blocked are the large myelinated ones that carry touch, proprioception, and motor impulses. This is what occurs when an arm or a leg "goes to sleep." The small amyelinated fibers are affected later. Yet, pain is usually the initial symptom of sciatica. Perhaps the precipitating factors are the edema and inflammation of nerve roots secondary not only to compression but also to irritation from electrochemical or autoimmunization mechanisms. The work of Smith and Brown[28] in which chondrolytic enzymes were injected into the disc space would tend to confirm this hypothesis. They report dramatic relief of pain in a high percentage of patients with sciatica, after chymopapain was injected into the disc, even though the ruptured or bulging disc could hardly have degenerated enough so soon after the injection to have taken pressure off the nerve. This prompt relief of pain could be due to a change in chemistry or to some other factor than easing of pressure, for which the relief would appear to be too dramatic. Another interesting fact in this work is that there is roentgenographic evidence of disc space narrowing within a few weeks and yet relatively little pain is experienced from the narrowing. The pain which these patients do experience, according to Smith and Brown,[28] is mild and purely in the spine and not down the legs. The fact that disc spaces can be seen to narrow in a matter of weeks and yet not produce severe pain would reinforce the belief that disc narrowing as seen on roentgenogram is not a very important aspect in the production of clinical symptoms. An interesting comparison to note here is that in cases of disc space infection pain and especially muscle spasm are very prominent findings. The disc space tends to disintegrate and collapse down. Yet, in patients injected with chymopapain a slightly similar process must be going on and pain is relieved. In patients who have had previous surgery, tying down of the nerve by scar tissue can definitely cause pain. Strangulation of the root by contracting scar tissue and intraneural fibrosis is very likely to cause sciatica.

Differential diagnosis

In making the diagnosis in cases of back pain, there are several other causes of backache besides degenerative changes in the disc or synovial joints that must be considered.

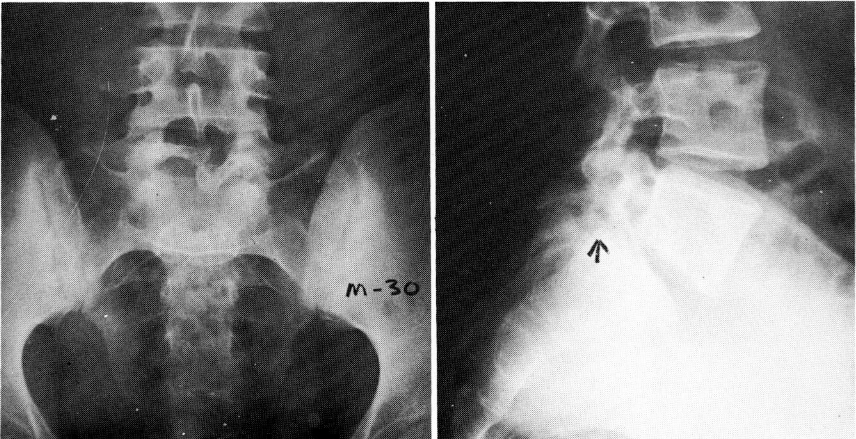

Fig. 4-8. This patient was first seen at age 24 with a backache. Spondylolisthesis was noted and was considered to be the cause of his pain. Only after several years did sclerosis show up in the sacroiliacs. This, along with diminished chest expansion, proved the disease to be Marie-Strümpell arthritis, the real cause of his pain. We had considered doing a spinal fusion on him because of his spondylolisthesis before we discovered the real cause of the pain.

Marie-Strümpell arthritis

This condition can be especially difficult to diagnose. The young, 20- to 35-year-old, male is the most likely candidate. (See Fig. 4-8.) The ratio is nine males to one female. In all probability this condition represents a variety of rheumatoid arthritis. There is quite a definite hereditary tendency. The condition usually starts in the low back with pain radiating out onto the buttocks. There are stiffness and flattening of the lumbar curve. The finding of diminished chest expansion is especially helpful in the diagnosis. The presence of only 1 inch or less of chest expansion in a young male may be considered pathognomonic. Roentgenographic and laboratory tests are often of no help in revealing the early case. Response to antiarthritics, especially phenylbutazone, is a very helpful sign and is often the premise on which the diagnosis must be made. Changes in the sacroiliac joints are usually the first roentgenographic signs, but these come at least a year and often years after the onset of symptoms.

Gout

Occasionally gout does cause backache, although in my experience it is not so frequent a cause as has been reported. History of other joint involvement, hyperuricemia, and especially response to uricosuric drugs are of value in making the diagnosis.

Osteoporosis

This disease is especially common in the female, starting ten or fifteen years after the menopause. Osteoporosis is often painful and there need not be evidence of a compression fracture in order for there to be pain. Generally, the pain from osteoporosis is more in the thoracolumbar area or upper lumbar area.

Compression fractures

Roentgenography will usually rule out fracture except in the osteoporotic person where the initial roentgenogram may appear negative for a fracture; then a later x-ray film, after two or three weeks, may show definite compression of one or more of the vertebral bodies. Frequently it is difficult to be sure that a compressed vertebra does not harbor metastatic carcinoma. A bone scan is very valuable in these cases, since, if the compression is the result of metastatic malignancy, other vertebral bodies besides the compressed one will usually be involved and can be seen on the scan.

Disc space infection

These patients usually have very severe back muscle spasm and severe pain, far out of proportion to the roentgenographic or laboratory findings. Laboratory tests are often negative. A history of disc surgery or of bacteremia is significant. Bone scan is a good diagnostic procedure. The roentgenogram will not become positive for a few weeks, and I have seen one case where it was two months after disc surgery before changes in the disc space characteristic of infection could be seen.

Charcot spine

This disease (Fig. 4-9) is uncommon now. Roentgenograms show very severe changes, out of proportion to the rather mild symptoms.

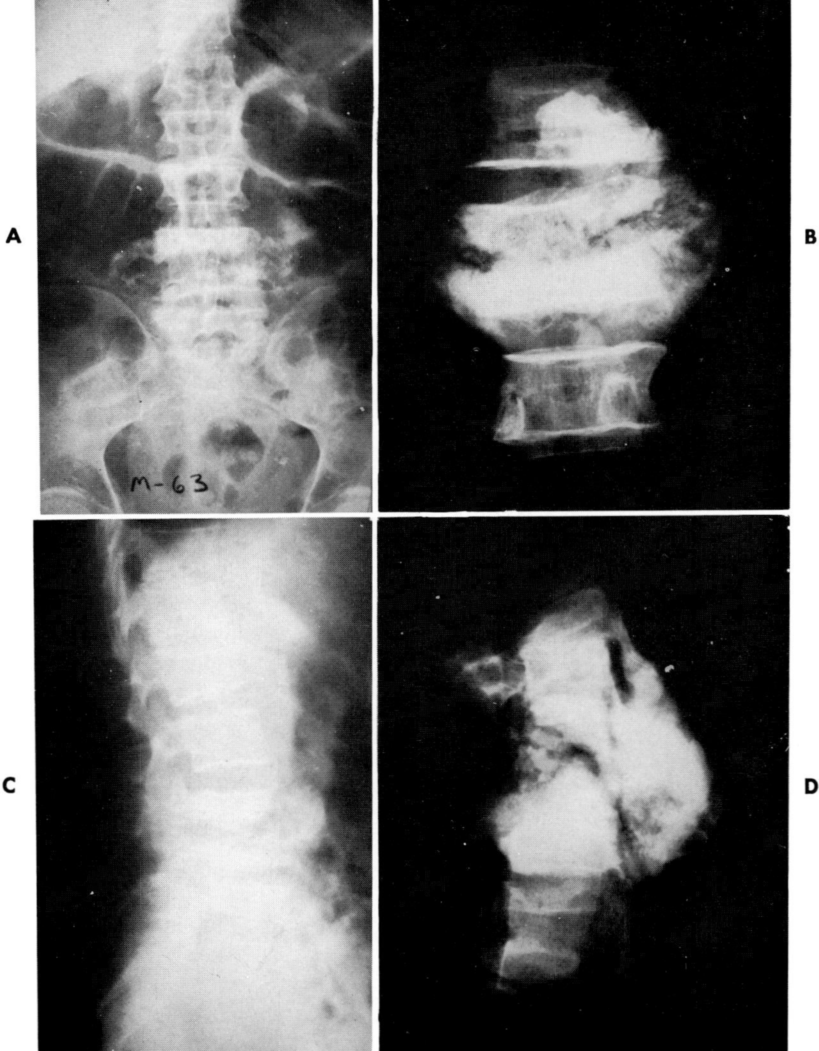

Fig. 4-9. A and **B,** Anteroposterior roentgenograms of a 63-year-old male, showing Charcot's spine. He had only mild back trouble. **C** and **D,** Roentgenograms of the same patient, but taken from the cadaver. He had died from cardiovascular disease. Note the severe changes in the spine; yet he had a paucity of symptoms.

Peptic ulcer

These patients usually have pain at the thoracolumbar area or higher. If there is a history of peptic ulcer and on examination of the spine there is no tenderness, no limitation of back motion, no pain on bending, and no relief by rest, suspect peptic ulcer as being the cause of pain.

Pancreatitis

This disease may cause pain in the upper lumbar area, often one-sided. There may be pain on deep percussion but no local tenderness, no relief by bed rest, and no limitation of back motion.

Aneurysm of the aorta

This condition sometimes produces deep aching pain, often one-sided, that is not relieved by bed rest, shows no limitation of back motion, and no local tenderness. Palpation and auscultation over the abdomen may reveal the aneurysm, as may roentgenograms of the abdomen. Occasionally an aortogram will be necessary to make the diagnosis.

Diverticulitis

This condition may cause deep aching pain that is not relieved by rest and is usually one-sided. There is no limitation of motion and there is no tenderness in the low back.

Retroperitoneal fibrosis

This disease can cause a dull, constant pain in the low back and may produce hydronephrosis. It is not related to back motion or bed rest. It may be caused by the drug Sansert.

Obstruction of the common iliac arteries

Intermittent claudication may be present in this condition. Pulses in the legs are reduced.

Prostatic cancer

Deep pain low in the back in males over age 60 can indicate this disease. In a male of this age group with bilateral sciatica cancer of the prostate must seriously be considered.

Metastatic malignancy to the spine

This condition must be at least considered in almost every case. The older the person, the greater the likelihood. Careful history and physical examination with roentgenograms will usually rule it out. Alkaline phosphatase studies should be done, and a bone scan is of real value.

Multiple myeloma

This disease should be considered in the person who is past 40. The disease is twice as frequent in males as in females. Anemia and increased sedimentation rate are usually present. The protein electrophoresis may show characteristic changes and, coupled with a bone marrow study, will detect most cases. Bence Jones protein will be present in advanced cases about 64% of the time, but in cases where the diagnosis is in doubt, it has proved of little value. Roentgenograms may reveal the multiple bone lesions in the ribs, skull, or pelvis.

Cord tumor

Very often the initial symptom of cord tumor is backache. The electromyogram is of value but the myelogram usually gives the diagnosis.

Arachnoiditis of the cauda equina

Severe, aching pain in the back and down the legs is characteristic of this disease. A history of repeated myelograms and repeated surgery is often present. The electromyogram will frequently show characteristic changes. While further myelograms should be avoided if possible, characteristic changes will usually be seen on the myelogram.

Genitourinary disease

Renal infection rarely causes back pain but may cause flank pain. Severe chronic or acute prostatitis occasionally causes low back pain. Severe cystitis rarely

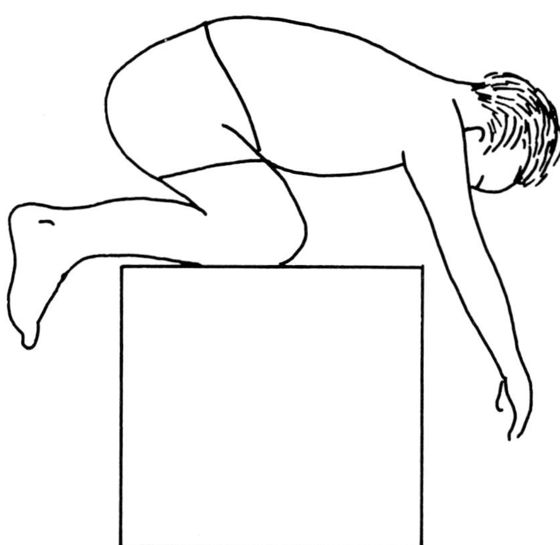

Fig. 4-10. The patient should kneel on a padded chair. Except in the very acute case or in cases with some other condition, such as hip disease, the patient will be able to touch the floor without more than minimal back pain.

causes back pain. The percentage of times that the genitourinary system can be incriminated for low back pain is very small.

Abnormal conditions of the female pelvis

Less than 2% of low back pain in females comes from the pelvic organs. If it is from the pelvic region, it is always worse during the menses. Retroversion of the uterus may rarely cause pain. In this condition the pessary test is of help. Acute inflammatory disease does cause a deep ache in the back, as does endometriosis.

Primary sacroiliac joint disease

Tuberculous infection of the sacroiliac joints is a rarity nowadays. Marie-Strümpell arthritis may start in the sacroiliacs. Occasionally there is some sacroiliac pain in the postpartum period, and osteitis condensans ilii may cause sacroiliac pain.

Psychogenic disease

There is no doubt that this condition is a frequent complicating factor that must be considered.

Malingering

In cases where the patient has prospects of monetary gain, the doctor must always keep this in mind. There is no doubt that on the average the patient who is being paid while he is ill will be longer in getting back to work. Most of the time this attitude cannot be considered downright malingering. The following are some tests that can be used as a help in revealing the patient whose back condition is strongly affected by emotional problems or the one who is malingering.

The Burns test. In this test the patient is asked to kneel on a firm stool (Fig. 4-10). The stool should be padded with a folded blanket or pillow. If a chair is used, an ordinary kitchen type chair is best. The back of the chair should be either to his right or to his left. Ask him to bend over and touch the floor. He may sit down so that his buttocks touch his heels if necessary, but he should touch the floor with his fingertips. If he does not have severe hip joint disease or very acute lumbago, he will be able to touch the floor. The examiner should stand in front of him so that the patient can fall against him if the patient is psychoneurotic and decides to fall forward to give a very convincing demonstration of how "bad off" he is. If a patient complaining of chronic lumbago cannot be persuaded to touch the floor, his is either partially or completely an emotional problem or he is a malingerer. This is a good test and in my experience very reliable.

The flip test. This test was described by Michele[18] in 1958.

> The mechanics of the flip sign are as follows. The patient is instructed to sit squarely on the examining table with his legs dangling off its side and to hold his

back as erect as possible [Fig. 4-11]. The arms hang at the sides of the body or may be used by the patient for supplemental fixation against the table or the side of the thigh to be tested [sic]. The examiner places the open palm of one hand against the distal thigh (suprapatellar area) of the affected extremity, depressing the thigh against the table, and his other hand under the heel cord so that the heel rests in the palm [Fig. 4-12]. The affected limb is then gradually extended at the knee. In cases of genuine sciatic tension no resistance or complaints are noted until the 45 degree arc is reached, but continuance of elevation past that point is attended with an acute reversal of the lumbar lordosis, and the patient tends to fall backward, frequently needing to brace himself against the table with his hands to prevent a complete backward fall on the table [Fig. 4-13].

In cases of genuine sciatic nerve tension, when the flip sign is positive, it is noted that the individual is unable to sit erect on the table with both knees fully extended. There is either a flexion attitude of the knee of the affected extremity or a reversal of the lumbar spine with backward flexion position of the trunk to avoid the pain associated with nerve root tension. The simulator, with a negative flip sign [Fig. 4-12], rarely evidences any difficulty in sitting on the table in an erect position, with both knees fully extended [Fig. 4-14].*

Testing of ability to bend forward in the sitting position. This test can be used for the person who is simulating inability to bend forward. In a sitting position with hips and knees normally flexed, even a person with a totally stiff back will be able to bend forward to where his head is nearly level with his knees unless he has hip joint disease or a very acute spinal condition.

List. If the patient who is showing a list is seated on a stool and asked to bend forward, a genuine list will remain, but a simulated one will disappear as he bends forward and touches the floor with his fingertips. This test will be used infrequently.

Plantar flexion of foot test. It is well known that in the case of sciatica if the leg is brought up in straight leg position to the point just before pain is experienced,[3] pain will be produced by dorsiflexing the ankle on the extended knee. If the pain is made worse by plantar flexing the ankle under the same circumstances, then this is presumptive evidence that at least to this extent there is an emotional overlay or deliberate malingering.

The flexed thigh test. We know that the straight leg test may cause pain in the patient with lumbago or sciatica. After performing the straight leg test, the knee is flexed as it is brought up toward the abdomen. It is not pushed hard so as to cause movement of the lumbar spine. If the patient complains of severe pain on this maneuver it may, except in the very acute case, be considered an indication of exaggeration, either conscious or unconscious. The conclusion does not hold true if the patient has trouble in the hip joint.

The Hoover test. The patient is flat on his back on the examining table. He is asked to lift his painful leg in an extended position—in other words, do straight leg raising. At the same time the examiner places the palm of his hand under the patient's other heel. If the patient is making a genuine effort to lift his leg he will push down on the opposite heel. If he is pretending to do a straight leg raising and not trying, he will not press down on the opposite heel.

*From Michele, A. A.: The flip sign in sciatic nerve tension, Surgery **44**:940, 1958.

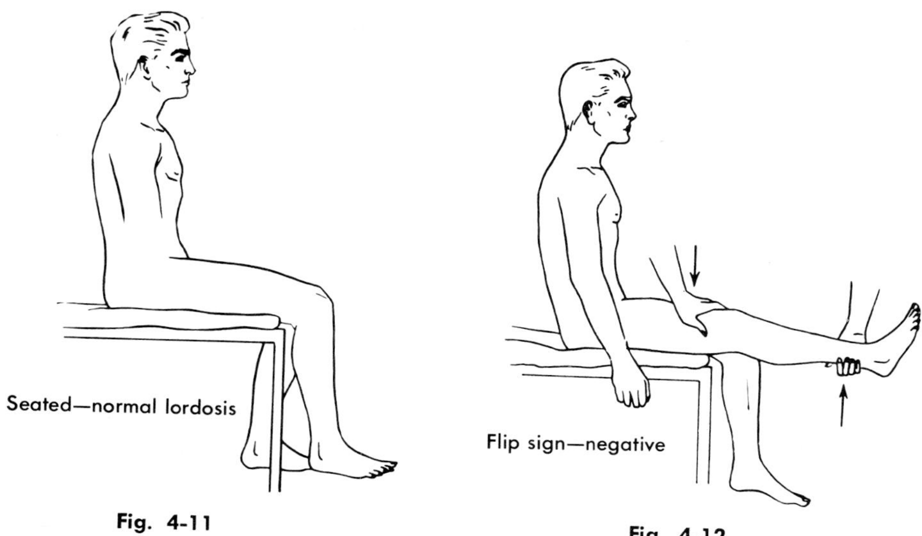

Fig. 4-11

Fig. 4-12

Fig. 4-11. Patient sitting erect on the examining table, legs dangling off the table. (From Michele, A. A.: Surgery **44:**940, 1958.)

Fig. 4-12. Patient with negative flip sign, knees extended and spine erect. (From Michele, A. A.: Surgery **44:**940, 1958.)

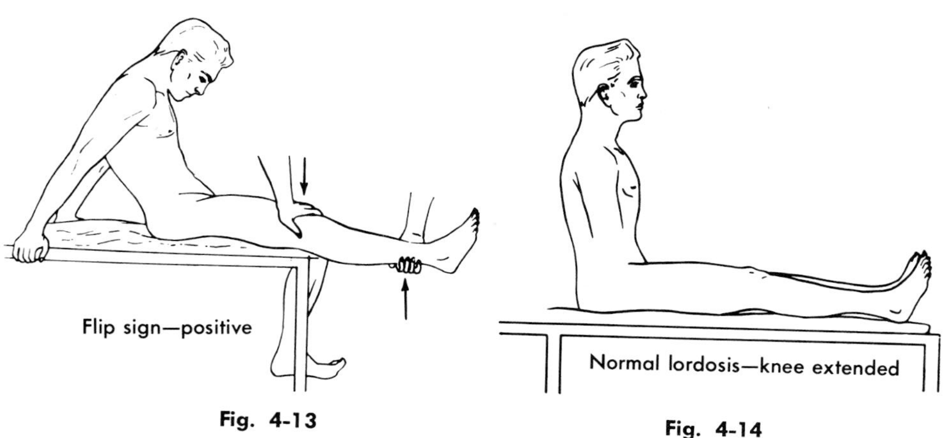

Fig. 4-13

Fig. 4-14

Fig. 4-13. Positive flip sign is present when the examiner, pressing the distal thigh against the table with one hand and with the other gradually elevating the heel with extension of the knee, produces a reversal of the lumbar lordosis with backward flexion of the trunk. (From Michele, A. A.: Surgery **44:**940, 1958.)

Fig. 4-14. Confirmatory test for negative flip sign: spine erect, both knees extended. (From Michele, A. A.: Surgery **44:**940, 1958.)

Treatment (conservative)

In the treatment of low back conditions we must recognize that disc degeneration is a more or less normal physiological process. There is the occasional person who in the course of his degenerative process develops back pain and sciatica of such a severe and disabling nature that surgery is indicated. But the vast majority of people will get over their attacks and be able to live reasonably normally. Conservative treatment consists, then, principally of teaching the person how to care for his back and training him in proper exercises.

Drugs may be ordered in the form of muscle relaxers and analgesics as indicated. Physical therapy may be used, but in our practice the principal function of physical therapy has been for training in exercises. Corsets are occasionally ordered, as are heel lifts to level the pelvis. Injection of trigger points with Xylocaine and hydrocortisone is of definite value.

It goes without saying that each patient is carefully examined and roentgenograms of the low back are taken. As a routine we make large anteroposterior and lateral records on 14- by 17-inch plates. A spot lateral focusing over the lumbosacral joint is taken, as are 45-degree lateral oblique views of the lumbosacral

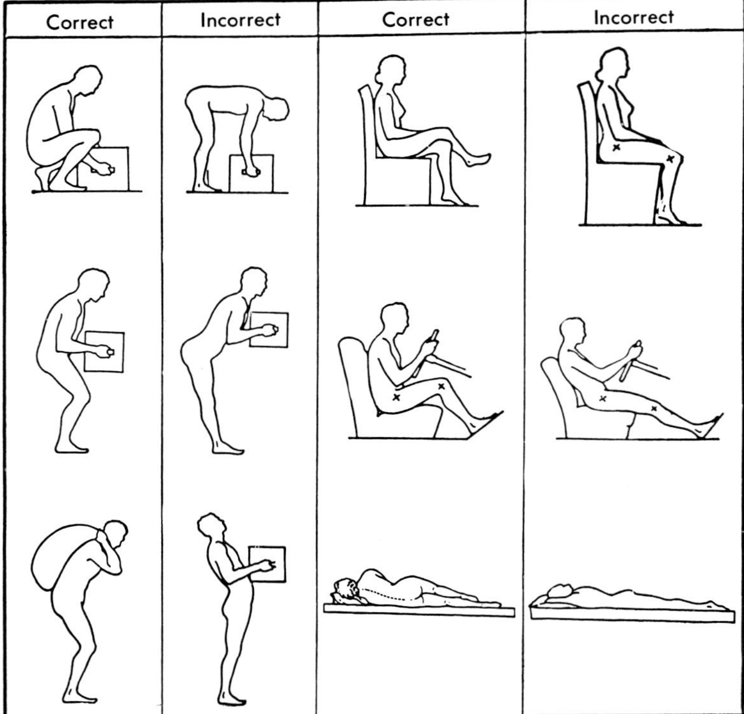

Fig. 4-15. Correct methods of lifting, sitting, and sleeping are illustrated. (From Williams, P. C.: The lumbosacral spine, New York, 1965, McGraw-Hill Book Co. Used by permission of publisher.)

area, and a 20-degree caudocephalad view, sometimes called the Ferguson view. Every effort is made to rule out other causes of low back pain: Marie-Strümpell arthritis, tumor, disc infection, abdominal or pelvic disease, etc.

If the patient comes in with an acute attack of lumbago, perhaps all bent over or listed to one side, we examine him, give him 100 mg. of Demerol, and have him go to the x-ray laboratory for a spine series, then to Physical Therapy. At Physical Therapy he is given hot packs and massage. Assuming that the roentgenograms have revealed a basically normal low spine, we use manipulations. These can be gentle; and if they are given at this time, after he is well relaxed with Demerol as well as perhaps an injectable muscle relaxer and has had hot packs, the manipulations may be of great benefit to him. This is the only situation in which we use manipulations, but we do find them to be valuable here. There is no doubt that some practitioners use manipulation very effectively.

As the patient gets over his acute attack, we then train him in exercises and instruct him in the routine care of his back. (See Fig. 4-15.)

Routine care of the back

We have a series of instructions that are given to every patient in the form of a printed sheet. The patient is told to read them over carefully; then the doctor goes over each instruction with him, explaining each one. The patient is then told to take the instruction sheet with him and read it further and to bring it with him the next time he comes to the doctor.

The instructions given the patients are as follows: (Most of these are rather standard.)

1. Sleep alone or in a king-sized bed.
2. Use a firm, level bed. It need not be hard.
3. Sleep on your side with the knees drawn up. *Do not* sleep on your abdomen or on your back. If you must sleep on your back, use a rolled up blanket or a pillow under your knees.
4. In getting out of bed, turn over on your side, draw up your knees, then swing your legs over the edge.
5. Do not sit with the legs straight out on an ottoman or footstool.
6. When you are driving, hitch your car seat forward.
7. When riding in a car, not driving, on long trips, use a low (2- or 3-inch) footstool if you are a short person.
8. Sit with the buttocks "tucked under" so that the hollow of the back is eradicated.
9. Avoid deep sofas.
10. Avoid stooping or lifting. If you must lift, bend your knees. (See Fig. 4-15.)
11. Do not bend forward with the knees straight. Always squat.
12. Do not lift loads in front of you above the waistline.
13. Never bend backward.

14. Avoid long standing as much as possible but, if unavoidable, place one foot on a low footstool.
15. Always stand and walk with the buttocks "tucked under," toes straight ahead.
16. Try to form a crease across the upper abdomen by holding the chest up and forward, elevating the front of the pelvis. Learn to live twenty-four hours a day with the hollow in the lower part of your back reduced to a minimum.
17. Women should avoid very high heels.

Exercises

In the early acute phase no exercises are started except possibly a very gentle type of isometric abdominal setting exercise. Basically, we use the Williams[30] exercises, starting gradually and building up. We usually use Williams' 1-B rather than 1.

Williams' 1-B and 2 can be performed even by a patient with quite acute lumbago or sciatica. The physical therapist trains the patient in these, trains him on the day we see him, and gives him one or two more training periods, a week apart.

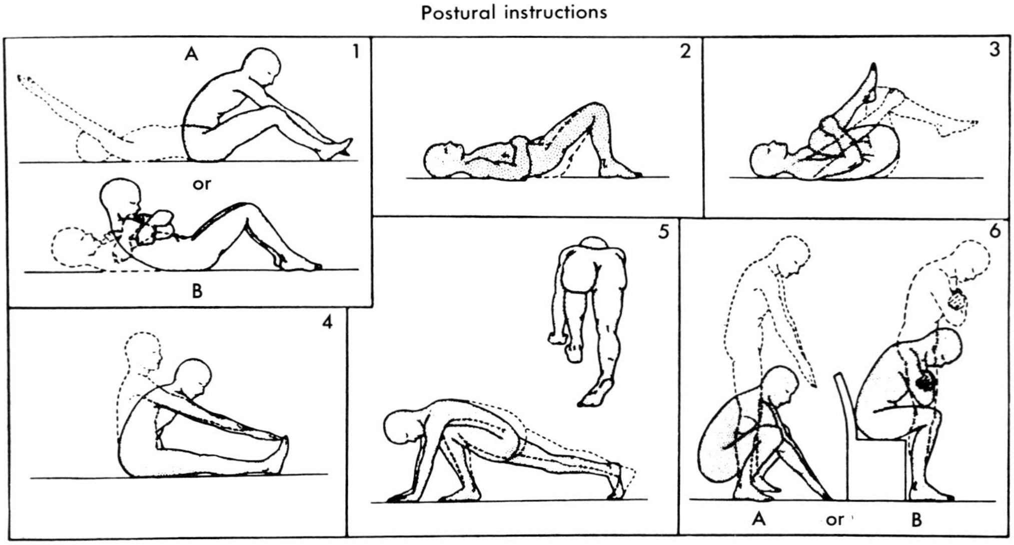

Fig. 4-16. We ordinarily start a patient on exercises 1-B, 2, and 3. Start very cautiously in the acute case and increase as pain subsides. Persistence is important. We go on to exercise 5 when the back is nearly free of symptoms. Exercise 4 is reserved for young persons who have become free of back symptoms and who still have good, flexible discs that will not be injured by the rather severe flexion of the lumbar spine. Exercise 6 is used only occasionally, and it should be used with caution in older persons who have arthritic knees. (From Williams, P. C.: The lumbosacral spine, New York, 1965, McGraw-Hill Book Co. Used by permission of publisher.)

It is most important to have these printed cards, showing the exercise you wish to give your patients (Fig. 4-16). When you have your own therapist, of course, this does not apply. But you might be surprised to learn what your patient gets if you order simply "Williams' exercises" in a department that is not used to your routine.

The success of exercises varies directly with the enthusiasm of the doctor and the physical therapist. An enthusiastic team that believes in the exercises and impresses the patient with their value will have remarkably better success in relieving the patient of his backache.

Williams' exercises 1-B, 2, and 3 are the most important. Williams' number 5 (the one in which the hip flexor is stretched) is, in my opinion, an important exercise also.

In the older patient with osteoporosis we use another exercise. In this one he sits up, flexes his spine by tightening the abdominals, and then flexes the hip. In other words it is a hip flexor exercise done in a sitting position with weights on the knees.

After back surgery the patient is placed on isometric abdominal setting and isometric gluteal tightening routines, as in other back conditions, but in addition he is put on hyperextension exercises of the lumbar spine. In back surgery, the sacrospinalis has been cut to some extent and exercises of the sacrospinalis are of value.

Corsets

The question of when to use a brace or corset has often been raised. Norton and Brown[25] showed that a lumbar brace may actually increase the motion of the lumbar area when the patient bends forward. Morris and colleagues[21] showed that a regular cast or corset increased the motion in the lumbosacral area on ordinary walking and mild bending. However, gross motions and extremes of motion are limited by a corset. Then how does a corset help? We know that it does help, because so many patients tell us that it does. Many women will tell us that just a little soft girdle helps them very much. These girdles certainly cannot restrict motion to any extent.[1]

Brown and associates[2] and also Morris and co-workers[21] performed the following experiment: Vertebral bodies in young persons were loaded to the breaking point. They were found to break when between 1000 and 1300 pounds were loaded. Yet the lumbar spine is often subjected to much more pressure than this on very heavy lifting because of the leverages of the lumbar spine. However, we must remember that the vertebral column is not out by itself but is inside the body, which in the act of lifting becomes a semirigid cylinder. When one tightens the muscles of his abdomen, the trunk becomes an even more rigid cylinder. When one performs the Valsalva maneuver, this also occurs. Morris and associates showed that by simply doing a Valsalva maneuver the weight on the lowest lumbar vertebra is lessened by as much as 30%. This phenomenon occurs because there is an actual pushing up on the diaphragm by the abdominal contents, which lifts some of the weight off the lumbar spine.

They[21] had a volunteer swallow a bulb and thus illustrated that intra-abdominal pressure is increased with the tightening of muscles without a corset but is increased more with a corset. With a corset there is more for the abdominal muscles to push against; therefore, there is more upward push on the thorax.

Nachemson and Morris[23a] then put a pressure gauge in the fifth lumbar disc. When an inflatable corset was inflated around the abdomen, the load on this fifth disc was reduced by as much as 25%. If it is the disc that is causing the trouble and we can lessen the pressure on this disc, the patient will feel better. Often this lessening is not very much but is enough to make the difference between pain and no pain. This effect is probably the reason that the tight girdle helps. It has been noted by many of us that wrestlers and weight lifters often wrap their abdomens before wrestling; this gives their abdominal muscles something to push against. There is a report that fighter pilots were found to be getting fractures in the vertebrae while pulling out of a dive but that with abdominal compression this could be prevented.

I believe that it is for the above reasons that the abdominal exercises help so much. They increase the strength of the muscles so that the torso acts as a semi-rigid cylinder, somewhat like a six-ply tire instead of a loose rubber bag. Strong abdominal muscles also may reduce lordosis a little.

Dr. Frank Raney, Jr.,[26] performed another experiment, in which he showed that with abdominal compression the spinal column in the lumbar area is actually elongated, thus tightening the ligaments and the annuli between the vertebrae.

The above information has certainly changed my ideas of how a corset helps. It may also explain why corsets do not seem to increase the incidence of successful fusion in arthrodesis of the low back, since corsets do not actually limit motion in this area and may, in fact, increase the motion in the lumbosacral joint. They may, however, act as a reminder against gross motions.

While corsets have a definite place in the treatment of low back pain, in recent years I have tended to get away from the large rigid corsets and use smaller ones. We formerly felt that if we were going to immobilize the lower spine, a corset must be rigid and extend at least from the lower thoracic area to the trochanters. Since we really do not immobilize the spine very much with these rigid corsets, we might as well use a corset that gives the patient the most comfort. Long heavy corsets with steel stays in the back often give less actual comfort to the painful back than the discomfort of wearing them, so the smaller girdle is more desirable. The obese person has a somewhat different situation and if he is improved by a support, he usually does better with a light brace such as a MacAusland brace.

Shoe lifts

While it is true that all population studies indicate that shortness of one leg, up to 1½ inches, that the patient has had most of his life does not predispose to low back trouble, we do feel that for a person who already has back trouble, leveling off the pelvis is of value.[6] We usually do not level it off completely immediately; but if, for example, the patient has ¾ inch of shortening on one side, we would make a ½-inch difference in the heel height between the shoes by taking ¼ inch off one side and adding that amount on the other. Later perhaps we would go to the complete correction.

Traction

The person whose sciatica has become so severe that ambulatory treatment will no longer suffice is admitted to the hospital for traction. We use pelvic traction with a total of 20 pounds weight. The head is elevated 25 degrees, and the knees and feet are cranked up about 7 or 8 inches each. The patient is allowed bathroom privileges for bowel movement only and is allowed to release the weight, level out the bed, and curl up on his side if he desires to. He is given enough sedation and muscle relaxant so that he will be content to relax and ignore the passage of time.

As to whether traction is better than plain bed rest, there is certainly an argument. I have felt that traction forces the patient to be quieter and certainly has some placebo effect. Numerous patients who have been ordered to bed at home for two weeks and have made no improvement have then gone ahead and improved very well in the hospital in traction.

If the patient is improving after two weeks of traction, I usually send him home with a hospital bed to continue the traction for another two weeks. If no improvement is made after two weeks of traction, we must decide whether to let him go home and live with his trouble longer or proceed with preparation for surgery. We almost never do a myelogram on the patient with a suspected ruptured disc unless he is ready to have surgery.

The electromyogram is of real value in diagnosing the presence of nerve root compression or irritation and establishing its location. We use the discogram[15] as a diagnostic aid to a limited extent, principally in cases of spondylolisthesis in patients between the ages of 30 and 45. When a spinal fusion has been decided upon and there is a question as to whether to extend the fusion to include the L4 interspace, if the myogram is negative at this L4 space and the discogram is reasonably normal, one can safely do an L5 to S1 fusion, leaving the L4 space open. I use the words "reasonably normal" because at this age few are absolutely normal.

Laminectomy and removal of the nucleus pulposus is used most often by me in cases of intractable sciatica. The place of chemonucleolysis is promising but, as of this writing, not yet established.

We find ourselves doing fewer spinal fusions for disc disease in recent years than previously. For example, we no longer believe that the presence of a narrowed disc space at L5 in the presence of a herniated disc at L4 is an indication for spinal fusion if laminectomy is to be done. Likewise we no longer consider the presence of an asymmetrical vertebra an indication for fusion. We would not, however, do a laminectomy on a patient with spondylolisthesis or spondylolysis without fusing.

I have noted recently that we have been operating on an increasing number of elderly patients with severe sciatica. Some of these have frankly ruptured discs, and one female in particular who was past 75 actually had an extruded disc. She had been disabled for several months before we finally operated on her. She made a rapid and uneventful recovery. The elderly seem to tolerate back surgery very well and should be given the benefits of surgery for their intractable sciatica the same as younger persons are. However, most of the patients who come to surgery at an advanced age have a lot of "washboarding," and the discs seem almost to be calcified. The blocking of the subarachnoid space results from a buildup at the disc space with choking off of the spinal canal. Decompression is very successful in these cases, and the surgeon must be sure to decompress well out along the course of the nerve, past its exit through the foramen.

Summary

Whatever our approach to treatment, it is clear that low back pain represents various stages of a more or less normal physiological process which in the majority of cases has a favorable prognosis. It is reasonable that therapeutic management should be tailored to the severity of the clinical manifestations. It is my opinion that if the patient can cut down some of his more vigorous activities, follow a set of rules for care of the low back, persistently carry out exercises that will keep his pelvic flexors and abdominal muscles strong, keep his weight down, and use harmless, nonaddicting drugs as necessary, the vast majority of those who suffer from the syndrome can live comfortable lives.

References

1. Bartelink, D. L.: The role of abdominal pressure in relieving the pressure on the lumbar intervertebral discs, J. Bone Joint Surg. **39-B:**718, 1957.
2. Brown, T., Hansen, R. J., and Yorra, A. J.: Some mechanical tests on the lumbosacral spine with particular reference to intervertebral discs; a preliminary report, J. Bone Joint Surg. **39-A:**1135, 1957.
3. Deyrle, W. M.: Sciatica; etiology and treatment, Clin. Orthop. **4:**166, 1954.

3a. Farfan, H. F.: Mechanical failure of the intervertebral joints. Paper read at the annual meeting of the Canadian Orthopaedic Association, June 18 to 23, 1967.

4. Farfan, H. F., and Sullivan, J. D.: The relation of facet orientation to intervertebral disc failure, Canad. J. Surg. **10:**179, 1967.
5. Ferguson, A. D.: The clinical and roentgenographic interpretation of the lumbosacral spine, Radiology **22:**548, 1934.
6. Ford, L., and Goodman, F. G.: X-ray studies of the lumbosacral spine, Southern Med. J. **10:**1123, 1966.
7. Friberg, S., and Hirsch, C.: Anatomical and clinical studies on lumbar disc degeneration, Acta Orthop. Scand. **19:**222, 1949.
8. Hansen, H. J.: Pathologic-anatomical interpretation of disc degeneration in dogs, Acta Orthop. Scand. **20:**280, 1951.
9. Hirsch, C.: An attempt to summarize past and recent facts and thoughts about low back pain, The Spectator, July, 1966.
10. Hirsch, C., and Schajowicz, F.: Studies on structural changes in the lumbar annulus fibrosus, Acta Orthop. Scand. **22:**184, 1953.

11. Hult, L.: The Munk Fors investigation, Acta Orthop. Scand., supp. 16, 1954.
12. Hult, L.: Cervical, dorsal, and lumbar spine syndromes, Acta Orthop. Scand., supp. 17, 1954.
13. Knutsson, F.: The vacuum phenomenon in the intervertebral discs, Acta Radiol. **23:**173, 1942.
14. Knutsson, F.: The instability associated with disk degeneration in the lumbar spine, Acta Radiol. **25:**593, 1944.
15. Lindblom, K.: Eine anatomische Studie über lumbale Zwischenwirbelscheibenprotrusionen und Zwischenwirbelscheibenbrüche in die Foramina intervertebralia hinein, Acta Radiol. **22:**711, 1941.
16. Lindblom, K.: Diagnostic puncture of intervertebral disks in sciatica, Acta Orthop. Scand. **17**(supp. 4):231, 1948.

16a. Macnab, Ian: Personal communication, January, 1968.

17. Mensor, M. C., and Duvall, G.: Absence of motion at the fourth and fifth lumbar interspaces in patients with and without low back pain, J. Bone Joint Surg. **41-A:**1047, 1959.
18. Michele, A. A.: The flip sign in sciatic nerve tension, Surgery **44:**940, 1958.
19. Morgan, F. P., and King, T.: Primary instability of the lumbar vertebrae as a common cause of low back pain, J. Bone Joint Surg. **39-B:**6, 1957.
20. Morris, J. M.: Biomechanics of the spine. In Disorders of the spine, University of California School of Medicine, Continuing Education in Health Sciences, lecture series, Nov. 17 and 18, 1967.
21. Morris, J. M., Lucas, D. B., and Bresler, B.: The role of the trunk in the stability of the spine, J. Bone Joint Surg. **43-A:**327, 1961.
22. Nachemson, A.: The effect of forward leaning on lumbar intradiscal pressure, Acta Orthop. Scand. **35:**314, 1965.
23. Nachemson, A.: In vivo discometry in lumbar discs with irregular nucleograms, Acta Orthop. Scand. **36:**418, 1965.

23a. Nachemson, A., and Morris, J. M.: In vivo measurements of intradiscal pressure; discometry, a method for the determination of pressure in the lower discs, J. Bone Joint Surg. **46-A:**1077, 1964.

24. Naylor, A.: The biophysical and biochemical aspects of intervertebral disc herniation and degeneration, Ann. Roy. Coll. Surg. Eng. **31:**91, 1962.
25. Norton, P. L., and Brown, T.: The immobilizing efficiency of back braces: their effect on the posture and motion of the lumbosacral spine, J. Bone Joint Surg. **39-A:**111, 1957.
26. Raney, F. L., Jr.: Exhibit shown at the meeting of the American College of Surgeons, Chicago, October, 1947.
27. Scott, J. C.: Stress factor in the disc syndrome, J. Bone Joint Surg. **37-B:**107, 1955.
28. Smith, L., and Brown, J. E.: Treatment of lumbar intervertebral disc lesions by direct injection of chymopapain, J. Bone Joint Surg. **49-B:**502, 1967.
29. Splittoff, C. A.: Roentgenographic comparison of patients with and without backache, J.A.M.A. **152:**1610, 1953.
30. Williams, P. C.: The lumbosacral spine, New York, 1965, McGraw-Hill Book Co.

5. Herniated lumbar intervertebral disc

Fred C. Reynolds, M.D.
Stanley F. Katz, M.D.

Putti[129] in 1927 said of sciatica: "Amongst painful diseases, sciatica occupies a foremost place by reason of its prevalence, its production by a great variety of conditions, the great disablement it may produce, and its tendency to relapse, all of which have long ago led to its recognition as one of the great scourges of humanity. It has been known as long as medicine has been studied but it has only been recognized as a clinical entity since the Italian physician, Domenico Cotugno, gave a description of it in 1764."*

Putti felt that his knowledge of this condition had progressed to the point that a differential diagnosis was relatively easy, and he says, "Since the time of Cotugno, chiefly through the efforts of neurologists, the symptomatology of sciatica has been increasingly well defined, and today we may say that we have the complete clinical picture and the differential diagnosis is easy." Despite the fact that a considerable mass of additional information has been compiled by various investigators since 1927, for me at least the differential diagnosis is still not always easy. Careful observation allows fairly accurate elimination of those cases in which the pathological changes are extraspinal with the possible exception of the degree of psychogenic involvement. Neuropsychological evaluation, reenforced by recently developed diagnostic aids such as (1) the differential spinal anesthetic used at Duke University Medical Center[3] and (2) the utilization of electroencephalography to verify responses to peripheral stimulation (devised by a local neurologist), has increased the reliability of separating the functional from the organic.

So that we may have a clear picture of where we stand today, it seems wise to review past observations. The voluminous nature of these, however, prohibits a complete review. Therefore, I will cover only those that seem pertinent to me.

Following Cotugno, Valleix in 1841, according to Danforth and Wilson,[39] further defined the clinical picture of sciatica and described tender spots along the course of the sciatic nerve, which became known as Valleix's spots. Virchow,[155]

*From Putti, V.: The Lady Jones Lecture: Pathogenesis of sciatic pain, Lancet **2**:53, 1927.

1857, seems to have been the first to describe a fractured disc. This autopsy finding was in a patient who died following severe injury. From additional studies Virchow described gross and microscopic details of the intervertebral disc, calling the larger clear cells that he found in the nucleus pulposus "physolipherous cells." Observed in his autopsy dissection was a tumor of the base of the skull, the cells of which resembled cells found in the intervertebral disc. He, therefore, named this tumor a "physolipherous enchondroma," which probably is the first description of a ruptured disc.

Von Luschka[156] in 1858 was apparently the first to describe a posteriorly protruded disc but attached no clinical significance to this autopsy finding. Lasègue[99] in 1864 described the straight leg raising test that still bears his name. Londorzey, in 1875, is said by Danforth and Wilson to have noted changes in skin temperature and muscle atrophy associated with some cases of sciatica. Babinski, they report, pointed out the frequent absence of the Achilles reflex on the involved side.

Brissaud, also from Danforth and Wilson, described the inclination of the spine associated with sciatica and coined the term "sciatic scoliosis." He recognized that the inclination was at times away from the side of pain, and at other times toward that side.

As far as I can tell, Goldthwait[61] was the first to attempt to explain the clinical picture of low back pain with or without sciatica as based upon anatomical conditions of the lower lumbar spine. It was his opinion that anomalies of the fifth lumbar transverse process—either enlargement, deformity, or sacralization—could cause pressure on the fifth lumbar root. These observations developed into the then popular concept that sciatica in certain cases was due to abnormality of the transverse process of the fifth lumbar vertebra, and stimulated use of the operation of resection of the transverse process, which later was advocated by Bauman[16] and others. Goldthwait also pointed out the frequency of an asymmetrical development of facets, suggesting that this might at times produce the clinical picture of low back pain and sciatica. As far as I know, it has not been demonstrated by laboratory study that asymmetry of the facets imparts a rotational strain to the disc unit. However, it seems likely that such is the case. If so, this could result in earlier disc degeneration. Goldthwait[61] in 1911 described a case of paraplegia in which the patient exhibited no evidence of abnormalities to explain the condition. Exploration was carried out by Cushing who failed to find anything to account for the sciatica and paraplegia. Goldthwait felt that it must have been the result of a ruptured intervertebral disc. He speculated that perhaps this might be the cause of other cases of sciatica with neurological changes.

During this time the diagnosis of lumbago gradually changed to sacroiliac and lumbosacral strains and sprains. Proponents of the above considerations as the cause of low back pain and sciatica were numerous. Hibbs[75] recommended spinal fusion for lumbosacral strains. Smith-Petersen[142] discussed lumbosacral and sacroiliac strains and devised a method of fusion of the sacroiliac joint for the treatment of resistant sacroiliac strains. In certain instances both the lumbosacral and the sacroiliac joints were fused on the painful side, and finally there was the trisacral fusion of Chandler.[25] Key[90] in 1924 described the pictures of low back pain and sciatica and ascribed most of these to strains or sprains of the lumbosacral joint. Whitman,[159] also in 1924, called attention to the horizontal position of the sacrum in some patients with severe lordosis and low back pain. He felt that this horizontal position contributed to weakness of the spine, with or without spondylolisthesis, and recommended spinal fusion for those patients who resisted conservative treatment.

At the 1924 meeting of the American Orthopaedic Association, a symposium on low back pain and sciatica contained the following discussions: (1) the horizontal sacrum, by Whitman; (2) resection of the transverse process, by Bauman; (3) sacroiliac and lumbosacral sprains, by Smith-Petersen; and (4) anatomy of the lumbosacral region, by Danforth and Wilson.[39] The latter authors observed from anatomical studies that in the lumbar spine the size of the nerve roots increases as one goes down, so that the fifth lumbar root is the largest. On the other hand, the foramen through which this root emerges from the spine is the smallest. The size of this foramen could be decreased further by the position of the facets; particularly was this noted in hyperextension. From these anatomical studies they concluded that the origin of sciatica must be the lumbosacral area of the spine. They found no evidence that it would be possible for sciatica to arise from any condition in the sacroiliac joint. They called attention to anomalies of the facets as a possible cause of decrease in the size of the intervertebral foramen, and the production of pain.

In 1926 Schmorl[135] published autopsy studies on over 5,000 spines and contributed to the detailed anatomy of the intervertebral disc. In one series of 3,000 spines he observed in 38% a rupture of one or more intervertebral discs into a vertebral body, and in 15% there was at least one posterior protrusion of the intervertebral disc into the spinal canal. However, in neither instance did he ascribe clinical significance to these findings. During the early part of this century, there were isolated reports from a number of neurosurgeons—Bucy,[23] Dandy,[38] and others—concerning operative findings of a large fibrocartilaginous mass producing spinal cord or nerve root compression. These usually were diagnosed as enchondroma.

In 1933 Ghormley[59] described what he termed the "facet syndrome"; in this he felt that arthritic changes in the facets or a narrowing of the intervertebral foramen as a result of these changes was the etiology of many cases of sciatica. Those cases that did not respond to conservative treatment were submitted to operation for excision of facets and spinal fusion.

In 1934 Freiberg and Vinke[49] described the "piriformis syndrome," in which sciatica was produced by inflammation and spasm of the piriformis muscle, with irritation of the sciatic nerve. In 1932 Williams[161] called attention to the narrowing of the lumbosacral junction in many cases of low back pain and sciatica and indicated that the important factor is degenerative change in the posterior portion of the lumbosacral disc. This was further elaborated upon in 1933 and 1937[162, 163] when he reported a study of 1,000 cases of low back pain and sciatica.

In 1935 Ober[121] described "Ober's syndrome," which was production of low back pain and sciatica from a tight fascia lata; the operation of fasciotomy was developed for its cure.[122] Heyman, in 1934[71] and again in 1939[73] and 1941,[74] described a posterior fascial stripping operation in the treatment of low back pain and sciatica. It was his feeling that in some of these cases there was definite abnormality in the soft tissues, as well as tight fascia in the spine, which could act very much as a tight plantar fascia does in producing pain at bony attachments. Biopsy material removed at this fascial stripping operation failed to show evidence of inflammation or other changes that would support a diagnosis of fibrositis or myositis, but he believed the fascia to be thickened.

In 1938 Steindler and Luck[144] described the alleviation of low back pain and sciatica by the injection of procaine into tender trigger spots. They postulated that in these patients sciatica was a referred pain.

Mixter and Barr[119] in 1934 demonstrated that rupture of the intervertebral disc into the spinal canal with nerve root compression could produce the clinical picture of low back pain and sciatica and that surgical removal of this ruptured disc material could relieve these symptoms.

Since that time the literature on the disc is abundant.

Concerning the disc unit, it appears that the anatomist Vesalius,[152] in 1555, first described the intervertebral disc. However, little was added until von Luschka[156] in 1858 gave an accurate description of the intervertebral disc and discussed its embryological development.

Fick,[46] in 1904 and again in 1911, contributed to the anatomical knowledge of the disc and ascribed to the disc the function of allowing motion of the spine. Among other isolated observations made by the early workers was that of Kolliker,[97] who in 1859 noted that the central portion of the disc of a 1-year-old child contained notochordal cells. In 1878 Lowe[109] found that the entire nucleus pulposus of the rat was formed by notochordal cells. Geist[58] observed that the twenty-three discs make up approximately one-fourteenth of the total height of an adult and one-fourth of the movable portion of the spine. Geist's measurements indicated that in the cervical region the discs make up 40% of the spine, 20% in the dorsal region, and 33⅓% in the lumbar area. Williams[161] seems to have been one of the first to ascribe low back pain and sciatica to alterations of function of the disc unit. He felt that the disc was important in keeping the vertebrae apart and maintaining proper alignment of the facets. In addition he observed that degenerative changes in the disc occur on the concave side of any spinal curve regardless of its cause.

In 1932 Keyes and Compere[93] conducted an extensive study on the development and structural characteristics of the intervertebral disc—a study that is still valid.

The annulus fibrosus may be described as a dense fibrous structure, firmly attached to the adjacent vertebral bodies. Arrangement of its fibers into layers, running in oblique direction, imparts an elastic-like function to this structure. No elastic fibers have been found in either the annulus or the nucleus. The annulus completely surrounds the fibrogelatinous, incompressible nucleus pulposus which, according to Hirsch and co-workers,[81] is made up of a three-dimensional network of collagen fibers enmeshed in a mucoprotein gel. Changes in position and shape of the nucleus are made possible by corresponding changes in the annulus.

Roofe,[133] Pedersen and associates,[126] and others have traced nerves in the long ligaments and in the annulus, but none have been found in the nucleus.

The intervertebral discs not only permit movement of the spine by virtue of their ability to yield locally to strain but also aid in returning the spine to the upright position. Further, they act as shock absorbers. This is not because either the nucleus or the annulus is elastic in the way a rubber ball or cushion is elastic but because the nucleus behaves as a liquid; and although it is incompressible, it may change its shape and position because of the elastic-like action of the annulus fibrosus. When pressure is released, it tends to return to its original shape and position. Hirsch[77] has studied both static and dynamic loading of the disc, recording vibrations within the disc as a result of the forces. He observed that after static loading the dynamic force necessary to reach the elastic limit of the disc was considerably reduced, suggesting that this may be a factor in disc prolapse when an individual is carrying a load and is subjected to a mild but sudden additional force.

The semiliquid nucleus also distributes pressure equally throughout the disc, so that in flexion of the spine it aids in protecting the bony margins of the vertebra from direct pressure unless the movement is carried beyond the point where the nucleus ceases to function. This wide range of movement can occur only in forward or backward bending, because of the restraint of facets, and here the disc may be flattened and the margins of the vertebrae subjected to great pressure.

In considering the physiology of the intervertebral disc, I am impressed by the following statement of Beadle.[17] "The whole intervertebral disc thus becomes a unit, a living unit, in the spinal system. It is a unit whose function is to control the continuous and infinitely varied cross-currents of tension, torsion, pressure and mechanical shock which interplay with one another as injurious agencies during every moment of life."*

Hirsch[77] states that the intervertebral joints and ligaments have no supporting function. They limit the extent of movement of the elastic pilar, the spine, as regards both direction and magnitude.

Inman and Saunders[84] believe that the disc is capable of drawing in water by osmosis to increase its power of resisting loading forces. In 1937 Barr and coworkers[10] loaded cadaver spines until the disc bulged laterally. They found that when the pressure was increased the disc suddenly ruptured with prolapse of nuclear material. The original height of the disc was not then restored. However,

*From Beadle, O. A.: The intervertebral disc, Medical Research Council, Special Report Series, No. 161, London, 1931, His Majesty's Stationery Office.

Freiberg was unable to cause a rupture of a normal disc by loading, the vertebrae giving way before this occurred.

Hirsch and colleagues[81] ascribed to aging an increase in the amount of collagen, while the ratio of collagen to polysaccharide decreases: "This implies that the protein moiety will occupy a larger number of polar groups of the polysaccharide, leaving fewer for other linkage and the binding of water."*

These authors have found the nucleus is made up of "1) collagen fibrils; 2) a polysaccharide component; 3) a protein component attached to the polysaccharide; and 4) water. In the natural state these substances form a three dimensional lattice gel system, in which cell bodies and intercellular material can be distinguished. The latter contains a dense collagen embedded in a matrix of ground substance which holds large amounts of chondroitin sulphate, water and salt."*

In degeneration large collagen bundles completely devoid of mucoid material may be seen.

At birth the disc contains approximately 88% water, which is steadily lost during life, so that at the age of 70 it contains only about 69%. Hendry[70] reports that "in a normal disc most of the fluid is held by imbibition or the property of a gel, but in degeneration fluids are retained mainly by osmotic properties."†

Coventry and associates[32] feel that by the end of the second decade there is a reduction of cells, with dehydration of the disc; in the third decade fissures form in the annulus, and in the fourth decade pigmentation is found with increased vascularity of posterior annulus. Lindblom[103] recently has demonstrated disc degeneration on the concave side of rat tails when they were tied in a U, confirming the postulation of Williams and others that prolonged pressure may result in disc degeneration.

As has been shown, changes take place within the disc throughout life. These changes are a normal aging process, which appears first on the concave side of all spinal curves. In some, the process is more rapid so that degenerative changes appear in earlier life. Whether this is caused by environment or heredity, or both, is not known. Many authors have postulated excessive pressure on the disc unit from the upright position as a cause of back pain and sciatica. It seems to me, however, that just the opposite is true in that the erect spine is better adapted to resist strain than a horizontal one. At any rate there occurs a crack in the cartilaginous plates, with loss of fluid and nuclear material into the vertebral body, or fissures develop in the annulus, sufficiently large to alter its function or allow escape of fluid and nuclear material; thus there is permanent alteration of function of the disc unit, since it does not properly transmit pressure from segment to segment and

*From Hirsch, C., Paulson, S., Sylven, B., and Snellman, O.: Biophysical and physiological investigations on cartilage and other mesenchymal tissues, Acta Orthop. Scand. **22**(supp. 10-14): 175, 1953.

†From Hendry, N. G. C.: The imbibition characteristics of normal and abnormal intervertebral discs; Proceedings of British Orthopaedic Association, Autumn, 1954, J. Bone Joint Surg. **37-B:**164, 1955.

does not allow normally controlled movement. Unusual stress and strain is placed upon all the surrounding supporting structures. This results in lipping or spur formation on the edges of the adjacent vertebral bodies, increased density of bone next to the cartilaginous plates, narrowing of the disc space with alteration of function of the apophyseal joints, followed by erosion of the articular cartilage, and degenerative changes in these joints. Or, in other words, we find development of the picture of degenerative arthritis of the spine. According to the studies of Rissanen,[132] degenerative changes in the intraspinous ligaments correlate well with changes in the disc but are more marked after profound disc degeneration. He describes the ligament changes as fatty degeneration, proliferation of small blood vessels, and changes in staining characteristics as a result of cavitation and eventual rupture.

Kohler[96] devised a method of injecting contrast media into the ligaments so that they could be studied by x-ray. He found evidence of change suggesting degeneration after age 50 and about equally distributed between patients with symptoms and those without. By x-ray examination the correlation of ligament degeneration with disc degeneration was not too good.

However, Knutsson[94] felt that by utilizing motion films he could demonstrate excess motion in a diseased disc before other x-ray evidence of degeneration was present.

These changes in the disc may cause low back pain with or without sciatica. Hirsch[76] injected hypertonic saline into the disc, intraspinous ligaments, and apophyseal joints. He observed that with injection of the joints a well-localized unilateral pain resulted, which spread over the sacroiliac and gluteal area and finally before disappearing involved the trochanteric area. Injection of the ligamentum flavum, intraspinous and supraspinous ligaments, produced pain but not of lumbago type. Injection of disc produced real lumbago and the full pattern of low back pain. Should posterior rupture with nerve root compression occur, this may also produce low back pain, sciatica, or both.

Verbrugge[150] has used disc puncture with instillation of cortisone in the disc to reduce the patient's symptoms and reports that many patients obtained sufficient relief to avoid surgery.

More recently, Garvin and co-workers[57] have described dissolution of the disc by papain instilled within the nucleus. This was followed by subsidence of symptoms in most patients. The disc space rapidly narrows but does not fuse. Just how long before it stabilizes is not yet known. Time may prove this to be a very useful substitute for surgery.

The place of surgery in the treatment of symptoms produced by altered function of a disc unit, without nerve root compression, that have resisted conservative therapy is stabilization of this segment. The place of surgery in the treatment of symptoms produced by nerve root compression that has resisted treatment is to relieve the compression. Spinal fusion at the time of decompression is of little value in my opinion.

References

1. Adson, A. W.: Diagnosis and treatment of tumors of the spinal cord, Northwest Med. **24:**309, 1925.
2. Adson, A. W., and Ott, W. O.: Results of the removal of tumors of the spinal cord, Arch. Neurol. Psychiat. **8:**520, 1922.
3. Ahlgren, E. W., Stephen, R., Lloyd, E. A. C., and McCollum, D. E.: Diagnosis of pain with a graduated spinal block technique, J.A.M.A. **195:**813, 1966.
4. Aitken, A. P., and Bradford, C. H.: End results of ruptured intervertebral discs in industry, Amer. J. Surg. **73:**365, 1947.
5. Armstrong, J. R.: The causes of unsatisfactory results from the operative treatment of lumbar disc lesions, J. Bone Joint Surg. **33-B:**31, 1951.
6. Ayers, C. E.: Lumbo-sacral backache, New Eng. J. Med. **200:**592, 1929.
7. Badgley, C. E.: The articular facets in relation to low-back pain and sciatic radiation, J. Bone Joint Surg. **23:**481, 1941.
8. Barker, L. F.: On the diagnosis and treatment of the maladies grouped under the designation "sciatica," Int. Clin. **1:**1, 1930.
9. Barr, J. S.: "Sciatica" caused by intervertebral-disc lesions; a report of forty cases of rupture of the intervertebral disc occurring in the low lumbar spine and causing pressure on the cauda equina, J. Bone Joint Surg. **19:**323, 1937.
10. Barr, J. S.: Ruptured intervertebral disc and sciatic pain, J. Bone Joint Surg. **29:**429, 1947.
11. Barr, J. S.: Low-back and sciatic pain: results of treatment, J. Bone Joint Surg. **33-A:** 633, 1951.
12. Barr, J. S., Hampton, A. O., and Mixter, W. J.: Pain low in back and "sciatica" due to lesion of the intervertebral disks, J.A.M.A. **109:**1265, 1937.
13. Barr, J. S., and Mixter, W. J.: Posterior protrusion of the lumbar intervertebral discs, J. Bone Joint Surg., **23:**444, 1941.
14. Bärsony, T., and Koppenstein, E.: Calcinosis intervertebralis, Fortschr. Roentgenstr. **41:**211, 1930.
15. Batts, M., Jr.: Rupture of the nucleus pulposus; an anatomical study, J. Bone Joint Surg. **21:**121, 1939.
16. Bauman, G. I.: The cause and treatment of certain types of low back pain and sciatica, J. Bone Joint Surg. **6:**909, 1924.
17. Beadle, O. A.: The intervertebral disc, Medical Research Council, Special Report Series, No. 161, London, 1931, His Majesty's Stationery Office.
18. Borski, A. A., and Smith, R. A.: Ureteral injury in lumbar-disc operation, J. Neurosurg. **17:**925, 1960.
19. Bradford, F. K.: Certain anatomic and physiologic aspects of the intervertebral disc, Southern Surg. **10:**623, 1941.
20. Breck, L. W., and Basom, W. C.: The flexion treatment for low-back pain; indications, outline of conservative management and a new spine-fusion procedure, J. Bone Joint Surg. **25:**58, 1943.
21. Brown, L. T.: Beef bone in stabilizing operations of the spine, J. Bone Joint Surg. **4:**711, 1922.
22. Brown, L. T.: Conservative treatment of backache, J. Bone Joint Surg. **14:**157, 1932.
23. Bucy, P. C.: Chondroma of intervertebral disc, J.A.M.A. **94:**1552, 1930.
24. Calvé, J., and Galland, M.: The intervertebral nucleus pulposus; its anatomy, its physiology, its pathology, J. Bone Joint Surg. **12:**555, 1930.
25. Chandler, F. A.: Spinal fusion operations in the treatment of low back and sciatic pain, J.A.M.A. **93:**1447, 1929.
26. Chandler, F. A.: Trisacral fusion, Surg. Gynec. Obstet. **48:**501, 1929.
27. Cloward, R. B., and Bucy, P. C.: Spinal extradural cyst and kyphosis dorsalis juvenalis, Amer. J. Roentgen. **38:**681, 1937.
28. Clymer, G., Mixter, W. J., and Voella, H.: Experience with spinal cord tumors during the past ten years, Arch. Neurol. Psychiat. **5:**213, 1921.

29. Colonna, P. C., and Friedenberg, Z. B.: The disc syndrome; results of the conservative care of patients with positive myelograms, J. Bone Joint Surg. **31-A:**614, 1949.
30. Compere, E. L., and Keyes, D. C.: Roentgenological studies of the intervertebral disc, Amer. J. Roentgen. **29:**774, 1933.
31. Congdon, R. T.: Spondylolisthesis and vertebral anomalies in skeletons of American aborigines; with clinical notes on spondylolisthesis, J. Bone Joint Surg. **14:**511, 1932.
32. Coventry, M. B., Ghormley, R. K., and Kernohan, J. W.: The intervertebral disc: its microscopic anatomy and pathology, J. Bone Joint Surg. **27:**105, 233, 460, 1945.
33. Craig, W. M., and Walsh, M. N.: Diagnosis and treatment of low back and sciatic pain caused by protruded intervertebral disk and hypertrophied ligaments, Minnesota Med. **22:**511, 1939.
34. Craig, W. M., and Walsh, M. N.: Neuro-anatomical and physiological aspects and significance of sciatica, J. Bone Joint Surg. **23:**417, 1941.
35. Crawford, A. S., Mitchell, C. L., and Granger, G. R.: Surgical treatment of low back pain with sciatic radiation: preliminary report on 346 cases, Arch. Surg. **59:**724, 1949.
36. Dandy, W. E.: Loose cartilage from intervertebral disk simulating tumor of the spinal cord, Arch. Surg. **19:**660, 1929.
37. Dandy, W. E.: Concealed ruptured intervertebral disks: plea for elimination of contrast media in diagnosis, J.A.M.A. **117:**821, 1941.
38. Dandy, W. E.: Recent advances in the diagnosis and treatment of ruptured intervertebral disks, Ann. Surg. **115:**514, 1942.
39. Danforth, M. S., and Wilson, P. D.: The anatomy of the lumbosacral region in relation to sciatic pain, J. Bone Joint Surg. **7:**109, 1925.
40. DeSaussure, R. L.: Vascular injury coincident to disc surgery, J. Neurosurg. **16:**222, 1959.
41. Deucher, W. G., and Love, J. G.: Pathologic aspects of posterior protrusions of the intervertebral disks, Arch. Path. **27:**201, 1939.
42. Donohue, W. L.: Pathology of the intervertebral disc, Amer. J. Med. Sci. **198:**419, 1939.
43. Echols, D. H.: Surgical treatment of sciatica: results 3 to 8 years after operation, Arch. Neurol. Psychiat. **61:**672, 1949.
44. Elsberg, C. A.: Experiences in spinal surgery: observations upon 60 laminectomies for spinal disease, Surg. Gynec. Obstet. **16:**117, 1913.
45. Farrell, B. P., and MacCracken, W. B.: Spine fusion for protruding intervertebral discs, J. Bone Joint Surg. **23:**457, 1941.
46. Fick, R.: Handbuch der Anatomie und Mechanik der Gelenke. In Bardeleben, editor: Handbuch der Anatomie des Menschen, vol. II, Part 1, Stuttgart, 1904, Gustav Fischer Verlag, p. 1.
47. Foerster, O.: The dermatomes in man, Brain **56:**1, 1933.
48. Ford, L. T.: The intervertebral disk: diagnosis. In American Academy of Orthopaedic Surgeons, Instructional Course Lectures, Ann Arbor, 1954, J. W. Edwards, vol. 11, pp. 108-117.
49. Freiberg, A. H., and Vinke, T. H.: Sciatica and the sacroiliac joint, J. Bone Joint. Surg. **16:**126, 1934.
50. Friberg, S.: Low back and sciatic pain caused by intervertebral disc herniation, Acta Chir. Scand. **85**(suppl. 64):1, 1941.
51. Friberg, S.: Anatomical studies of lumbar disc degeneration, Acta Orthop. Scand. **17** (supp. 4):224, 1948.
52. Friberg, S., and Hirsch, C.: On late results of operative treatment for intervertebral disc prolapses in the lumbar region, Acta Chir. Scand. **93:**161, 1946.
53. Friberg, S., and Hirsch, C.: Anatomical and clinical studies on lumbar disc degeneration, Acta Orthop. Scand. **19:**222, 1949.
54. Friberg, S., and Hult, L.: Comparative study of abrodil myelogram and operative findings in low back pain and sciatica, Acta Orthop. Scand. **20:**303, 1951.
55. Gama, C.: Neuralgic pain wrongly ascribed to posterior hernia of intervertebral discs; report of 2 cases, J. Int. Coll. Surg. **13:**578, 1950.

56. Gardner, W. J., Wise, R. E., Hughes, C. R., O'Connell, F. B., Jr., and Weiford, E. C.: X-ray visualization of the intervertebral disk with a consideration of the morbidity of disk puncture, Arch. Surg. **64:**355, 1952.
57. Garvin, P. J., Jennings, R. B., Smith, L., and Gesler, R. M.: Chymopapain: a pharmacologic and toxicologic evaluation in experimental animals, Clin. Orthop. **41:**204, 1965.
58. Geist, E. L.: The intervertebral disk, J.A.M.A. **96:**1676, 1931.
59. Ghormley, R. K.: Low back pain with special reference to the articular facets, with presentation of an operative procedure, J.A.M.A. **101:**1773, 1933.
60. Ghormley, R. K., Bickel, W. H., and Dickson, D. D.: Study of acute infectious lesions of intervertebral disks, Southern Med. J. **33:**347, 1940.
61. Goldthwait, J. E.: The lumbosacral articulation: an explanation of many cases of "lumbago," "sciatica" and paraplegia, Boston Med. Surg. J. **164:**365, 1911.
62. Grant, F. C.: Operative results in intervertebral discs, J. Neurosurg. **1:**332, 1944.
63. Grant, F. C.: Operative results in intervertebral disks, Ann. Surg. **124:**1066, 1946.
64. Greenwood, J., Jr., McGuire, T. H., and Kimbell, F.: A study of the causes of failure in the herniated intervertebral disc operation; an analysis of sixty-seven reoperated cases, J. Neurosurg. **9:**15, 1952.
65. Gurdjian, E. S., and Webster, J. E.: Lumbar herniations of the nucleus pulposus, Amer. J. Surg. **76:**235, 1948.
66. Hadley, L. A.: Bony masses projecting into the spinal canal opposite a break in the neural arch of the fifth lumbar vertebra, J. Bone Joint Surg. **37-A:**787, 1955.
67. Hampton, A. O.: Iodized oil myelography; use in the diagnosis of rupture of the intervertebral disk into the spinal canal, Arch. Surg. **40:**444, 1940.
68. Hampton, A. O., and Robinson, J. M.: The roentgenographic demonstration of rupture of the intervertebral disc into the spinal canal after injection of Lipiodol, with special reference to unilateral lumbar lesions accompanied by low back pain with "sciatic" radiation, Amer. J. Roentgen. **36:**782, 1936.
69. Hansen, H. J.: A pathologic-anatomical interpretation of disc degeneration in dogs, Acta Orthop. Scand. **20:**280, 1950-1951.
70. Hendry, N. G. C.: The imbibition characteristics of normal and abnormal intervertebral discs; Proceedings of British Orthopaedic Association, Autumn, 1954, J. Bone Joint Surg. **37-B:**164, 1955.
71. Heyman, C. H.: Thoughts on the relief of sciatic pain, J. Bone Joint Surg. **16:**889, 1934.
72. Heyman, C. H.: Spinal cord compression associated with scoliosis, J. Bone Joint Surg. **19:**1081, 1937.
73. Heyman, C. H.: Posterior fasciotomy in the treatment of back pain, J. Bone Joint Surg. **21:**397, 1939.
74. Heyman, C. H.: The relief of low-back pain and sciatica by release of fascia and muscle, J. Bone Joint Surg. **23:**474, 1941.
75. Hibbs, R.: An operation for progressive spinal deformities, New York J. Med. **93:**1013, 1911.
76. Hirsch, C.: An attempt to diagnose the level of a disc lesion clinically by disc puncture, Acta Orthop. Scand. **18:**132, 1948-1949.
77. Hirsch, C.: Studies on the mechanism of low back pain, Acta Orthop. Scand. **20:**261, 1951.
78. Hirsch, C.: Reaction of intervertebral discs to compression forces, J. Bone Joint Surg. **37-A:**1188, 1955.
79. Hirsch, C. and Nachemson, A.: New observations on the mechanical behavior of lumbar discs, Acta Orthop. Scand. **23:**254, 1954.
80. Hirsch, C., and Schajowicz, F.: Studies on structural changes in the lumbar annulus fibrosus, Acta Orthop. Scand. **22:**184, 1953.
81. Hirsch, C., Paulson, S., Sylven, B., and Snellman, O.: Biophysical and physiological investigations on cartilage and other mesenchymal tissues, Acta Orthop. Scand. **22**(supp. 10-14):175, 1953.
82. Hirsch, C., Snellman, O., Sylven, B., and Paulson, S.: Biophysical and physiological in-

vestigations on cartilage and other mesenchymal tissues. **II.** The ultrastructure of bovine and human nuclei pulposi, J. Bone Joint Surg. **38-A:** 333, 1950.

83. Horwitz, T.: Lesions of the intervertebral disk and ligamentum flavum of lumbar vertebrae; an anatomic study of 75 human cadavers, Surgery **6:**410, 1939.
84. Inman, V. T., and Saunders, J.: Referred pain from skeletal structures, J. Nerve Ment. Dis. **99:**660, 1944.
85. Inman, V. T., and Saunders, J.: Anatomico-physiological aspects of injuries to the intervertebral disc, J. Bone Joint Surg. **29:**461, 1947.
86. Johnson, R. W.: Posterior luxations of the lumbosacral joint, J. Bone Joint Surg. **16:** 867, 1934.
87. Joplin, R. J.: The intervertebral disc: embryology, anatomy, physiology and pathology, Surg. Gynec. Obstet. **61:**591, 1935.
88. Keegan, J.: Dermatome hypalgesia associated with herniation of intervertebral disk, Arch. Neurol. Psychiat. **50:**67, 1943.
89. Keegan, J.: Diagnosis of herniation of lumbar intervertebral disks by neurologic signs, J.A.M.A. **126:**868, 1944.
90. Key, J. A.: Low back pain as seen in an orthopedic clinic, Amer. J. Med. Sci. **168:**526, 1924.
91. Key, J. A.: Intervertebral disk lesion and low-back pain. In American Academy of Orthopaedic Surgeons, Instructional Course Lectures, Ann Arbor, 1954, J. W. Edwards, vol. 11, p. 99.
92. Key, J. A.: The intervertebral disk: anatomy, physiology and pathology. In American Academy of Orthopaedic Surgeons, Instructional Course Lectures, Ann Arbor, 1954, J. W. Edwards, vol. 11, pp. 101-107.
93. Keyes, D. C., and Compere, E. L.: The normal and pathological physiology of the nucleus pulposus of the intervertebral disc; an anatomical, clinical, and experimental study, J. Bone Joint Surg. **14:**897, 1932.
94. Knutsson, F.: The instability associated with disk degeneration in the lumbar spine, Acta Radiol. **25:**593, 1944.
95. Knutsson, F.: Lumbar myelography with water-soluble contrast in cases of disc prolapse, Acta Orthop. Scand. **20:**294, 1951.
96. Kohler, R.: Contrast examination of lumbar interspinous ligaments, Acta Orthop. Scand. (supp. 55), 1962.
97. Kolliker, A.: Ueber die Beziehungen des Chorda dorsalis zur Bildung der wirbel der Selachier und einiger andern Fische, Verh. Ges. Phys.-Med. Ges. Wurzburg **10:**193, 1860.
98. Kuhns, J. G.: Conservative treatment of sciatic pain in low-back disability, J. Bone Joint Surg. **23:**435, 1941.
99. Lasègue, C. H.: Considérations sur la sciatique, Arch. Gén. Méd. **2:**558, 1864.
100. Lindblom, K.: Protrusions of disks and nerve compression in the lumbar region, Acta Radiol. **25:**195, 1944.
101. Lindblom, K.: Diagnostic puncture of intervertebral disks in sciatica, Acta Orthop. Scand. **17**(supp. 4):231, 1948.
102. Lindblom, K.: Technique and results of diagnostic disc puncture and injection (discography) in the lumbar region, Acta Orthop. Scand. **20:**315, 1951.
103. Lindblom, K.: Intervertebral disc degeneration considered a pressure atrophy, J. Bone Joint Surg. **39-A:**933, 1957.
104. Love, J. G.: Protrusion of the intervertebral disk (fibrocartilage) into the spinal canal, Proc. Staff Meet. Mayo Clin. **11:**529, 1936.
105. Love, J. G.: Low back and sciatic pain, Surg. Clin. N. Amer. **19:**943, 1939.
106. Love, J. G.: Protruded intervertebral disks with a note regarding hypertrophy of ligamenta flava, J.A.M.A. **113:**2029, 1939.
107. Love, J. G.: Removal of protruded intervertebral disks without laminectomy, Proc. Staff Meet. Mayo Clin. **14:**800, 1939.
108. Love, J. G., and Walsh, M. N.: Protruded intervertebral disks; a report of 100 cases in which operation was performed, J.A.M.A. **111:**396, 1938.
109. Lowe, L.: Zur Kenntniss der Saugethierchorda, Arch. Mikrosk Anat. **16:**597, 1879.

110. Marble, H. C., and Bishop, W. A.: Intervertebral disc injury; analysis from an industrial standpoint, J. Industr. Hyg. Toxicol. **27:**103, 1945.
111. McKay, H. W., Baird, H. H., and Justis, H. R.: Management of ureteral injuries, J.A.M.A. **154:**202, 1954.
112. Meyerding, H. W.: Spondylolisthesis, J. Bone Joint Surg. **13:**39, 1931.
113. Meyerding, H. W.: Low backache and sciatic pain associated with spondylolisthesis and protruded intervertebral disc: incidence, significance and treatment, J. Bone Joint Surg. **23:**461, 1941.
114. Middleton, G. S., and Teacher, J. H.: Injury of the spinal cord due to rupture of an intervertebral disc during muscular effort, Glasgow Med. J. **76:**1, 1911.
115. Milward, F. J., and Grout, J. L. A.: Changes in the intervertebral discs following lumbar puncture, Lancet **2:**183, 1936.
116. Minot, C. C.: The notochord and its ultimate fate; laboratory textbook of embryology, Philadelphia, 1910, P. Blakiston's Son & Co.
117. Mixter, W. J.: Rupture of the lumbar intervertebral disk; an etiologic factor for so-called "sciatic" pain, Ann. Surg. **106:**777, 1937.
118. Mixter, W. J., and Ayer, J. B.: Herniation or rupture of the intervertebral disc into the spinal canal, New Eng. J. Med. **213:**385, 1935.
119. Mixter, W. J., and Barr, J. S.: Rupture of the intervertebral disc with involvement of the spinal canal, New Eng. J. Med. **211:**210, 1934.
120. Munro, D., and Harding, W. G.: Lumbar puncture; its potential role in production of injuries to intervertebral disk, J.A.M.A. **119:**482, 1942.
121. Ober, F. R.: Back strain and sciatica, J.A.M.A. **104:**1586, 1935.
122. Ober, F. R.: Fasciotomy for sciatic pain, J. Bone Joint Surg. **23:**471, 1941.
123. O'Connell, J. E. A.: Protrusions of the lumbar intervertebral discs; a clinical review based on 500 cases treated by excision of the protrusion, J. Bone Joint Surg. **33-B:**8, 1951.
124. Odell, R. T., Conrad, M., and Key, J. A.: Removal of lumbar intervertebral disks: postoperative results. In American Academy of Orthopaedic Surgeons, Instructional Course Lectures, Ann Arbor, 1954, J. W. Edwards, vol. 11, pp. 126-129.
125. Pease, C. N.: Injuries to the vertebrae and intervertebral disks following lumbar puncture, Amer. J. Dis. Child. **49:**849, 1935.
126. Pedersen, H. E., Blunck, C. F. J., and Gardner, E.: The anatomy of the lumbosacral posterior rami and meningeal branches of spinal nerves (sinu-vertebral nerves), J. Bone Joint Surg. **38-A:**377, 1956.
127. Peet, M. M., and Echols, D. H.: Herniation of the nucleus pulposus; a cause of compression of the spinal cord, Arch. Neurol. Psychiat. **32:**924, 1934.
128. Petter, C. K.: Methods of measuring the pressure of the intervertebral disc, J. Bone Joint Surg. **15:**365, 1933.
129. Putti, V.: The Lady Jones Lecture: Pathogenesis of sciatic pain, Lancet **2:**53, 1927.
130. Ramsey, R. H.: Conservative treatment of intervertebral disk lesions. In American Academy of Orthopaedic Surgeons, Instructional Course Lectures, Ann Arbor, 1954, J. W. Edwards, vol. 11, pp. 118-120.
131. Reynolds, F. C.: The intervertebral disk: surgical technique. In American Academy of Orthopaedic Surgeons, Instructional Course Lectures, Ann Arbor, 1954, J. W. Edwards, vol. 11, pp. 121-125.
132. Rissanen, P. M.: The surgical anatomy and pathology of the supraspinous and interspinous ligaments of the lumbar spine with special reference to ligament ruptures, Acta Orthop. Scand., Supp. 46, p. 1, 1960.
133. Roofe, P. G.: Innervation of annulus fibrosus and posterior longitudinal ligament, Arch. Neurol. Psychiat. **44:**100, 1940.
134. Sandoz, I., and Hodges, C. V.: Ureteral injury incident to lumbar disk operation, J. Urol. **93:**687, 1965.
135. Schmorl, G.: Die pathologische Anatomie der Wirbelsaüle, Verh. Deutsch. Orthop. Ges. **21:**3, 1926.

136. Scott, J. C.: Stress factor in the disc syndrome, J. Bone Joint Surg. **37-B:**107, 1955.
137. Shinners, B. M., and Hamby, W. B.: The results of surgical removal of protruded lumbar intervertebral discs, J. Neurosurg. **1:**117, 1944.
138. Shinners, B. M., and Hamby, W. B.: Protruded lumbar intervertebral discs; results following surgical and non-surgical therapy, J. Neurosurg. **6:**450, 1949.
139. Smith, A. DeF: Posterior displacement of the fifth lumbar vertebra, J. Bone Joint Surg. **16:**877, 1934.
140. Smith, A. DeF., Deery, E. M., and Hagman, G. L.: Herniation of the nucleus pulposus; a study of 100 cases treated by operation, J. Bone Joint Surg. **26:**821, 1944.
141. Smith, L., and Brown, J. E.: Treatment of lumbar intervertebral disc lesions by direct injection of chymopapain, J. Bone Joint Surg. **49-B:**502, 1967.
142. Smith-Petersen, M. N.: Arthrodesis of the sacroliac joint; a new method of approach, J. Orthop. Surg. **3:**400, 1921.
143. Spurling, R. G., Mayfield, F. H., and Rogers, J. B.: Hypertrophy of the ligamenta flava as a cause of low back pain, J.A.M.A. **109:** 928, 1937.
144. Steindler, A., and Luck, J. V.: Differential diagnosis of pain low in the back; allocation of the source of pain by procaine hydrochloride method, J.A.M.A. **110:**106, 1938.
145. Steindler, A.: The spine; non-disk sciatica. In American Academy of Orthopaedic Surgeons, Instructional Course Lectures, Ann Arbor, 1956, J. W. Edwards, vol. 13, pp. 61-70.
146. Stookey, B.: Compression of the spinal cord due to ventral extradural cervical chondromas, Arch. Neurol. Psychiat. **20:**275, 1928.
147. Sylven, B.: On the biology of nucleus pulposus, Acta Orthop. Scand. **20:**275, 1951.
148. Toumey, J. W., Poppen, J. L., and Hurley, M. T.: Cauda equina tumors as a cause of the low-back syndrome, J. Bone Joint Surg. **32-A:**249, 1950.
149. Verbiest, H.: Further experiences of the pathological influence of a developmental narrowness of the bony lumbar vertebral canal, J. Bone Joint Surg. **37-B:**576, 1955.
150. Verbrugge, J.: Personal communication, 1950.
151. Vesalius, A.: De humani corporis fabrica, Padua, 1543.
152. Vesalius, A.: De humani corporis fabrica tibri septem, Basileae, 1555, J. Operinum, p. 71.
153. Viets, H. R., and Domenico Cotungno: His description of the cerebrospinal fluid, with a translation of part of his De ischiade nervosa commentarius (1764) and a bibliography of his important works, Bull. Inst. Hist. Med. **3:**710, 1935.
154. Viner, N.: The lipiodol test for patency of the cerebrospinal canal in a case of sciatica with unusual features, Arch. Neurol. Psychiat. **13:**767, 1925.
155. Virchow, R.: Untersuchunger über die Entwickelung des Schädelgrundes, Berlin, 1857, G. Reimer.
156. Von Luschka, H.: Die Halgelenke des menschlichen Körpers. IV, Berlin, 1858, G. Reimer.
157. Von Muralt, R. H.: Ueber einige Beobachtungen von Bandschelbenvorfallen bei lumbosakralen Assimilationswirbeln, Acta Orthop. Scand. **18:**88, 1949.
158. Waugh, O. S., Cameron, H. F., Scarrow, H. G., and Howarth, J. C.: Follow-up on lumbar disc lesions, Canad. Med. Ass. J. **61:**607, 1949.
159. Whitman, A.: An anatomic variation of the lumbo-sacral joint; its diagnosis and treatment, J. Bone Joint Surg. **6:**808, 1924.
160. Wiberg, G.: Back pain in relation to the nerve supply of the intervertebral disc, Acta Orthop. Scand. **19:**211, 1949.
161. Williams, P. C.: Reduced lumbosacral joint space, J.A.M.A. **99:**1677, 1932.
162. Williams, P. C.: Lesions of the lumbosacral spine, J. Bone Joint Surg. **19:**690, 1937.
163. Williams, P. C., and Yglesias, L.: Lumbosacral facetectomy for post-fusion persistent sciatica, J. Bone Joint Surg. **15:**579, 1933.
164. Willis, T. A.: Anatomical variations and roentgenographic appearance of the low back in relation to sciatic pain, J. Bone Joint Surg. **23:**410, 1941.
165. Young, H. H.: Non-neurological lesions simulating protruded intervertebral disk, J.A.M.A. **148:**1101, 1952.

6. Pathogenesis of symptoms in discogenic low back pain

Ian Macnab, M.B., Ch.B.

In order to understand the pathogenesis of symptoms derived from degenerative disc disease, it is necessary to have a clear concept of the mechanical changes that may arise from breakdown of an intervertebral disc. The intervertebral disc consists of three major parts: the annulus fibrosus, the nucleus pulposus, and the hyaline cartilage plate. Up to the age of 30, the nucleus pulposus is gelatinous. The annulus (Fig. 6-1) acts like a coiled spring, pulling the vertebral bodies together against the elastic resistance of the nucleus pulposus, with the result that when the spine is sectioned sagittally, the unopposed pull of the annulus makes the nucleus bulge. This has been called "turgor" of the nucleus in the past; in actual fact, it is a manifestation of the springlike action, the compressing action, of the annulus fibrosus. This makes for a very good coupling unit, provided all the structures remain intact.

The nucleus pulposus acts like a ball bearing and, in flexion and extension, the vertebral bodies roll over this incompressible gel, while the posterior joints guide and steady the movements. However, once degenerative changes involve any one of the components of the disc, such as inspissation of the nucleus pulposus, tear of the annulus, or rupture of the hyaline cartilage plate—once these changes occur, the smooth action is lost and the movement between the adjacent segments becomes uneven, excessive, and irregular.

This is the stage of segmental instability. Normally, on flexion of the spine, the discal borders of the vertebral bodies become parallel above the fifth lumbar vertebra. This is the maximum range of flexion permitted. In the stage of segmental instability, excessive degrees of flexion and extension are permitted and a certain amount of backward and forward gliding movement occurs as well (Figs. 6-2 and 6-3).

One problem posed in motion studies is the fact that when the patient is in pain the associated muscle guarding does not permit adequate flexion and extension roentgenograms to be taken. However, there are two other radiological changes that

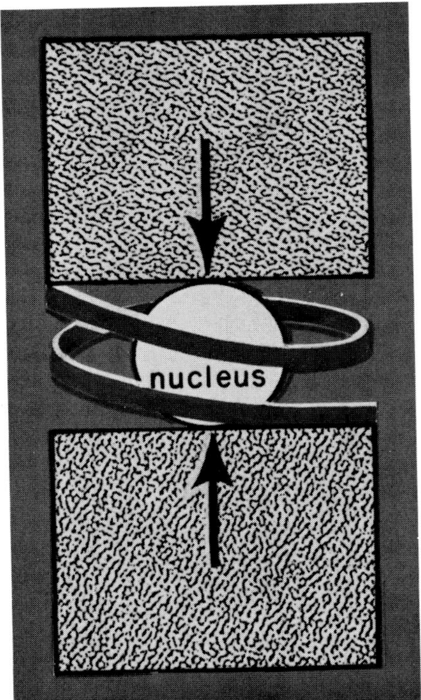

Fig. 6-1. Disc structure. The annulus acts like a coiled spring pulling the vertebral bodies together against the elastic resistance of the nucleus pulposus.

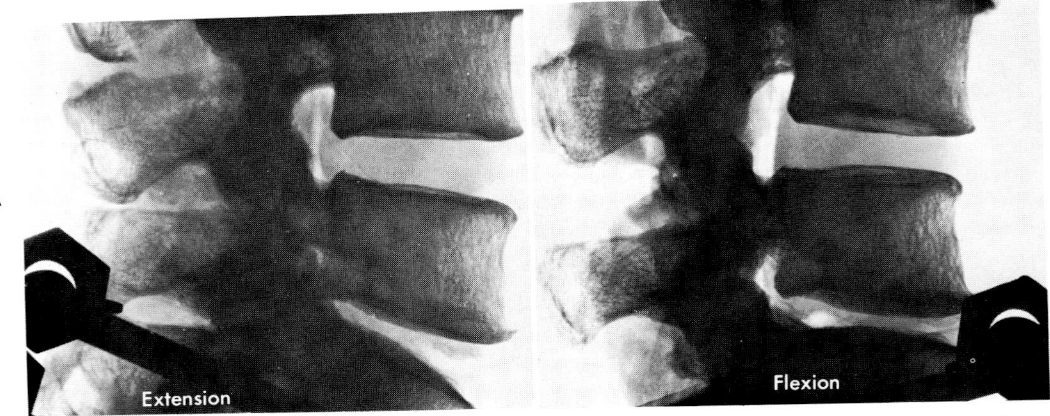

Fig. 6-2. A, X-ray film of excised specimen held in a vise in extension. **B,** When the spine is flexed, the vertebral body of L4 moves forward slightly in relation to the vertebral body of L5. The anterior portion of the disc is now narrower than the posterior portion and this does not normally occur. This is the earliest abnormality associated with disc degeneration that can be recorded on x-ray.

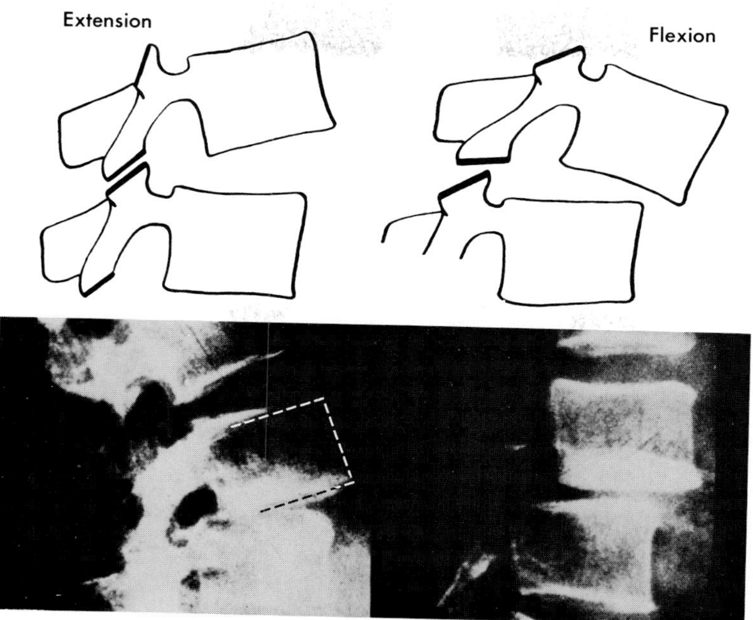

Fig. 6-3. A gross degree of backward and forward shift of the vertebral body of L4—a horizontal pistonlike movement—is associated with marked segmental instability.

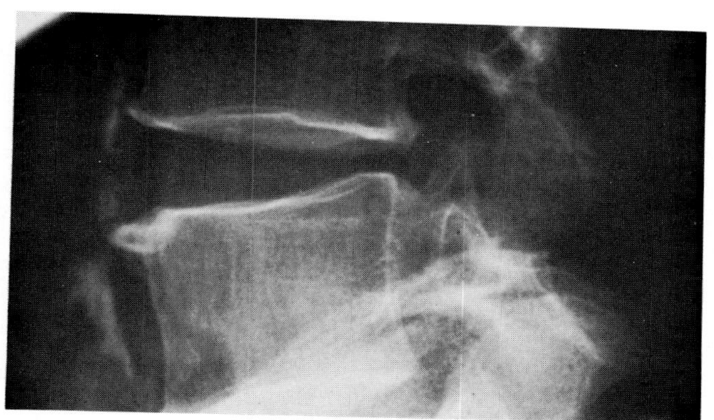

Fig. 6-4. The traction spur. The osteophyte is seen to project horizontally from the vertebral body and arises about 2 mm. away from the discal edge of the vertebral body.

are indicative of instability: the Knuttson phenomenon of air in the disc and the traction spur.

The traction spur differs anatomically and radiologically from other spondylophytes in that it projects horizontally and develops at a point about 2 mm. above the vertebral body edge (Fig. 6-4). It owes its development to the manner of at-

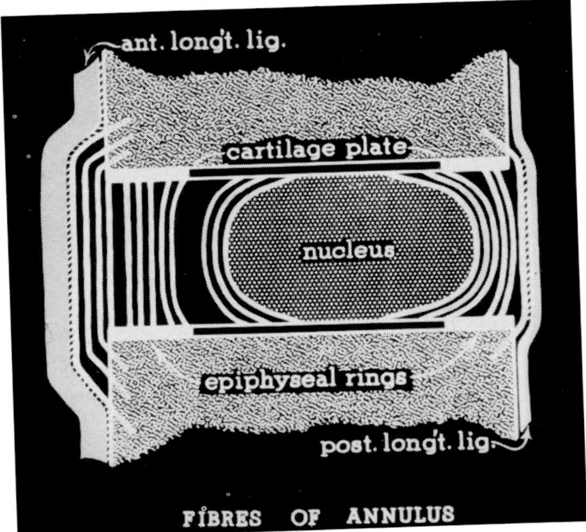

Fig. 6-5. The annulus fibers are divided into three groups: the cartilage fibers run from one cartilaginous plate to the other, the middle group run from one epiphyseal ring to the other, and the outermost group are attached between the epiphyseal ring and the anchoring ring. Their attachment anteriorly to the sides of the vertebral bodies is therefore about 2 mm. away from the discal edge of the vertebral body.

tachment of the annulus fibers, which are divided into three groups: the cartilaginous fibers, the epiphyseal fibers, and the outermost annulus fibers (Fig. 6-5). With abnormal movements, an excessive strain is applied to the outermost fibers, and it is here that the traction spur develops. It is the small traction spur that is clinically significant in that it is probably indicative of present instability, whereas the large traction spur indicates that the segment has been unstable at some time in the past but may indeed be stable at the time the roentgenogram is taken because of fibrotic changes occurring within the disc.

Segmental instability by itself is probably not painful, but the spine is vulnerable to trauma. A forced and unguarded movement falling on the wobbly segment may produce a posterior joint strain or a posterior joint subluxation, and repeated injuries may indeed result in osteochondral fractures and loose bodies within the posterior joints.

Disc degeneration in a stage of segmental instability produces symptoms by virtue of predisposing to ligamentous and joint strains. The telltale signs on x-ray are the Knuttson phenomenon, abnormal movements, and the traction spur.

The next stage of disc degeneration is segmental hyperextension. Extension of the lumbar spine is limited by the anterior fibers of the annulus. When degenerative changes cause these fibers to lose their elasticity, the involved segment or segments may hyperextend. (See Fig. 6-6.) This tendency will be exaggerated if the

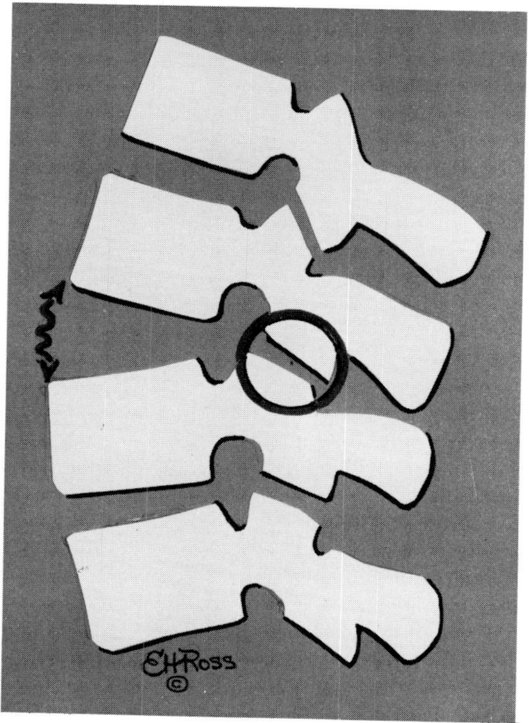

Fig. 6-6. Segmental hyperextension. With degeneration of the anterior fibers in the annulus, the resistance to hyperextension is lost and the posterior joints may be pushed beyond their normal range and indeed may be held in forced hyperextension with a normal stance.

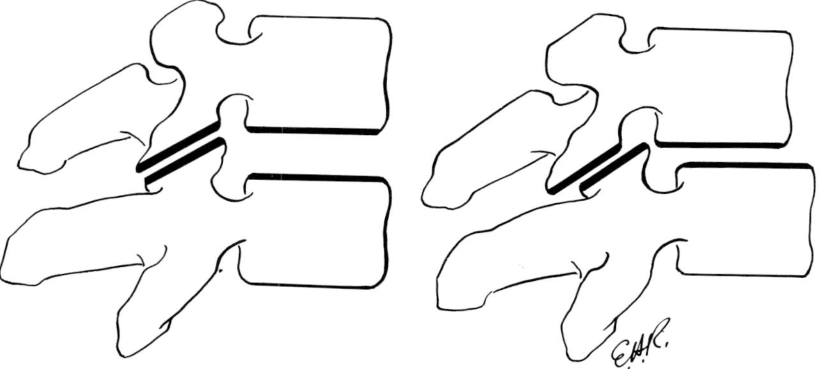

Fig. 6-7. As the intervertebral discs lose height, the posterior joints subluxate and the vertebral body moves, not only downward but backward as well, because of the inclined plane of the posterior joints.

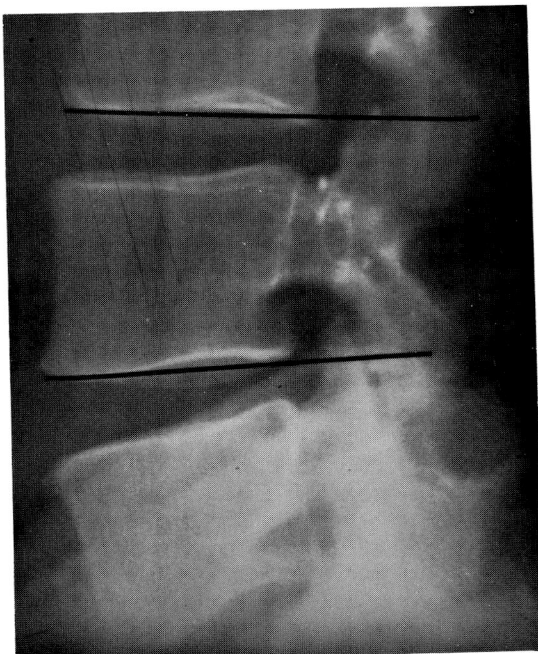

Fig. 6-8. The joint body line. Note how the tip of the superior articular facet of L5 passes above the joint body line. Subluxation of the posterior joints is present at this level.

patient has weak abdominal muscles and tight tensors, is overweight, or wears high heels. When this type of degenerative change occurs, the related posterior joints in normal posture are held in hyperextension. There is no safety factor of movement, and the extension strains of everyday living push the joints past their physiologically permitted limits and are painful. Eventually the posterior joints may subluxate.

A similar change may be seen in the next stage of disc degeneration: disc narrowing. As the intervertebral discs lose height, the posterior joints must override and subluxate (Fig. 6-7). Evidence of this can be seen on routine x-ray examination. Normally, on the lateral view above the level of L5, the tip of the superior articular facet just reaches a line extending back from the undersurface of the vertebral body above it. I have termed this the "joint body line." With extreme degrees of subluxation, the superior articular facet will impinge against the pedicle above; intermediate degrees of subluxation can be recognized when the tip of the superior articular facet passes above the joint body line (Fig. 6-8). In the anteroposterior view normally, as Lee Hadley pointed out, a lazy S can be drawn from the transverse process over the posterior joints. With minor degrees of subluxation, this line is interrupted (Fig. 6-9). With gross subluxation, the tip of the superior articular facet becomes squared off where it impinges against the pedicle

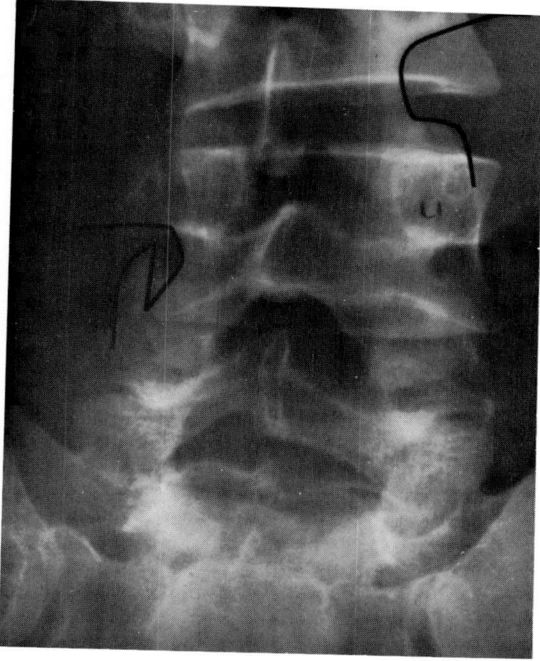

Fig. 6-9. X-ray film showing interruption of Hadley's line, due to subluxation of the posterior articular facets of L4 and L5 on the right. The normal configuration is shown at the L3-L4 level on the left.

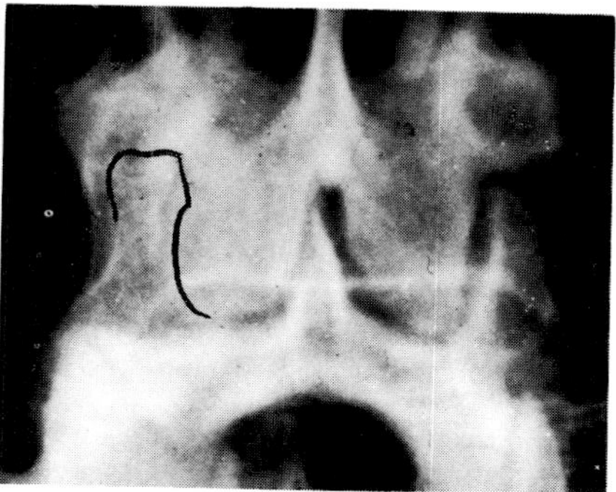

Fig. 6-10. Gross subluxation of posterior articular facets. Notice how the tip of the articular facet on the right impinges against the pedicle above and is flattened and squared off at the tip.

(Fig. 6-10). In the oblique view, a line of sclerosis can be seen on the lamina, produced by impingement of the subluxated inferior articular facet.

With chronic posterior joint subluxation, the facets assume the position normally adopted on extreme extension and, as in segmental hyperextension, the extension strains of everyday living put the joints beyond their physiologically permitted limits and may produce pain. The pain experienced may be either local back pain or local pain with referred pain (reflex pain) in sciatic distribution, without root irritation. Or indeed it may be true root pain due to root compression. Root compression is seen in association with disc degeneration *as distinct from disc herniation* under the following circumstances.

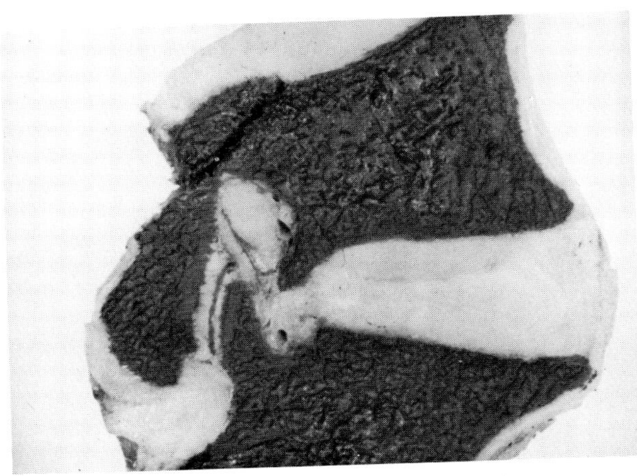

Fig. 6-11. Section of lumbar spine showing relationship of the nerve root to the tip of the superior articular facet.

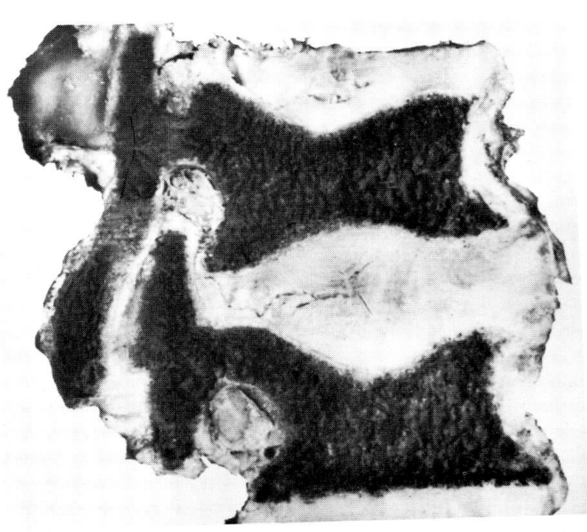

Fig. 6-12. With gross subluxation of the posterior joints, the nerve root may be impinged as shown in this specimen by the tip of the articular facet and compressed between the facet and the pedicle above.

Facet impingement

The nerve roots, as they emerge through the foramen, lie in close relation to the tip of the superior articular facet. With gross degrees of subluxation, the nerve root may be compressed between the tip of the superior articular facet and the pedicle above. (See Figs. 6-11 and 6-12.)

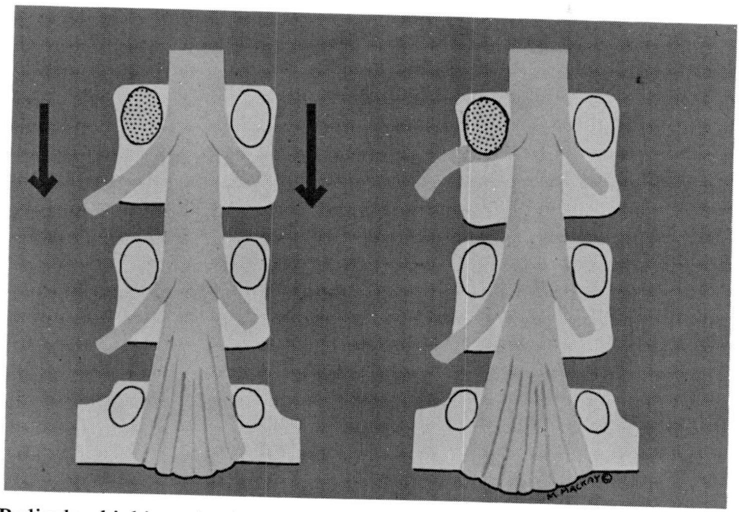

Fig. 6-13. Pedicular kinking. As the intervertebral disc narrows, shown diagrammatically here as narrowing on one side, the pedicle may descend on the nerve root and kink it as it emerges through the foramen.

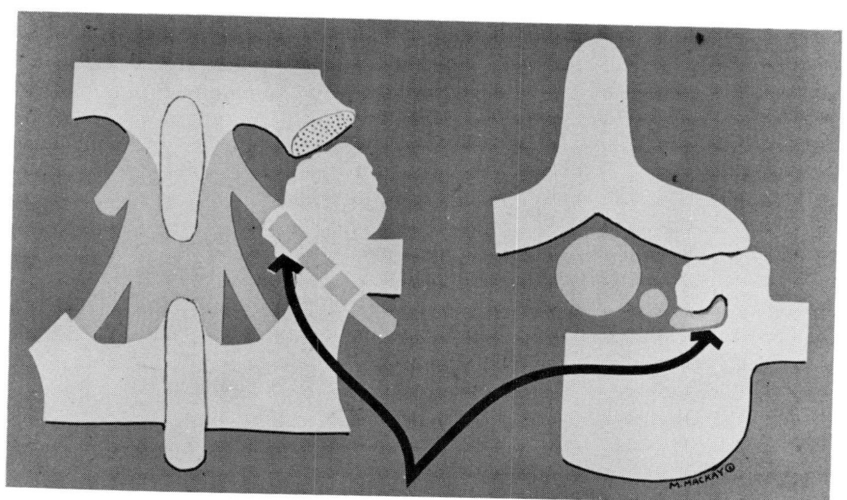

Fig. 6-14. Segmental spinal stenosis. The spinal canal is narrowed, and the nerve root is jeopardized as it courses through the subarticular gutter prior to its emergence through the intervertebral foramen.

Pedicular kinking

The nerve roots of the cauda equina normally course obliquely downward and outward. After their emergence from the intervertebral foramen, they are firmly held by the muscle masses. As the intervertebral bodies approach one another, the pedicles descend like a guillotine on the nerve roots and may kink them as they emerge through the foramen (Fig. 6-13).

Segmental spinal stenosis

A segmental spinal stenosis can be produced by a combination of shingling or overlapping of the laminae, buckling of the ligamentum flavum, and disc collapse with a diffuse annular bulge. Narrowing of the spinal canal is more pronounced if these changes are combined with a subluxation of the posterior joints, which are enlarged by diffuse osteophytic outgrowths. In such instances, the nerve roots are trapped in the subarticular gutter as they loop around the pedicle to emerge through the foramen. (See Fig. 6-14.) The myelogram characteristically shows "waisting" of the oil column rather than a discrete indentation. This myelographic appearance may be interpreted mistakenly as evidence of a disc herniation of a central type. Moreover, the demonstration of a diffuse bulge of a disc at operation may be mistaken as evidence of a disc protrusion. Excision of this bulging mass of disc, however, does nothing to relieve a nerve root entrapment that has taken place distal to the disc as the nerve passes into the intervertebral foramen.

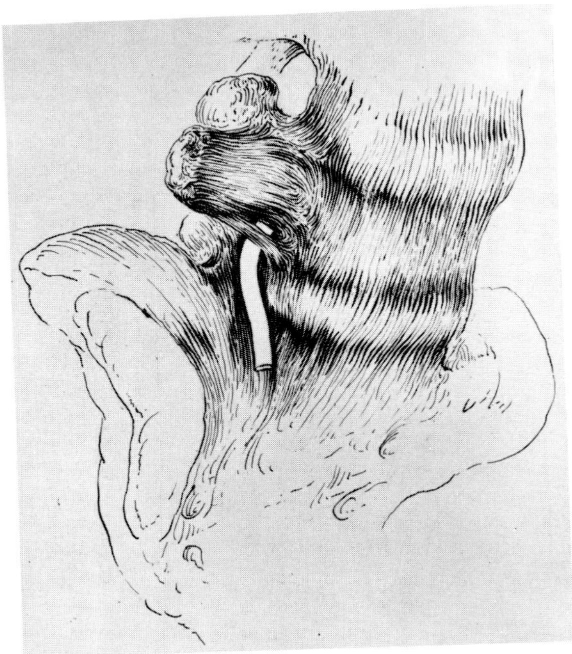

Fig. 6-15. The corporo-transverse ligament with the nerve root running underneath it.

Extraforaminal entrapment of the nerve root

There is a strong ligamentous band that runs from the transverse process to the vertebral body (Fig. 6-15). Though this is not described in standard textbooks on anatomy, it was a constant finding in my dissections and I called it the corporo-transverse ligament. At the lumbosacral level, the fifth root courses between this ligament and the ala of the sacrum. With disc collapse, the edge of the ligament descends on the nerve root and traps it against the ala of the sacrum (Fig. 6-16). A lateral diffuse bulge of the disc may also engulf the nerve root after it has emerged from the foramen (Fig. 6-17).

The telltale signs on x-ray study then, at this stage of disc degeneration, are interruption of the joint body line on the lateral roentgenogram, subluxation of the posterior joints on the oblique view, and interruption of Hadley's line on the antero-posterior view. These x-ray findings confirm subluxation of the facets which may also, on occasion, trap the nerve root in the foramen. Gross narrowing of an intervertebral disc at the same level as the nerve root involvement is suggestive of pedicular kinking. This diagnosis becomes more suspect if the myelogram proves to be negative. Pedicular kinking of the nerve root can be confirmed by selective nerve root infiltration. The nerve root, outlined by an injection of contrast material (Fig. 6-18), can be seen to run obliquely past the pedicle and to enter the subarachnoid space. With pedicular kinking, when more contrast material is injected, it is found that the contrast material will course down the sciatic nerve,

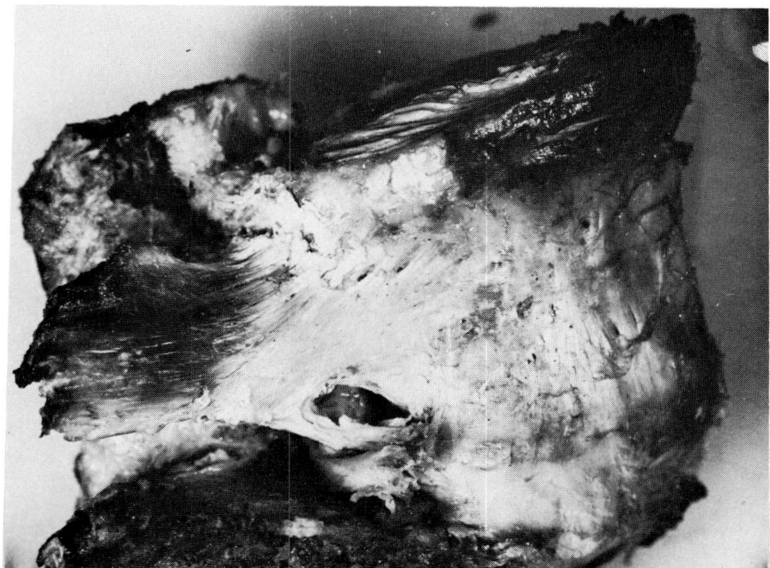

Fig. 6-16. Specimen showing fifth lumbar nerve root kinked by the edge of the corporo-transverse ligament.

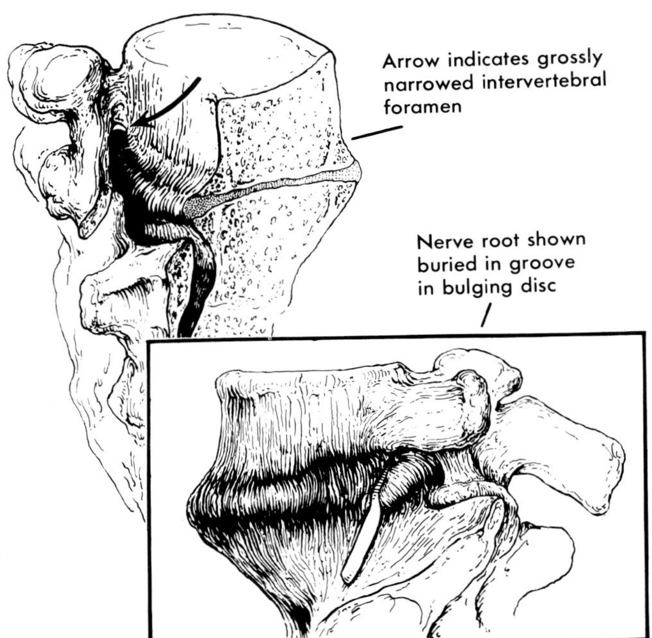

Fig. 6-17. Drawing of specimen to show the fifth lumbar nerve root engulfed, after it has emerged from the foramen, by a lateral bulge of the disc. (From Macnab, I.: J. Bone Joint Surg. **36-B:**319, 1954.)

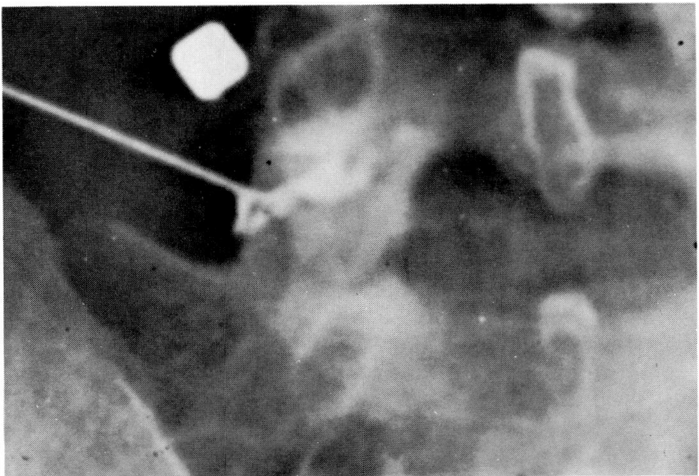

Fig. 6-18. The nerve root has been injected with 1 ml. of oil-soluble radiopaque material. It can be seen to turn a right angle around the pedicle, instead of running the normal oblique course into the spinal canal.

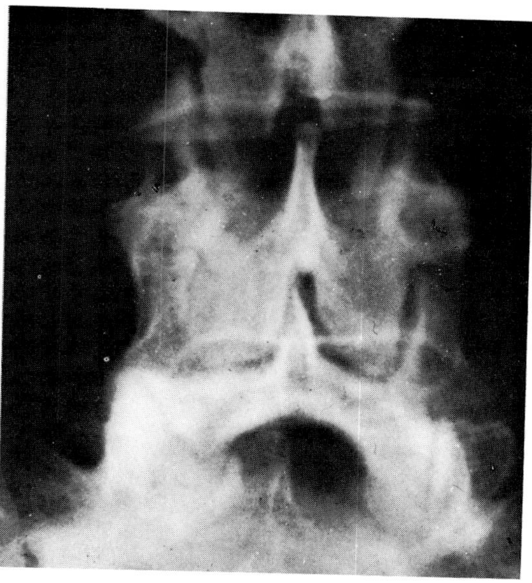

Fig. 6-19. Note the very narrow interlaminar space at L4-L5 contrasted with the wide interlaminar space at L3-L4. Note also that the middle edge of the posterior facets encroaches upon the midline. This is a very good example of segmental spinal stenosis involving the right side of the spinal canal more markedly than the left because of the gross changes in the posterior joints on the right. In this instance, there was a combination of facet impingement and subarticular entrapment of the nerve roots.

rather than run into the subarachnoid space; the obstruction created by the pedicle is sometimes clearly shown. Complete relief of symptoms on injection of the nerve root now with a local anesthetic confirms the site of the lesion. Segmental spinal stenosis is demonstrated by a narrowing of the interlaminar space on the anteroposterior view. This narrowing is best shown by tomography. Segmental spinal stenosis should be highly suspect if narrowing of the interlaminar space is combined with posterior joint subluxation and osteoarthritis. (See Fig. 6-19.)

Repeated damage to the posterior joints, especially when associated with subluxation, will lead to degenerative changes. This is the true osteoarthritis of the spine. Gross lipping of the vertebral bodies, often erroneously referred to as osteoarthritis of the spine, is merely a manifestation of disc degeneration. It is, in fact, a healing phase. Marked lipping may be present without associated degenerative changes in the posterior joints. On the other hand, minimal changes in the discs may be associated with severe damage to the posterior joints. It is not surprising, therefore, that a patient with severe back pain may show a normal roentgenogram. By the same token, it is not surprising that gross changes may be seen on the routine x-ray film, without the patient having had any back pain at all. Straight x-ray studies cannot tell the whole story.

The terms "disc degeneration" and "disc herniation" have in recent years been used so loosely as to almost lose their significance. A disc herniation is a specific lesion that may occur during the course of disc degeneration and give rise to symptoms because of pressure of disc material on the posterior longitudinal ligament or on a nerve root. Disc degeneration, alone, may also produce sciatica without involving any nerve root pressure. Admittedly, in the latter stages of disc degeneration, under certain circumstances, nerve root compression may indeed be produced, but the manner of production of root irritation is entirely different from that seen with disc herniation.

Summary of pathogenesis of symptoms in disc degeneration

Type I. Segmental instability. Pain is due to repetitive ligamentous strain. Acute episodes may precipitate a posterior joint subluxation. The pain may be experienced locally or may be referred down the leg in sciatic distribution without involvement of nerve roots.

Type II. Segmental hyperextension. Pain is due to a chronic hyperextension strain of the posterior joints.

Type III. Chronic posterior joint subluxation associated with disc narrowing. There is pain due to a chronic hyperextension strain of the posterior joints. Occasionally, root compression may result from impingement of the nerve root by the superior articular facet as the nerve root courses through the foramen.

Type IV. Posterior joint arthritis. This is secondary to mechanical instability induced by disc degeneration in the large majority of cases. A primary posterior joint arthritis may occur but it is very rare. This type of lesion gives rise to local and/or referred pain.

Type V. Root irritation. Root irritation may result from disc herniation, spinal stenosis, foraminal entrapment of the nerve root, pedicular kinking of the nerve root, or extraforaminal engulfment of the nerve root by a lateral bulge of the disc or by a lateral osteophyte.

References

1. Hadley, L.: Apophyseal subluxation, J. Bone Joint Surg. **18:**428, 1936.
2. Knuttson, F.: The instability associated with disk degeneration in the lumbar spine, Acta Radiol. **25:**593, 1944.

7. Anterior disc excision and interbody spine fusion for chronic low back pain

J. Leonard Goldner, M.D.
Donald E. McCollum, M.D.
James R. Urbaniak, M.D.

The design of a program for the management of lumbosacral pain with or without sciatica must be based on etiological factors. Pain syndromes severe enough to require surgical treatment may be due to disease or injury within the intervertebral disc, to instability or abnormality of the bony vertebral body, or to alteration of the ligamentous and other supporting structures. The treatment of the low back syndrome must be varied according to the physical and emotional profile of the patient and the experience of the treating physician. In this country the most widely used surgical procedure for the relief of intractable low back pain and sciatica includes a posterior hemilaminectomy with decompression of the nerve root. When a disc problem is recurrent or when instability exists, removal of the intervertebral disc is supplemented by posterior or posterolateral spine fusion. These two types of treatment have been successful in providing relief for the majority of patients. However, during the past twenty years at Duke University Medical Center, we have encountered a large group of patients who have not responded to these standard surgical operations. Either the surgery performed was not sufficient to relieve all pain of the back or lower extremity or, because the diagnostic findings were inconclusive, the patient was not operated upon. In order to improve both our diagnosis and the end results, contrast discography[10] and anterior disc excision[7, 11, 12] with interbody spine fusion have been added to the treatment of the low back. The major value of this operative approach has been to provide a method of salvage treatment for the patient who has had one previous posterior operative procedure, or more, without obtaining either relief of pain or spinal stability.

Anterior discectomy and fusion has also been successful when used as a primary method of treatment in patients who had complaint of low back pain and in whom myelography showed no abnormality.

This study includes a review of 50 patients operated upon at Duke University Medical Center from February of 1964 to September of 1966. The follow-up period ranges from one to three years. The initial patients managed by the anterior fusion method were so treated because previous posterior surgery had failed or additional posterior surgical treatment was not felt likely to succeed.[13, 17, 20, 22] As our experience and our confidence in the procedure increased, a greater variety of back problems were considered suitable for this method of treatment. Guidelines were established in order to decide between anterior and posterior types of disc removal and spinal fusion.

History

The anterior approach for disc excision and interbody spine fusion was originally proposed for use in the treatment of spondylolisthesis.[1, 2] The procedure actually antedates the 1934 report of Mixter and Barr[19a] that described the posterior herniation of the ruptured disc. Apparently, Lane and Moore first discussed the transperitoneal approach for the removal of an intervertebral disc in the lumbar area.[11] They described the operative procedure and end results in 36 patients in whom they had placed heterologous bone between the adjacent lumbar vertebral bodies. Harmon[9] popularized the retroperitoneal transabdominal exposure and reported 30 cases in which this method had been used prior to 1950 and 737 patients treated by 1963. He used special instruments for making a circular hole across the interspace and into the opposing surfaces of the adjacent vertebral bodies. Other reports concerned primarily with degenerative intervertebral disc disease appeared between 1951 and 1963. Humphries and Hawk[13] reported findings in 30 patients in whom they had reinforced the bone graft with a compression plate. Subsequently Humphries discontinued use of this procedure.

Use of the anterior disc removal and interbody fusion for spondylolisthesis was first reported by Burns[1] in 1933. His report was followed by those of Jenkins[15] and Mercer[19] in 1936. Speed[23] reported 1 patient treated by this method in 1938 and Friberg[5] reported 4 patients in 1939. Since 1939 several reports of larger numbers of patients have been presented.[4, 14, 16] The literature indicates that most of these investigators were concerned with management of spondylolisthesis by the anterior discectomy and fusion, but few considered the method of treatment suitable for primary intervertebral disc disease or for the treatment of patients in whom previous efforts at posterior removal of the disc and posterior spine fusion had failed.[3, 24, 25]

The value of anterior interbody fusion has been questioned by many observers who noted the reported high incidence of pseudarthrosis and inconsistent results in the relief of pain. To be considered successful the operation must be performed in such a way that bony union occurs consistently rather than occasionally and that pain is relieved. The preoperative diagnosis and indications for operation must be clear and accurate. Treatment must be applied to the correct number of interspaces, and all diseased discs must be included in the fusion. Preoperative evaluation of the patient must take into account not only physical factors but emotional factors as well. Both must be treated in order to rehabilitate the patient successfully.

Comparison of anterior and posterior spine fusion

Several factors may be involved in recurrent or continued pain following posterior spine fusion. Recurrent extrusion of intervertebral disc fragments occasionally occurs beneath a solid posterior spine fusion. Bony overgrowth of the posterior fusion with encroachment upon the nerve root in the neural foramen may cause compression of the nerve root. Continued pain after successful posterior spine fusion may also be due to extensive fibrosis of the nerve roots from injury or multiple explorations. Dural cysts and sacculations may form beneath the posterior spine fusion and lead to progressive deterioration of nerve roots several years after posterior root exploration and spinal fusion has been done. Bony overgrowth may decrease the anterior and posterior diameter of the spinal canal and make future decompression more difficult.

Repair of a posterior pseudarthrosis is uncertain because of the poor blood supply of the fibrous union, the difficulty of maintaining compression and immobilization, and the occasional necessity of including an additional interspace in order to maintain a wide surface area for bone grafting. In the presence of sciatica the nerve roots must be reexamined at the time of repair of the pseudarthrosis, and more perineural fibrosis results. The posterior bone defect resulting from numerous efforts at complete nerve root decompression, foraminotomy, and sensory rhizotomy can jeopardize the success of an attempted fusion. The transverse processes are used for placement of bone grafts, but extensive soft tissue muscle dissection, considerable blood loss, and easy breakage of the transverse process make this procedure difficult. Posterior lateral fusion is useful, but in certain situations it will not accomplish as much as an anterior discectomy and fusion.

Anterior retroperitoneal exposure of the lumbar spine provides ready access to the intervertebral disc for complete removal of the nucleus pulposus. In the hands of those experienced with the procedure, anterior interbody spine fusion has a success rate as good as or slightly better than other types of combined discectomy and spine fusion. When pseudarthrosis develops following anterior interbody fusion, repair can be done again through an anterior approach, without difficulty, or the nonunion can be stabilized by posterior fusion. Recurrent protrusions of the discs do not occur posteriorly following anterior disc excision and spine fusion.

Frequently, following removal of a disc fragment that has extruded through the posterior longitudinal ligament the nerve root is decompressed; however, due to continued compression and instability within the intervertebral space, back pain continues. Anterior decompression and stabilization by interbody bone grafts relieves the discomfort arising from within the interspace. Anterior spine fusion may be used as a supplement to posterior spine fusion at any time in the program of treatment.

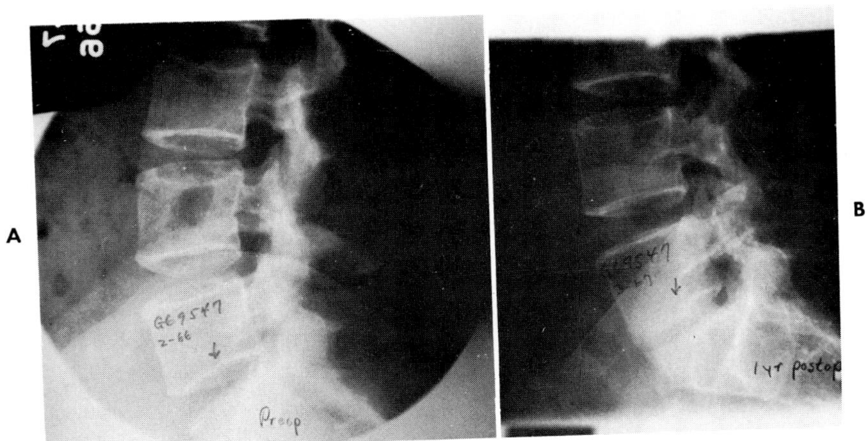

Fig. 7-1. A, Preoperative film shows narrowing of the lumbosacral joint of a patient with chronic low back pain of six years' duration; pain radiated to the buttocks but not to the posterior thigh nor calf. Myelogram and electromyogram were negative. Discogram showed a pattern normal at the L3 and L4 levels but abnormal at the lumbosacral joint. **B,** Lateral x-ray view one year after operation shows solid anterior interbody fusion. Pain was relieved, completely, and the patient returned to moderately heavy work after eight months. Arrows designate lumbosacral joint.

Choice of operative procedure

In the past ten years our management of acute and chronic back problems has included (1) laminectomy and discectomy through a posterior approach, (2) discectomy and posterior fusion, (3) discectomy and posterolateral fusion, and (4) anterior discectomy and interbody fusion. The results and complications have allowed us to establish guidelines for treatment. A flexible classification has resulted:

1. Protrusion of the intervertebral disc with nerve root compression. This classic syndrome, at any age, should be managed by excision of the intervertebral disc through a posterior approach without arthrodesis.

2. Degenerative disc disease in the lumbosacral interspace, which shows narrowing of the joint on x-ray and localized subchondral change in the vertebral bodies. In the absence of radiculopathy, and with a negative myelogram, most orthopaedic surgeons should manage this by posterior or posterolateral fusion. If the physician is experienced in the anterior interbody fusion, this procedure affords a more complete relief of pain and more rapid convalescence. (See Fig. 7-1.)

When degenerative changes with narrowing of the interspace occur at the lower two spaces without radiculopathy, anterior discectomy and interbody fusion lead to more rapid relief of symptoms and a higher success rate of fusion than a similar procedure through a posterior approach. Isolated narrowing between the fourth and fifth lumbar vertebrae has been managed more satisfactorily by anterior discectomy and fusion than by posterior fusion.

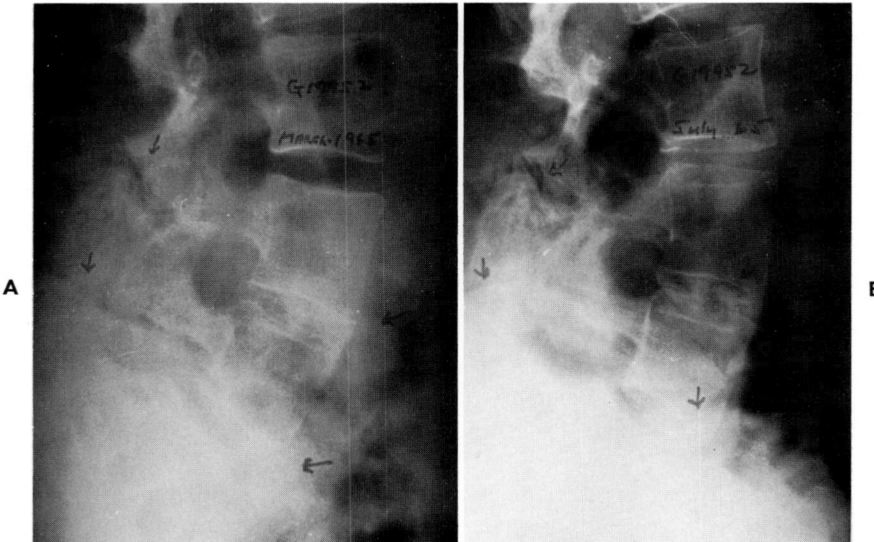

Fig. 7-2. A, After a second laminectomy for intervertebral disc disease, posterior spine fusion was attempted at two levels. Pseudarthrosis can be seen at both levels. Back and buttock pain persisted. Discogram was normal at the third lumbar interspace. **B,** Following anterior interbody spine fusion at the L4 and L5 levels, pain was considerably improved but not completely relieved. Spine fusion appeared to be solid, as seen on flexion and extension films. Posterior arrows designate two areas of pseudarthrosis; anterior arrows on right show anterior fusion.

3. Spondylolisthesis. Treated by conventional posterior arthrodesis, spondylolisthesis usually requires decompression of nerve roots at one level and inclusion of three posterior elements (with spinous processes, laminal arches, and facets). The rate of nonunion following a two-level posterior spine fusion is approximately 35%. Posterolateral fusion accompanied by decompression provides stabilization of the involved vertebral body and includes only two units rather than three, with a subsequent reduction in pseudarthrosis rate. However, nonunions do occur. The posterolateral spine fusion is preferable to the anterior interbody fusion in the young male with spondylolisthesis.

In the patient who has undergone an attempted posterior spine fusion and nerve root decompression for spondylolisthesis, pseudarthrosis at one or both levels may cause continued pain and can be demonstrated by the use of flexion and extension roentgenograms (Fig. 7-2). Anterior fusion at two levels will provide stability and will allow the posterior pseudarthrosis to heal. Pain may persist in spondylolisthesis despite a solid posterior fusion and may be caused by instability and motion of the vertebral body anteriorly. Anterior interbody fusion of the lumbosacral space will relieve pain by stabilizing the vertebral body of L5 and preventing further motion at the pars interarticularis.

We do not consider anterior interbody spine fusion to be the primary procedure of choice in spondylolisthesis. Posterior decompression and posterolateral transverse process fusion are more successful.

Anatomy and physiology of low back pain

Successful treatment of low back pain and radiculopathy requires careful analysis and pinpointing of the tissue involved in the pathological condition. The intervertebral disc, the supporting bony structures, and the supporting ligaments have differing sensory receptors. Experimental studies of Hirsch have shown myelinated nerve fibers in the annulus fibrosus. The supporting ligaments of the intervertebral space, the laminal arches, the facets, and the spinous processes all have sensory receptors. Painful stimuli originate from the synovium surrounding the facets and periosteum. Sensory nerve fibers are present in the vascular structures, in the nerves anterior to the vertebral bodies, and in the nerve chains on either side of the interspace.

The most frequent cause of back and lower extremity pain originates in the intervertebral disc. Direct stimulation of the sensory receptors located in the soft tissue between the vertebral bodies may produce pain; and bulging of the annulus may produce pressure on the highly innervated posterior longitudinal ligaments and, subsequently, on the nerve root.

Evidence of interspace pain caused by variations in pressure in the intervertebral space is seen frequently during discography. Few symptoms are caused by the injection of opaque media into a normal interspace, but injection into an abnormal disc immediately reproduces the patient's low back and leg pain. Additional evidence of interspace pain can be obtained from some patients who associate a "grating" sensation in the back with reproduction of their pain. The associated grating and reproduction of pain correlate with narrowing of the intervertebral space and diminished strength of the intervertebral disc bond. Other alterations of intervertebral disc material may result either in compression of the anterior aspect of the nerve root or in posterior irritation by thick ligamentum flavum or hypermobile laminal arch. Continued stretch of nerve roots fixed by fibrosis from previous trauma or surgical exploration may also cause pain.

The intervertebral disc changes its composition with age. Variations in age of the patient, mechanism of the injury, and area of the interspace involved may produce different clinical pictures. The disc syndrome in the adolescent has physical signs that differ considerably from those related to the adult disc syndrome. The soft bulging annulus and posterior longitudinal ligament cause different physical findings and a different myelographic picture and discogram from those produced by the firm calcified nodule or enlarging osteophyte in the older patient. Fragmentation of the nucleus pulposus and defects in the annulus fibrosus may result in hypermobility of both of these elements within the intervertebral space. The changes may produce a dull aching backache in one patient and moderate back pain and radiculopathy in another. Postural alterations and variations in muscle tone may cause changes in intervertebral pressure sufficient to cause back pain that can be relieved by change of position or recumbency.

Adequate treatment of the patient with the low back syndrome requires time and effort in order to determine the cause of pain. Not only may the intervertebral disc and the accompanying nerve root be involved. Alterations of posture, obesity, osteoporosis, systemic disease, loss of muscle tone, and emotional overlay also must be evaluated in order to arrive at an accurate diagnosis and proper treatment.

Diagnostic studies used for assessing back pain and radiculopathy

The preoperative assessment of 50 patients operated upon between February of 1964 and September of 1966 at Duke University Medical Center included a detailed history, a physical examination with emphasis on the musculoskeletal system, and multiple x-ray views of the lumbosacral spine. Details of previous operative procedures were obtained.

Electromyography provided helpful information in determining whether nerve root irritation was old or recent. Negative electromyographic findings were helpful in ruling out nerve root compression. The electromyogram was also helpful in recognizing the patient whose primary problem was that of a conversion hysteria or other emotional problem manifested by psychosomatic complaints.

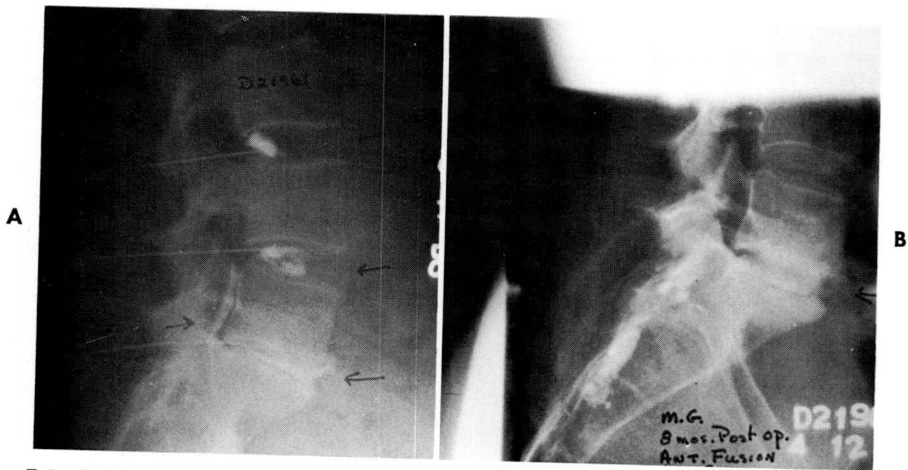

Fig. 7-3. A, Discogram done at three levels demonstrates three different patterns that are seen in intervertebral discs. The pattern at the third lumbar interspace shows the contour of a cotton ball, which is considered normal. The pattern at the fourth lumbar interspace is a bilocular one and is also considered normal. Pain was not reproduced with injection at these two levels. The lumbosacral interspace can be seen to fill completely with dye, and a leak through the posterior longitudinal ligament can also be seen. Pain was reproduced with injection of the lumbosacral joint. **B,** Pain was relieved by anterior discectomy and interbody spine fusion. No previous surgery had been done. The posterior arrow designates the dye after it leaked through the posterior longitudinal ligament.

Myelography was utilized as a diagnostic aid both in localizing the involved interspace and in ruling out nerve root compression by disc fragments. A large myelographic defect was considered a contraindication to anterior interbody fusion and an indication for posterior decompression. Defects produced by scar from multiple operative procedures made interpretation of the myelogram difficult. The defect from scarring is usually characteristic. Both the fluoroscopic interpretation of the dye pattern and multiple x-ray views are necessary for the correct interpretation of the myelogram.

Intervertebral discography was used occasionally in assessing the 50 patients in this series (Fig. 7-3, *A*). However, it proved so helpful that is it now used routinely when anterior interbody spine fusion is considered. Discography provides information not available from any other source. Routine spine films and myelogram may be negative, and the discogram may show a completely disorganized disc with reproduction of the pain on injection. The size, shape, and location of the opaque medium in the interspace can be determined by multiple rapidly exposed x-ray films. Abnormalities of intervertebral discs can be determined by configuration of the contrast material, demonstration of a leak through the posterior longitudinal ligament, and by the total volume accepted and the pressure necessary to inject the material. Reproduction of pain at the time of injection was considered a reliable index to disc abnormality.

There appeared to be close correlation between the abnormal discogram and reproduction of the patient's clinical back pain or sciatica. An abnormal interspace, which does not reproduce pain at the time of injection, is usually not the major cause of the patient's discomfort. Normal configuration of the dye pattern represents the space not involved in the pain syndrome. Correct interpretation of the discogram requires a knowledge of certain technical errors that may occur. Placement of the needle in the annulus rather than in the nucleus pulposus may produce an x-ray picture of a leak through the posterior longitudinal ligament. Most patients over the age of 50 will show a degenerative pattern with discogram, and it is in this group of patients that the reproduction of pain by the injection is of most importance. The speed and ease of discography are facilitated by use of the image intensifier to localize the needle placement prior to injection. Pain produced by injection of a diseased disc is diminished and much better tolerated by the patient if 0.5 ml. of local anesthetic is added to 1.5 ml. of the contrast material prior to injection. Reproduction of pain still occurs but lasts only sixty seconds if the anesthetic is mixed with the dye; pain may last for fifteen minutes if anesthetic is not included. Multiple rapid exposures with the cineradiograph at the time of injection are helpful in detecting subtle alterations in the interspace and in observing any leakage of the dye the moment that it occurs. We have seen no evidence that insertion of a needle into a normal intervertebral disc results in any subsequent abnormality. Discography of the lower three lumbar interspaces has provided information that was otherwise not available. Detection of changes at the interspace between the third and fourth lumbar vertebrae has necessitated inclusion of this level in the fusion at the time of initial surgery and has diminished the need for later surgery because of an unrecognized defect at this interspace. The information provided by the discogram has allowed exclusion of one lower interspace from the fusion procedure. Prior to the use of discography the lumbosacral disc was included in the procedure because of slight narrowing of the interspace or electromyographic evidence of involvement of the two nerve roots. Frequently discography has provided the only positive finding in patients with disabling chronic intermittent low back pain with or without sciatica, minimal physical findings, minimal x-ray change, and a negative myelogram.

Differential spinal anesthesia was utilized frequently as a diagnostic aid in the management of these patients. By serial injection of increasing concentrations of procaine into the subarachnoid space we have avoided surgical operations in patients with a marked psychogenic overlay or with a significant hysterical component to their illness. If the back and leg pains were partially relieved by low concentrations with a local anesthetic and completely relieved by higher concentrations, the pain was considered to be organic in origin. However, if the patient's pain was relieved by an initial injection of sterile saline and then persisted after a complete motor block, emotional factors were considered to be more likely. Once discography had been added as a routine diagnostic study, the use of differential spinal analgesia as a diagnostic test was less necessary. The positive discogram provided direct evidence of pain reproduction and intervertebral disc pathology. The differential spinal test is still valuable in assessing patients who have had multiple operative procedures, since discography cannot then be relied upon completely. A discogram done in an interspace previously operated upon may reproduce pain but is of little value otherwise.

Laminograms and lateral roentgenograms taken during flexion and extension of the spine provide information concerning the presence or absence of a pseudarthrosis. Bone density, trabecular pattern, and the height of the interspace are determined by detailed x-ray studies. Information obtained during the first six months after surgery is not so accurate as that obtained during the second six-month postoperative period.

Classification of 50 patients who underwent anterior interbody spine fusion

The 50 patients operated upon demonstrated several major patterns. Most of these patients had had previous surgery for management of intervertebral disc disease and had persistent pain. The different syndromes were classified into the following nine groups:

Group 1. Patients in this group complained of chronic recurrent low back pain and minimal unilateral sciatica. Examination usually showed a positive sciatic stretch test, a positive electromyogram, x-ray evidence of a narrow interspace with increased subchondral bone density, a negative myelogram, and a positive discogram at one or two of the three spaces tested. No previous surgery had been done.

Surgery in this group consisted of a retroperitoneal approach to the involved interspaces, removal of the intervertebral disc, and an anterior interbody spine fusion using rectangular autologous iliac bone grafts. The patients were mobilized rapidly and sitting was allowed at five days and walking allowed at seven days.

Group 2. Patients in this group had essentially the same clinical picture as those in Group 1; but two interspaces were involved on x-ray study, an electromyogram was positive for one root, and a discogram was positive at two interspaces. (See Fig. 7-4, *A*.) Both interspaces were included in the anterior fusion.

Group 3. These patients had undergone one or more posterior laminectomies

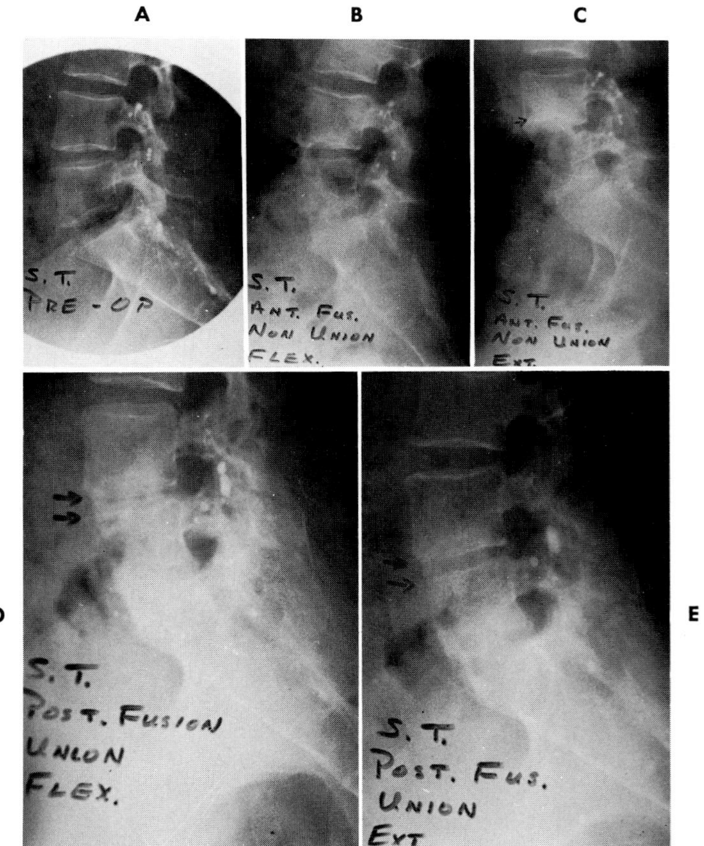

Fig. 7-4. A, Laminectomy had been performed twice on this patient at the L4 and L5 levels. Back pain and leg pain were both prominent in her symptoms, and discogram was abnormal at both the L4 and L5 levels. Myelogram showed a defect thought to be due to scar tissue. **B** and **C,** Following anterior interbody spine fusion, the patient's symptoms improved for approximately three months but then the back pain recurred. Flexion and extension films at this time showed motion between the bodies of L4 and L5. **D** and **E,** Following posterolateral fusion, the interbody spine fusion between L4 and L5 solidified and her back pain was relieved. The posterior spine fusion also appeared solid on flexion and extension.

for disc removal and had persistent low back pain with minimal sciatica. Electromyogram was usually positive and the myelogram showed no defect. Discogram was abnormal at the lower interspace and normal at the third and fourth lumbar interspaces. One level was included in the anterior interbody fusion. (See Fig. 7-5, *B*.) Excessive instability of the vertebral bodies and small persistent defects in the posterior longitudinal ligament were frequently observed at the time of surgery. No effort was made to expose the nerve roots from the anterior approach.

Group 4. These patients had undergone one or more previous laminectomies and simultaneous attempts at posterior spine fusion. Pseudarthrosis developed and persistent back pain without leg pain was present. The electromyogram usually showed old changes, straight leg raising tests were painful, myelography showed no large defect, and the differential spinal test indicated organic pain. (See Fig. 7-6.) Discography was done at the third lumbar interspace only. If the discogram appeared normal, then anterior fusion of the two lower levels was carried out. Residual disc material appeared degenerated.

Group 5. These patients showed essentially the same picture as those listed in Group 4 but gave a history of a febrile course after their previous surgery. Discography and myelography were not done in this group because of the prior infection. Relief of back pain and severe radiculopathy after anterior interbody fusion occurred within a few days. Cultures of interspace were negative.

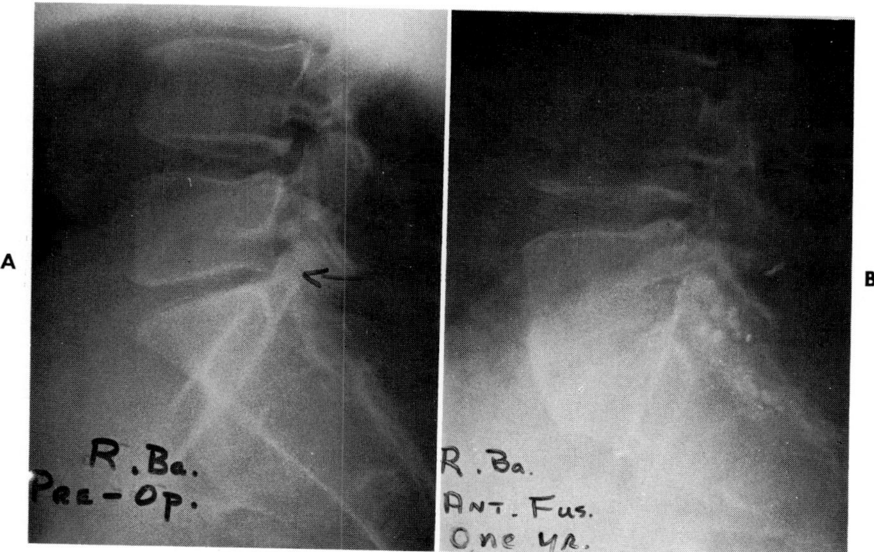

Fig. 7-5. A, Classic disc syndrome with low back pain, sciatica, positive straight leg raising, and a positive myelogram was confirmed by the narrowed appearance of the lumbosacral joint on the plain film. Following laminectomy, leg pain was relieved but back pain continued. **B,** The silver clip marking the level of the laminectomy is visible in the posterior elements. Anterior interbody spine fusion has been done and is solid twelve months after the surgery. Back pain was relieved, and the result was graded as excellent.

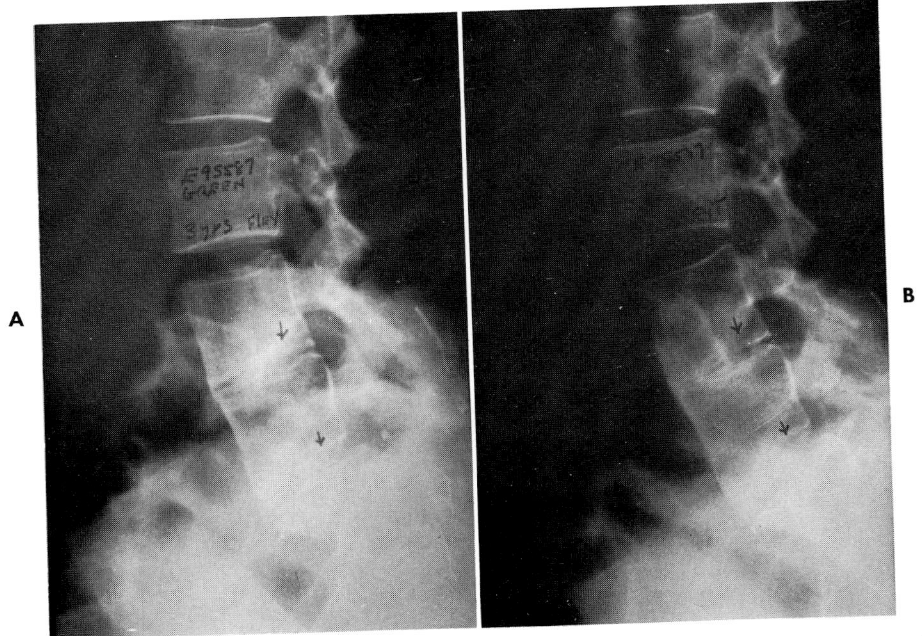

Fig. 7-6. Two previous laminectomies had been supplemented by an attempted posterior fusion. The braided wire used to stabilize the posterior elements can be seen. Pseudarthrosis resulted in continued back pain. Myelogram showed no significant defect, and discogram at the third lumbar interspace was normal. Following anterior interbody spine fusion at the L4 and L5 levels, back pain and leg pain were relieved. **A,** Flexion. **B,** Extension.

Group 6. This group of patients had had several posterior laminectomies with exploration of the lower two or three interspaces. Nerve root fibrosis and radiculopathy persisted. Bony instability and degenerative changes in the facet articulations and the vertebral bodies were usually seen on x-ray. (See Fig. 7-7.) The pars interarticularis frequently showed surgical defects and often the laminal arches had been removed. Treatment consisted of anterior removal of the remaining disc material, autologous bone grafting at two or three interspaces, and postoperative limitation of activity for several weeks. At six months, stress roentgenograms were taken. If pseudarthrosis was apparent at that time, then the spine was supplemented with a posterolateral fusion.

Group 7. These patients had undergone initial posterior laminectomy, nerve root decompression, and an attempt at posterior spine fusion. Anterior discectomy and interbody fusions were carried out at the lower two levels. Fusion was successful at one level but pseudarthrosis developed at the other, most frequently the upper level, and persistent pain was correlated with the nonunion. (See Fig. 7-4, *B* to *E*.) They were treated either by an attempt at refusion anteriorly or by posterolateral fusion.

Group 8. Patients in this group had undergone posterior laminectomy and

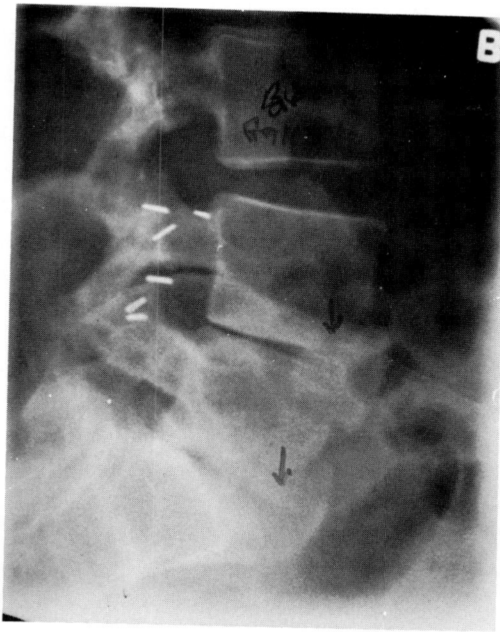

Fig. 7-7. Several previous laminectomies had been performed, and much bone had been removed from the posterior elements. Severe back and buttock pain persisted. After anterior disc excision and interbody spine fusion at two spaces, a solid bony union resulted. The functional result was rated as good at one year after the spine fusion.

nerve root decompression, attempts at posterior spine fusion, and other pain-relieving operations such as rhizotomy and cordotomy. The back pain was persistent and radiculopathy involved both thighs. Additional posterior surgery has been found to give little relief to this particular group of patients. Anterior discectomy and arthrodesis of the vertebral bodies will diminish low back pain, lessen radiculopathy, improve overall mobility of the spine, and diminish discomfort sufficiently to warrant this additional surgery.

Group 9. Spondylolisthesis must be considered separately from the degenerative disc problems. The defect in the pars interarticularis allows hypermobility of the vertebral body anteriorly, and nerve root compression occurs most often without myelographic defect. Treatment recommended will depend to some extent upon the age and sex of the patient, the presence of nerve root compression, and previous treatment. In general, anterior interbody spine fusion is not recommended as primary surgical treatment for spondylolisthesis. We have found several different patterns within the classification of spondylolisthesis:

Group 9-A. In this group are included males or females 14 to 30 years of age. A neural arch defect is demonstrable by x-ray, and the primary complaints are of back pain with thigh radiation which is aggravated by hyperextension of the lumbar spine. Treatment of this group of patients consists of surgical removal of the lateral portion of the posterior laminal arch, in order to decompress the nerve root in the area of the pars interarticularis defect, followed by posterolateral fusion of the transverse processes of the hypermobile vertebra to the transverse processes of the vertebra below. The fusion includes the facets, spinous processes, and remainder of the laminal arch. The young female in this age group may also be managed by a single-space anterior interbody fusion. Two young women in our series were treated in this way and obtained adequate relief of their complaints.

Group 9-B. Patients in this group had a grade I spondylolisthesis with subjective complaints of back pain but in addition findings of nerve root compression. The electromyogram usually showed changes in the L5 root. The myelogram was characteristically within normal limits. Discogram above the point of slippage was negative. Treatment consisted of decompression of the involved nerve root and arthrodesis of the transverse process of the fifth lumbar vertebra to the sacrum with inclusion of the posterior elements. In the event of failure of the posterior fusion, anterior interbody fusion was carried out at the lumbosacral joint in third- or fourth-decade patients.

Two patients in this group had been treated primarily by an anterior fusion of a single interspace with relief of back pain and leg pain for approximately three months. However, the back, buttock, and thigh pain recurred and local tenderness over the loose posterior element of the fifth lumbar vertebra was found on palpation. Posterior decompression and posterolateral fusion afforded complete relief of residual complaints.

Group 9-C. Patients in this group had spondylolisthesis that had been managed by posterior nerve root decompression at a single space and an attempt at posterior arthrodesis of the last two lumbar vertebrae to the sacrum. Pseudarthrosis had developed at one or more interspaces. These patients were treated successfully by anterior fusion of vertebral bodies with relief of pain and radiculopathy.

Group 9-D. One 22-year-old male with a grade I spondylolisthesis had been treated initially by anterior discectomy and interbody fusion of the lumbosacral joint. The pain was improved but he continued to have discomfort with extension. Stress x-ray studies showed a pseudarthrosis in the anterior fusion. Pain was relieved by posterior decompression and posterolateral transverse process fusion.

Group 9-E. Two of our patients with grade II spondylolisthesis had been treated by decompression of nerve roots and posterior fusion. Roentgenograms showed what appeared to be solid posterior fusion. At the time of anterior exploration continued motion of the displaced vertebra through the pars interarticularis and the intact intervertebral disc bond was demonstrated. Unless the transverse process or the pars interarticularis is included in the posterior fusion, the vertebral body may continue to be hypermobile in spondylolisthesis and cause pain.

Group 9-F. Anterior spine fusion should not be attempted in patients with greater than a grade II displacement. We attempted an anterior interbody spine fusion in one of our patients with grade III spondylolisthesis. Inadequate bone contact was obtained. There was much technical difficulty in inserting the graft. Solid union resulted; however, due to the technical difficulties, we recommend that this particular problem be managed initially by posterolateral spine fusion.

Surgical technique

A nasogastric tube is inserted after the patient is asleep to prevent abdominal distention. Anesthesia is induced by intravenous anesthetic followed by halothane that is supplemented with muscle relaxants. The Trendelenburg position displaces the abdominal contents proximally and reduces venous stasis in the lower extremities. The abdomen and iliac crest are prepared with soap, water and Betadine and the skin is covered with transparent adhesive dressing. To simplify evaluation of postoperative relief from pain the iliac bone graft is usually taken from the side opposite the radicular pain. The partial thickness graft is removed prior to exposure of the anterior lumbar spine in order to reduce operative time and blood loss. The abdominal approach and mobilization of the iliac vessels are done by a general surgeon.

The retroperitoneal approach to the vertebral bodies described by Harmon[7] has been used in 40 of the 50 patients reviewed. A transperitoneal approach is made when the patient has had multiple previous abdominal procedures. A left paramedian incision is made through the skin and superficial fascia, the anterior rectus sheath is opened, and the muscle is retracted laterally. The retroperitoneal space is entered inferiorly at the linea semilunaris, and the peritoneum is separated by blunt dissection from the undersurface of the posterior rectus sheath. Small peritoneal tears are repaired immediately. The rectus sheath is incised from the hemilunar notch to its superior border. The psoas muscle is identified, the iliac artery and vein are identified on the left side, and the left ureter is located. In exposure of the lower two lumbar spaces the ureter is left in its peritoneal bed and reflected to the right. If more than three interspaces are to be exposed, the ureter is retracted to the left side.

The sacral promontory is identified by palpation. The sympathetic nerves coursing over the sacral promontory are not disturbed, and the major sympathetic chains on either side of the lumbar vertebrae are carefully dissected and retracted laterally. Saline injection into the prevertebral fascia over the lumbar vertebrae makes the dissection of the sympathetic nerves easier.

The lumbosacral interspace is exposed by retracting the left iliac artery and vein to the left and the right iliac artery and vein to the right. Spiked retractors, driven into the body of the lumbar vertebrae, are helpful in maintaining exposure.

In exposure of the fourth lumbar interspace the left artery and vein and ureter are displaced to the right side of the spine and held in place by spiked retractors.

The anterior longitudinal ligament is elevated from the annulus as a flap with the base attached to the left. This flap when tagged with sutures affords additional retraction for the vessels. Hyperextension of the operating table brings the spine closer to the surface of the wound and affords better exposure of the interspace. The intervertebral disc and remainder of the annulus are separated from the cartilaginous plates[6] of the vertebrae with a thin osteotome. Once detached from the vertebral body above and below, the disc can be removed easily with a large pituitary rongeur and large curets. The space is cleaned out thoroughly, back to the posterior longitudinal ligament, before any bone is removed. In this way bleeding is minimal and dissection can be done under direct vision. Cartilage surfaces are removed from the vertebral bodies with an osteotome until bleeding bone is encountered. Vigorous bleeding may occur from the posterior aspect of the vertebral bodies and can be controlled by small amounts of bone wax.

When the soft tissue and cartilage have been removed from the interspace, a shallow notch is cut from the opposing surfaces of the vertebral body above and below. The dimensions of the notch are measured carefully with a caliper and a graft is cut from the iliac bone graft to fit tightly into this notch. The graft is made slightly larger than the notch so that firm impaction can be obtained. The lateral recesses of the intervertebral space are then packed with vertical struts of bone graft placed with the cortex outward around the periphery of the interspace. Any remaining defects are packed with cancellous bone.

Removal of the bone graft prior to carrying out the abdominal approach saves time, as the exposure of the anterior surface of the vertebral body is not lost once it is obtained. The patient should not be hyperextended until exposure of an anterior vertebral body is obtained because hyperextension places more tension upon the blood vessels and makes them more difficult to mobilize.

The electrocautery is valuable in obtaining hemostasis and can be used for incisions or dissections. Special care must be taken not to coagulate the fine sympathetic fibers coursing over the anterior aspect of the lumbosacral joint and the sacrum. The anterior surface of the first sacral segment must not be cauterized, and soft tissue should be stripped bluntly from the anterior surface of the fourth and fifth lumbar vertebrae before the cautery is used in these areas.

Following completion of the anterior fusion all layers are closed with absorbable suture and when necessary deep stay sutures have been left in place for ten to fourteen days. Estimated blood loss is replaced during the operative procedure. Frequently an additional transfusion is necessary during the first twenty-four hours after operation.

Postoperative management

A low negative pressure is connected to the nasogastric tube until active peristalsis occurs, usually at thirty-six hours. The patient is turned frequently and is given intermittent positive pressure breathing with bronchodilaters and wetting agents. The patients are most comfortable with the hips and knees in slight flexion, and the lateral recumbent position is allowed as soon as the patient desires.

In order to reduce the likelihood of deep thrombophlebitis, patients are given 500 ml. of hypertonic high-molecular dextran intravenously every other day until they are ambulatory. The decreased sludging produced by dextran appears to have been very effective in reducing the incidence of thrombophlebitis in these postoperative patients.

In order to preserve abdominal tone unilateral straight leg raising is begun on the third postoperative day and is continued indefinitely. A low back corset allows the patient to sit and walk more comfortably by the fifth postoperative day. Patients are advised to increase their activities gradually to the limit of tolerance but are not allowed to drive an automobile for three months. Daily walking and isometric abdominal and gluteal exercises are encouraged.

As a baseline, postoperative lateral x-ray study of the lumbosacral area is made. Approximately three months after surgery repeat lateral flexion and extension x-ray films are made with the patient standing. Roentgenograms are repeated at six and twelve months postoperatively. Laminograms are made only when pseudarthrosis is suspected. The average length of time required for solid interbody spine fusion with trabeculations across the interspace has been twelve months.

Early or immediate complications

Peritoneal tears. Peritoneal tears were frequent with the retroperitoneal approach. Immediate repair was carried out and no complications have been noted.

Venous bleeding. Eight patients had significant venous bleeding, requiring more than the usual blood replacement. This complication occurred more often in the early patients than in recent ones. Recognition of the variations of the branches of the iliac vein and ligation of large veins prior to dividing have diminished this kind of bleeding. Use of the cautery should be avoided close to the major vein and should not be relied upon for management of large branches.

Arterial bleeding. Five patients showed rapid arterial bleeding of sufficient degree to require more than the usual blood replacement. Control was obtained easily. No patients have developed false or true aneurysms or had significant delayed hemorrhage.

Excessive osseous bleeding. This complication occurred in 12 patients and was found to be most frequent when bone was resected in the posterior aspect of the vertebral body. Bleeding is more profuse in patients with osteoporosis. Small amounts of bone wax have been helpful in controlling the bleeding and no interference with fusion has been noted.

Sympathetic nerve interruption. Two patients showed clinical evidence of sympathectomy on the left side. One patient after a year still showed an increase in skin temperature on the left side as compared to the right. A second patient had a transient sympathectomy effect for several weeks, which then subsided.

Retrograde ejaculation. A careful sexual history was obtained from each male who underwent anterior interbody spine fusion. Transient impotence has been noted in 3 patients. Retrograde ejaculation was reported by 2 patients. These complications occurred early in the series of patients operated upon by either transperitoneal or retroperitoneal approach. During the past two years this complication has been prevented by careful avoidance of the sympathetic chain. Soft tissues over the sacral promontory are left intact and the cautery is not used in this area. The retroperitoneal approach allows an easier dissection of the lumbar and sacral sympathetics than does the transperitoneal approach.

Incisional hernia. One patient developed a postoperative hematoma and, four months after his surgery, an incisional hernia. Two efforts at repair were necessary before adequate obliteration of the fascial defect was obtained.

Delayed retroperitoneal hemorrhage. This complication occurred in 2 patients who showed evidence of continued blood loss for several hours after the operative procedure was completed. Adequate blood replacement and supportive measures were sufficient to restore blood volume without exploration of the fusion site.

Wound dehiscence. One patient developed a large retroperitoneal hematoma with a spontaneous opening of the incision on the sixth postoperative day. He was taken immediately to the operating room where the wound was explored and a hematoma estimated at 700 ml. of blood was removed. The wound was irrigated and closed and healed primarily.

Thrombophlebitis. Two patients developed deep thrombophlebitis that required anticoagulant therapy. The postoperative use of intravenous dextran was begun three years ago, and there have been no recognizable instances of thrombophlebitis since that time. Early active motion and early ambulation are also encouraged, to help prevent thrombophlebitis.

Lateral femoral cutaneous nerve paresthesias. A complication that occurred in 5 patients in this group was characterized by hyperesthesia for several weeks or hyperesthesia for several months after surgery. Avoidance of the anterior superior iliac spine at the time of removal of the bone graft has been successful in eliminating this complication.

Pseudarthrosis. Six patients developed symptomatic pseudarthrosis that produced back pain and leg pain. Motion on flexion and extension roentgenograms confirmed the diagnosis. When failure of fusion occurred in patients who had undergone a two-space fusion, the pseudarthrosis always involved the upper level. One patient developed a pseudarthrosis at the lumbosacral interspace and another patient developed pseudarthrosis at both the upper and the lower level. Of the 6 patients, 4 were operated on again, after a six- to twelve-month waiting period. Three of these had posterior spine fusions, at which time manipulation of the spinous processes showed motion. In these patients, posterolateral fusions were done using autologous bone grafting. Fusion occurred rapidly and pain was eliminated within three months. One patient was reoperated upon anteriorly, since only one interspace was involved and posterior surgery had been done previously. The remaining 2 patients had mild discomfort thought to be related to the pseudarthrosis. However, in these the pain was considered insufficient to warrant additional surgery.

Intervertebral disc degeneration. Four patients developed symptoms at the interspace above a solid fusion at the lower two vertebrae. These patients had good relief of back pain and leg pain for approximately six months after the fusion but then gradually had recurrence of back pain. Conservative treatment did not control their symptoms. At the time of exploration the nerve roots were involved by a bulging intervertebral disc. Nerve root decompression and posterolateral fusion afforded relief in all instances. None of these patients had had discography prior to the initial anterior fusion. Since we have begun to use discography more routinely, involvement of the third interspace has been recognized and treated at the time of the initial fusion.

Evaluation of functional results

Results of surgery were classified as based on an assessment of the degree of relief of back or lower extremity pain, which was rated as excellent, good, fair, slight or none, or worse. The rating of "return to gainful occupation" depended on return to original work, light work, or some other job and on the overall subjective and objective current condition of the patient.

A preliminary assessment of these 50 patients includes a one-year follow-up in 6 of them and two or more years' follow-up in the other 44 patients. The classification of results is shown below:

Excellent	15
Good	13
Fair	16
Poor	4
Same	2

The 2 patients who showed no improvement had multiple physical problems as well as emotional difficulties. Psychiatric treatment afforded some improvement in conjunction with surgical treatment, but the somatic complaints persisted. Both of these patients showed solid posterior fusion and physical complaints were not diminished by anterior disc excision and interbody fusion.

Conclusions

The retrospective study of these 50 patients has pointed out guidelines to aid in the diagnosis and to determine the selection of treatment in future patients.

1. A careful preliminary assessment of the patient, using all techniques available, is necessary. Intervertebral discography is valuable and frequently an essential diagnostic study in the preoperative evaluation of the patient.

2. Bony union was demonstrated by x-ray only twelve months after interbody spine fusion.

3. The presence of an anterior or posterior pseudarthrosis results in pain. A painful pseudarthrosis is an indication for additional surgery.

4. The treatment of choice for the patient with spondylolisthesis is posterior decompression and posterolateral spine fusion. If pain persists then, anterior interbody spine fusion can be used as a secondary procedure.

Summary

Follow-up study of the first 50 patients treated at Duke University Medical Center by anterior disc excision and anterior interbody spine fusion with autologous bone suggests that the procedure is useful in the management of patients with mechanical low back pain with or without radiculopathy. Anterior spine fusion was found most useful in the treatment of patients who had had previous posterior low back surgery without relief of radiculopathy or who had developed a pseudarthrosis following an attempt at spine fusion. Anterior discectomy and interbody fusion provide a physiological method of removing abnormal disc material and, at the same time, producing stability of the spine. The anterior approach does not supplant the posterior approach to the intervertebral disc, but it does supplement currently accepted methods of managing low back pain and radiculopathy. Anterior spine fusion affords a successful method for treatment of the patient who continues to have back pain after hemilaminectomy. The use of discography, followed by anterior spine fusion when indicated, is an effective procedure for the patient with intractable low back pain who is not a candidate for hemilaminectomy.

References

1. Burns, B. H.: An operation for spondylolisthesis, Lancet **1:**1233, 1933.
2. Capener, N.: Spondylolisthesis, Brit. J. Surg. **19:**374, 1932.
3. Fowler, S. B.: Personal communication, 1967.
4. Freebody, D.: Motion picture shown at Vancouver meeting of the American Orthopaedic Association, 1965.
5. Friberg, S.: Studies on spondylolisthesis, Acta Chir. Scand. **82** (supp. 55):1, 1939.
6. Goldner, M. Z.: Personal communication, 1964.
7. Harmon, P.: Results from treatment of sciatica due to lumbar disc protrusion, Amer. J. Surg. **80:**829, 1950.
8. Harmon, P.: Anterior extraperitoneal disc excision and vertebral body fusion, Clin. Orthop. **18:**169, 1961.
9. Harmon, P.: Anterior disc excision and fusion of the lumbar vertebral bodies, J. Int. Coll. Surg. **40:**572, 1963.
10. Hirsch, C.: An attempt to diagnose the level of a disc lesion clinically by disc puncture, Acta Orthop. Scand. **18:**132, 1949.
11. Hodgson, A. R., and Stock, F. E.: Anterior spine fusion for treatment of tuberculosis of the spine, J. Bone Joint Surg. **42-A:**295, 1960.
12. Hult, L.: Retroperitoneal disc fenestration in low-back pain and sciatica, Acta Orthop. Scand. **20:**342, 1951.
13. Humphries, A. W., and Hawk, W. A.: Anterior fusion of lumbar spine using an internal fixation device, J. Bone Joint Surg. **41-A:**371, 1959.
14. Ingebrigtsen, R.: Indications for anterior transperitoneal fusion in the treatment of spondylolisthesis, Acta Chir. Scand. **105:**172, 1953.
15. Jenkins, J. A.: Spondylolisthesis, Brit. J. Surg. **24:**80, 1936.
16. Laurent, L. E.: Spondylolisthesis, Acta Orthop. Scand., supp. 35, 1958.
17. Ley, E. B., and Thurston, W. D.: Retroperitoneal approach to lumbar disc, Rocky Mountain Med. J. **51:**121, 1954.
18. McCollum, D. E., and Stephen, C. R.: The use of graduated spinal anesthesia in the differential diagnosis of pain of the back and lower extremities, Southern Med. J. **57:**410, 1964.
19. Mercer, W.: Spondylolisthesis, Edinburgh Med. J. **43:**545, 1936.

19a. Mixter, W. J., and Barr, J. S.: Rupture of the intervertebral disc with involvement of the spinal canal, New Eng. J. Med. **211**:210, 1934.
20. Sacks, S.: Intervertebral disc excision and lumbar spine fusion by a transperitoneal approach, J. Bone Joint Surg. **43-B**:401, 1961.
21. Sacks, S.: Experiences with anterior transperitoneal lumbar spine fusions in 200 patients, in Ninth SICOT Congress: abstracts of papers, 1963, pp. 8-14.
22. Shanewise, R. P.: Anterior intervertebral lumbar spine fusions, Western J. Surg. **71**:212, 1963.
23. Speed, K.: Spondylolisthesis; treatment by anterior bone graft, Arch. Surg. **37**:175, 1938.
24. Stein, R. O.: Anterior spine fusion, Bull. Hosp. Joint Dis. **13**:322, 1952.
25. Stewart, D. Y.: The anterior disk excision and interbody fusion approach to the problem of degenerative disk disease of the lower lumbar spinal segments, New York J. Med. **61**:3252, 1961.

8. The multiply operated back

Mark B. Coventry, M.D.
Richard N. Stauffer, M.D.

The subtitle of this discussion might be "The Salvage of the Back Cripple." Spinal fusion was introduced as a method of treating certain conditions, especially in the low back, by Hibbs[9] and by Albee,[2] in the early 1900's. In 1934, Mixter and Barr[15] introduced laminectomy for disc protrusion. Laminectomy and spinal fusion alone or in combination are now being used extensively for patients with lumbar disc disease. It is inevitable, of course, that these procedures are not always successful, and one can postulate reasons for this. The problem obviously starts with the proper selection of the patient for the operation. Then one must consider the technical aspects of both disc and spinal fusion operations.

We shall discuss two studies done at the Mayo Clinic. We reviewed in detail 35 patients who had been operated on by one of us (M.B.C.) for pseudarthrosis of the lumbar part of the spine between 1946 and 1963. These findings will be presented later. Between January 1963 (when our study ended) and July 1966, Hoover[10] reviewed another 33 patients, in whom lateral fusion alone was done as a salvage procedure after spinal fusion or laminectomy or both. Over half of these had undergone attempts at fusion; the rest had had laminectomy alone. He reviewed another 34 patients in whom anterior lumbar fusion was done as a salvage operation after an unsuccessful spinal operation, similarly with or without attempt at fusion. It is on the experience gained in these selected patients that we will base the rest of this discussion.

Thus, as orthopaedists, we are confronted with the patient who consults us because of continued pain after disc removal, attempted lumbar fusion, or both. The pain may be in the back, in the sciatic distribution, or, as is most common, in both.

Evaluation of the patient who has had multiple back operations

Perhaps in no other problem in orthopaedics is it so important to consider the patient as a whole. The separation of organic from psychological complaints is indeed difficult. In our program for the patient who has had an unsuccessful back operation, we start with orthopaedic and medical evaluations and follow these with a neurological examination and a psychiatric evaluation. We then try immobilization in a brace or a cast or in bed. If there is no strong contraindication and if the pain is relieved in part by immobilization, then refusion is considered. Every effort must be made to find out why the original fusion was done. The reasons include (1) degenerated disc syndrome; (2) spondylolysis; (3) protruded intervertebral disc with localized degenerative changes, spondylolysis, or congenital changes; (4) long-standing, static, low back pain.

Proper roentgenograms are essential for evaluation of the solidity of the fusion. While the inadequacy of most methods is recognized, in fusions more than a year old one can usually see an area of pseudarthrosis if it exists. Between six and twelve months after the time of fusion, or thereafter, bending films are important; we have found the flexion-extension films to be superior to the lateral bending films because some rotation will often obscure accurate superimposition in the latter. Three-quarter views are sometimes of value.

The next step is the neurological examination. Here too, one must differentiate between the neurological findings that were present before the initial operation and the changes subsequent to it.

Psychiatric evaluation is a necessity in any patient who has undergone multiple operations. Not only does it sometimes uncover certain latent and obscure emotional problems but it also helps considerably in the future care of the patient. If we once take on the surgical treatment of such a patient, we will be responsible for many months of future care in many ways, including the ultimate insurance and industrial commission problems and the eventual rehabilitation of the patient. A good psychological background is invaluable. We precede our psychiatric consultation with a Minnesota Multiphasic Personality Inventory (MMPI), and then usually a single interview with a psychiatrist is sufficient for at least establishing a background. Additional interviews can be arranged if problems arise that need further clarification.

If an attempt at refusion is being considered seriously, the patient is then given a trial period of immobilization in a brace (such as that developed by Norton and Brown[16]), a cast, or a proper corset or even bed rest may be used. Arbitrarily, we use a three-month period of observation on this "rest" regimen. The patient then returns for further evaluation. If no strong contraindication has turned up and if the pain is relieved at least in part by the immobilization, then we are usually committed to an attempt at refusion.

If the neurosurgeon and orthopaedist work together on disc problems, the neurosurgeon is asked to see the patient. If the orthopaedist does his own disc surgery, he must be prepared at this time to make a decision as to whether or not nerve roots should be explored. This usually means another myelogram, in spite of the notorious indefiniteness of myelography after disc surgery. If sciatic pain is a prominent factor, one is usually compelled to perform myelography. If there is no root pain, it usually is not done.

In summary, then, the decision to reoperate on the patient is based on the appropriate answers to these questions: (1) Was the initial fusion truly indicated? (2) Is there reasonable certainty of pseudarthrosis? (3) Is the patient's pain relieved by rest (bed or brace)? and (4) Is the patient free of serious psychoneurotic traits?

Operation

Until 1963, at this institution most refusions were done posteriorly by some modification of the Hibbs-Albee technique. Since 1963, refusions have also been done posterolaterally, although on occasion the anterior approach has been used and, even more rarely, circumferential fusion has been attempted with both posterolateral and anterior approaches. There seems little doubt from our experience that the incidence of successful fusion is higher now that we are using the posterolateral approach rather than the posterior fusion only.

Some of the results reported after posterior fusion are shown in Table 8-1; these data relate to primary fusion operations, not those for refusion. Fusion has been reported to occur in 50% to 100% of the patients. At the Mayo Clinic, for one-level lumbar fusion the incidence of success is about 95% and for two-level fusion, about 85%. Perhaps this is chiefly of historical importance now because, although we continue to use a posterior graft for most one-level fusions, the posterolateral technique for two-level fusions is almost routine at the present.

Reoperation involves a few problems not present during the primary operation, not the least of which is extensive scarring with prolongation of the surgical time and increased blood loss.

In our review of attempted repair of pseudarthrosis between 1946 and 1963, there were 35 patients (21 women and 14 men) with a mean age of 41.4 years. These 35 patients had had a total of forty-nine previous attempts at fusion before they consulted us. In 3 of the women, two attempts at fusion were done at this

Table 8-1. Reported results after posterior lumbar fusion

				% of fusion	
	Year	*Cases (no.)*	*Method*	*L4-S1*	*L5-S1*
Cleveland and co-workers[5]	1948	357	"Clothespin" graft	83	96
King[13]	1944	44	Transarticular screw and Hibbs	90.9	
Smith[20]	1948	?	Transarticular screw and Hibbs	50	92
Boucher[4]	1959	175	Transarticular screw and Hibbs	86	100
McElvenny[14]	1963	?	Hibbs	70	95
Howorth[11]	1964	174	Transarticular screw and Hibbs	80	97

institution; another woman underwent four operations. Thus, our initial attempt at posterior fusion was unsuccessful in 4 of these 35 patients.

These patients were all observed for a minimum of three years after their last operation. A good result was absence of all or almost all of the pain. A fair result was represented by sufficient decrease in pain so that the patient was able to work. A poor result was one in which the pain was not relieved and the patient could not work. The results in these 35 patients are shown in Table 8-2. Back pain was relieved in 21 of 35 patients and leg pain, in 11 of 28. Note also that the results in men were considerably better than those in women. Overall, 60% of the patients had relief of back pain and 40% had relief of leg pain.

Posterolateral fusion

Since 1963, when this study was completed, we have been using posterolateral fusion for most pseudarthrosis repairs involving more than one level. Hoover's[10] study shows that 33 posterolateral fusions were used for salvage operation after fusion or laminectomy or both had been unsuccessful, and that fusion was achieved in 94% (this is the percentage of fusion and not the percentage of relief of symptoms). Symptomatic relief has not yet been evaluated in this group.

We use the posterolateral fusion in most pseudarthroses at this time. Seldom have the transverse processes, the facets, and the pars interarticularis portions of the laminae been involved by previous surgical procedures. Thus the bone of the bed for the graft is normal. If it is true that the healing of bone can be considered to be a contest between the osteogenic process and the mechanical strain imposed on it, then the lack of stress on the bone grafts placed laterally, as compared with those placed only posteriorly, may be one of the reasons why these grafts are more successful. The quantity of bone against which the graft is placed, its blood supply, and the fact that one can put a larger mass of grafts laterally may also contribute to success. The lateral approach was first described by Watkins[23] in 1953 but he exposed these areas laterally rather than from the midline. Truchly and Thompson[22] reported on their use of a modified Watkins approach in 43 patients. They used multiple, thin strips of bone rather than a single large block between the transverse processes. Of their patients, 93% achieved fusion, and 24 patients were treated for postoperative pseudarthrosis; 40 of the 43 grafts involved multiple interspaces. Adkins[1] extended the dorsal midline approach laterally and

Table 8-2. Results of fusion in 35 patients

	Good	*Fair*	*Poor*
Back pain	21	8	6
Leg pain*	11	9	8
Women (total, 21)	11	7	3
Men (total, 14)	10	1	3

*Seven patients with back pain had no leg pain.

utilized more or less the standard approach by simply stretching it. He placed tibial grafts as blocks between the transverse processes. Kelly[12] modified this by placing fibular bone between the transverse processes.

In our operation for posterolateral fusion, the region is approached through a midline incision in the standard fashion, but the incision is extended at least one level above so that less retraction force is necessary. More is involved than simply laying iliac bone onto transverse processes. Attention must be paid to the careful preparation of the lateral gutter, which extends from the tip of the transverse process to its base and then from the superior facet along the pars interarticularis to the inferior facet. If the facet is included in the fusion, the posterior half of the facet is removed and additionally blocked with bone. The inferior facet of the vertebra above the fusion must be left intact so that one does not interfere with the articulation of the vertebrae at this level. Bleeding is carefully controlled, and the segmental artery always present near the pars interarticularis is carefully observed and cauterized. The bone is decorticated and the iliac strips, removed through the same incision or through a separate one, are placed on the transverse process and extended medially to and including the base of the lamina and the facets. We frequently do not carry decortication and grafting further toward the midline because the additional posterior fusion on the laminae and spinous processes serves no special purpose. Furthermore, this area has been frequently involved in multiple laminectomies. Lateral fusion extends the operating time and more blood will be lost, but we have found that this is a small price to pay for the improved incidence in fusion.

Anterior fusion

A few words should be said about the use of anterior lumbar fusion. For a while this was thought to be the answer to our problems, but currently we use it less frequently and find the indication for it very limited. Least success with anterior fusion is obtained in the patient with no facets or posterior arches remaining after extensive neurological surgery. Anterior fusion removes the anterior annulus, which is its strongest part, and there is very little structural support of the spinal column if anterior grafting is done under these circumstances. Thus, we prefer not to do anterior fusion unless there seems to be no other alternative. At present, most backs can be salvaged with posterolateral fusion. Hoover's[10] data show that, among 34 patients treated by anterior fusion as a salvage procedure, fusion was achieved in only 68%. Glowing reports regarding anterior fusion have appeared in the literature[3, 6-8, 17-19, 21, 24] but critical review of the roentgenograms shows instances in which, at least according to our criteria, fusion is not truly solid. Also, we have had the disappointing experience of finding that a result that was good after one year may not be good after two years because some of these grafts remain avascular and crumble with the passage of time.

The very rare patient who has almost no neural arch posteriorly and who might best be treated by fusion may need circular (that is, lateral and anterior)

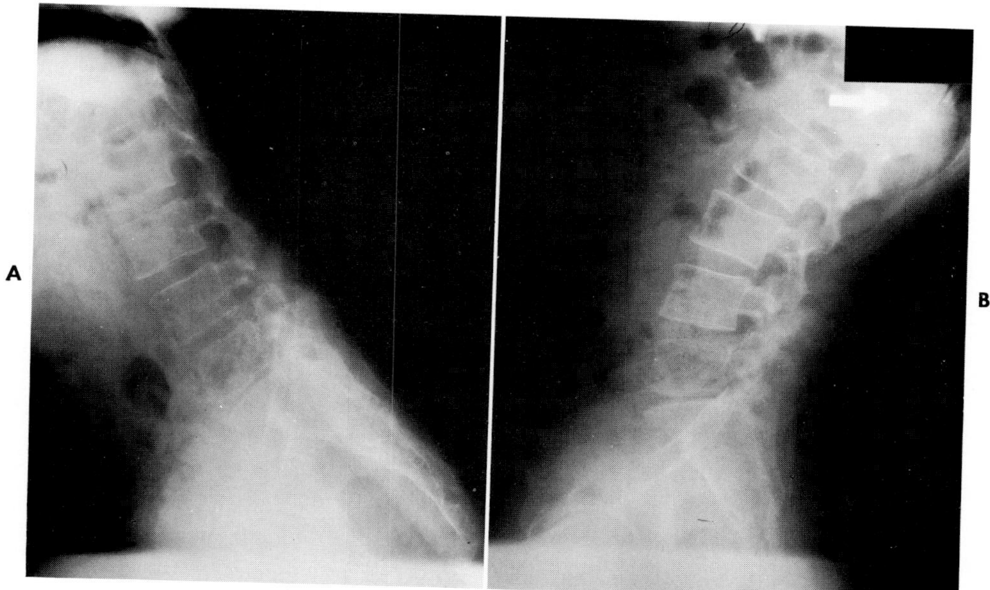

Fig. 8-1. Case 1. Lateral views of flexion, A, and extension, B, of lumboscral region, showing motion at L4-L5 interspace.

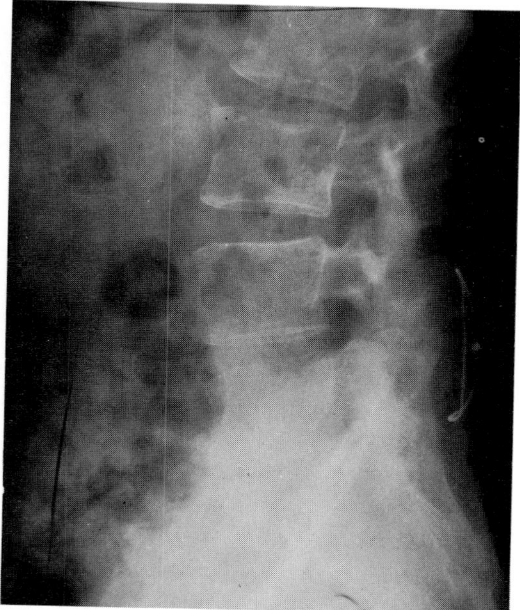

Fig. 8-2. Case 1. Lateral roentgenogram sixteen months postoperatively.

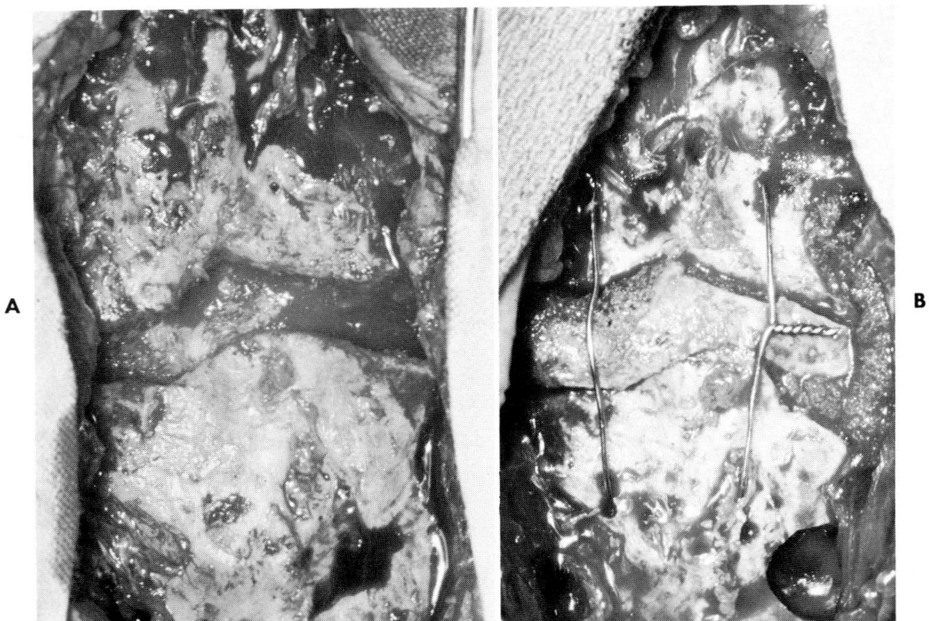

Fig. 8-3. Exposure and excision of fibrous pseudarthrosis before, **A,** and after, **B,** insertion of bone graft and stabilizing wire sutures in another patient with defect similar to that in Case 1.

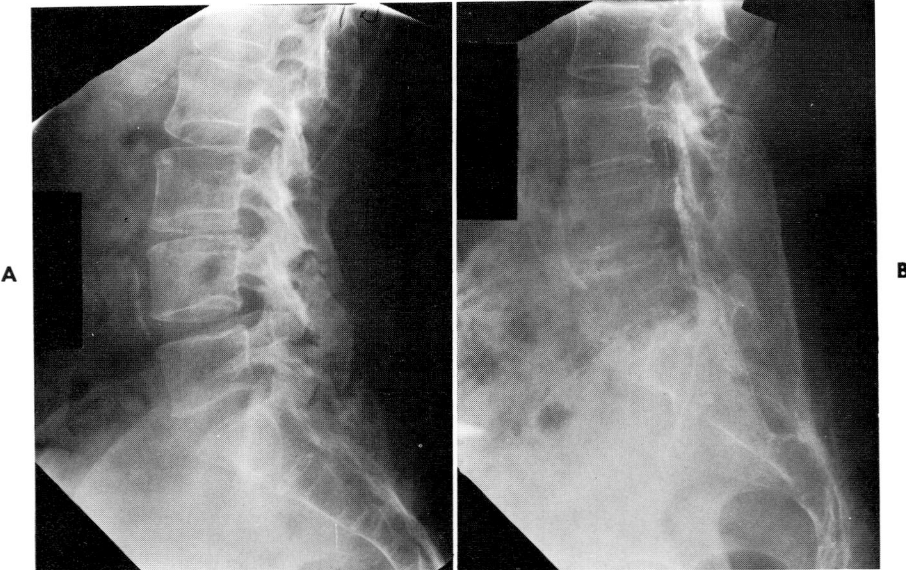

Fig. 8-4. Case 2. Lumbosacral region showing, **A,** obvious pseudarthrosis of L5-S level preoperatively and, **B,** apparently solid fusion seven years postoperatively.

fusion. We have done this in several patients, but our results have not yet been evaluated thoroughly.

Report of illustrative cases

Case 1. A 41-year-old laborer had had a previous fusion attempt of L4, L5, and the sacrum. Flexion and extension roentgenograms (Fig. 8-1) showed motion (pseudarthrosis). Repair was by posterior graft to the area of pseudarthrosis which was at L4 and L5 only. Sixteen months postoperatively, fusion was solid (Fig. 8-2); the pain has been relieved, and the patient is back at work doing manual labor. This result is good.

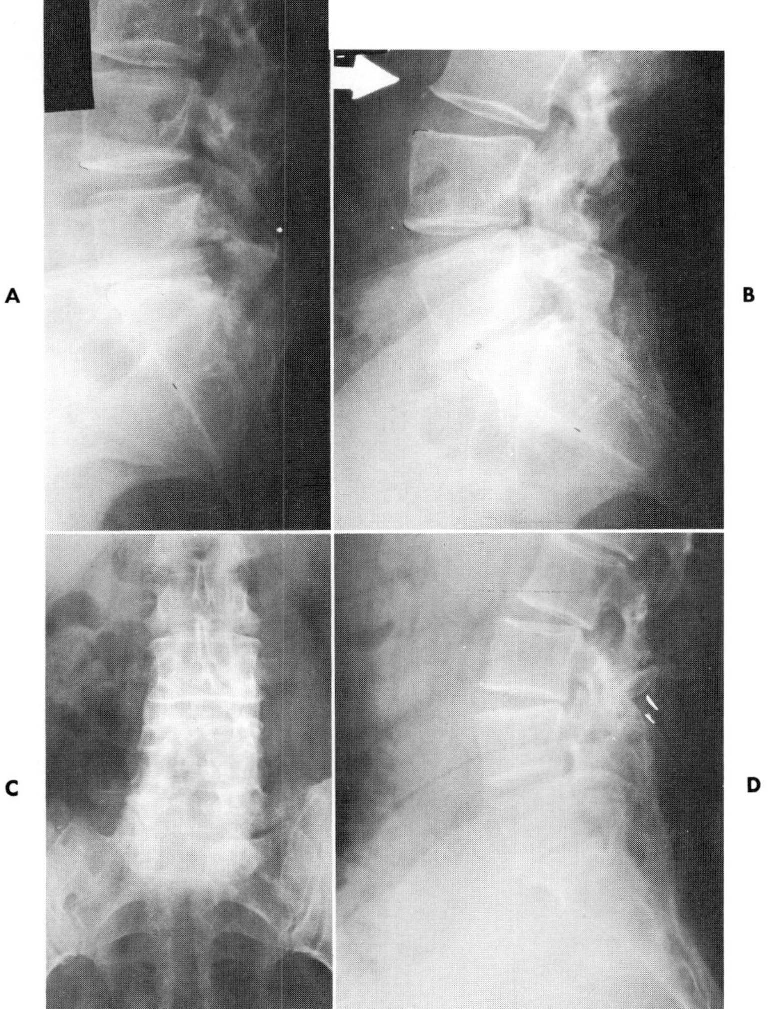

Fig. 8-5. Case 3. **A,** Flexion, and, **B,** extension roentgenograms of lumbosacral region preoperatively, showing motion at both L4-L5 and L5-S interspaces. **C,** Anteroposterior, and, **D,** lateral views eight years postoperatively, showing apparently solid fusion.

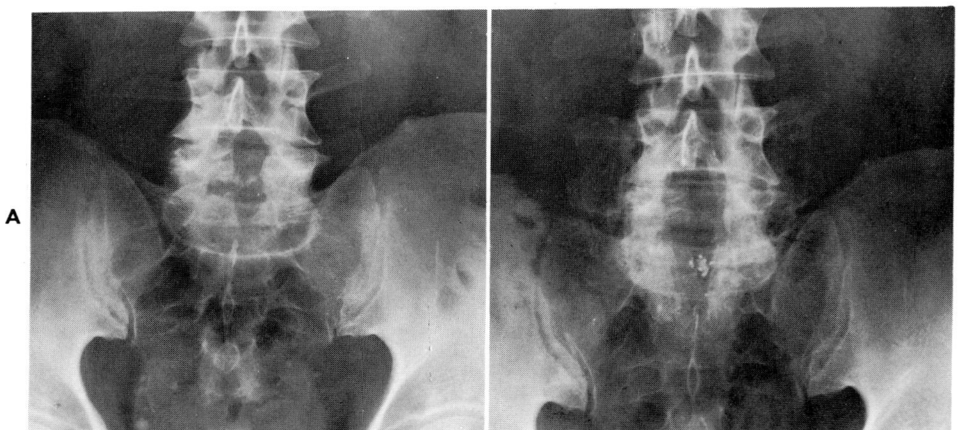

Fig. 8-6. Case 4. Lumbosacral region preoperatively, **A,** and seven months after lateral fusion of L4 to sacrum, **B.**

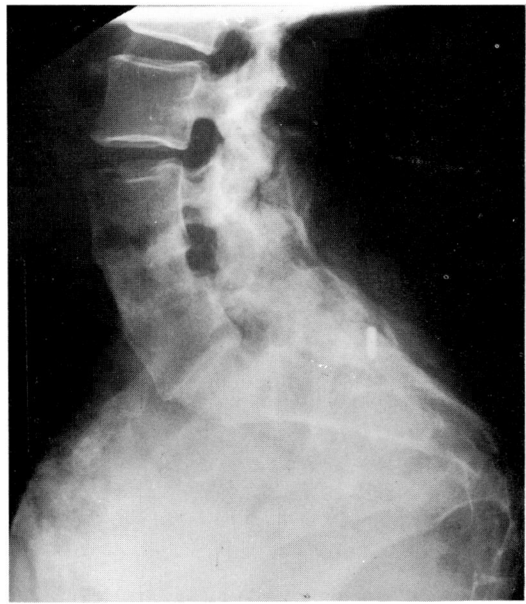

Fig. 8-7. Case 5. Lumbosacral region one year after anterior interbody fusion of L4-L5 and L5-S1.

In a similar problem in another patient, the pseudarthrosis was excised and bone was grafted; the graft was held by wire sutures (Fig. 8-3). This technique can be used when there is fibrous union and only one level is involved.

Case 2. A 44-year-old housewife and schoolteacher had undergone attempted fusions (elsewhere) from L2 to S1. We found the L2-L3 fusion to be solid. L3-L4 and L4-L5 were grafted posteriorly (Fig. 8-4). Pain was relieved for two years and then returned. This patient has a personality disorder and is a narcotics addict. This result is poor.

Case 3. This 50-year-old housewife had undergone previous laminectomy (elsewhere) at L4 and L5 with attempted fusion of L4-L5 and L5-S1. Pseudarthrosis was apparent on examination here (Fig. 8-5, *A* and *B*). After exploration of the nerve roots and an attempt at refusion of L4-L5 and L5-S1 here, fusion was solid at these levels (Fig. 8-5, *C* and *D*). The leg pain was relieved; the back pain was 50% better, and this degree of relief allowed her to be as active as she wished although she still complained of pain.

Case 4. A 45-year-old factory worker had had two previous laminectomies (elsewhere). During operation for laminectomy and posterolateral fusion at the Mayo Clinic, disc protrusion was found at L4. Lateral fusion was attempted at L4, L5, and S (Fig. 8-6). Seven months postoperatively, the fusion was solid and the partial foot drop was improving. Back pain was minimal and there was no leg pain; the patient was back at work. This result is good.

Case 5. In this 37-year-old housewife, three previous attempts had been made (elsewhere) at fusion from L4 to sacrum, and extensive laminectomies had been performed. Anterior fusion was attempted here (L4-L5 and L5-S1), and the fusion was solid one year postoperatively (Fig. 8-7). There was no back or leg pain. This result is good.

Conclusions

The results of two studies at the Mayo Clinic as to incidence of success of spinal fusion and relief of pain in patients who have had previous back operations have been presented. The basic problem is the selection of patients for reoperation. This must be done with extreme care. When this selection has been made, every effort should be exerted to effect a technically sound fusion. Our recent experience indicates that the posterolateral fusion on the transverse processes and in the lateral gutters of the laminae will give a higher incidence of fusion than will any other specific technique. If fusion is successful, one may expect relief of back pain in 60% of cases and relief of leg pain in 40%. In most of our patients there had been only one previous attempt at fusion, but some had had many previous operations. One patient with seven former operations (four for disc removal and three for fusion) now had a successful fusion and, although the leg pain continued to be troublesome, the back pain was relieved. Another patient who had undergone eight previous attempts at fusion had a solid fusion after the ninth attempt; in spite of this, the patient's pain continued. These extreme instances illustrate the difficulty in selecting the right patient for reoperation.

References

1. Adkins, E. W. O.: Lumbo-sacral arthrodesis after laminectomy, J. Bone Joint Surg. **37-B:**208, 1955.
2. Albee, F. H.: Transplantation of a portion of the tibia into the spine for Pott's disease: a preliminary report, J.A.M.A. **57:**885, 1911.
3. Batchelor, J. S.: Anterior interbody spinal fusion, Guy's Hosp. Rep. **112:**61, 1963.

4. Boucher, H. H.: A method of spinal fusion, J. Bone Joint Surg. **41-B:**248, 1959.
5. Cleveland, M., Bosworth, D. M., and Thompson, F. R.: Pseudarthrosis in lumbosacral spine, J. Bone Joint Surg. **30-A:**302, 1948.
6. Cloward, R. B.: Lesions of the intervertebral disks and their treatment by interbody fusion methods: the painful disk, Clin. Orthop. **27:**51, 1963.
7. Connor, A. C., Rooney, J. A., and Carroll, J. P.: Anterior lumbar fusion: a technique combining intervertebral and intravertebral body fixation, Surg. Clin. N. Amer. **47:**231, 1967.
8. Harmon, P. H.: Anterior excision and vertebral body fusion operation for intervertebral disk syndromes of the lower lumbar spine: three- to five-year results in 244 cases, Clin. Orthop. **26:**107, 1963.
9. Hibbs, R. A.: An operation for Pott's disease of the spine, J.A.M.A. **59:**433, 1912.
10. Hoover, N. W.: Methods of lumbar fusion, J. Bone Joint Surg. **50-A:**194, 1968.
11. Howorth, B.: Low backache and sciatica: results of surgical treatment. I. Spine fusion only. II. Removal of nucleus pulposus and spine fusion, J. Bone Joint Surg. **46-A:**1485, 1964.
12. Kelly, R. P.: Intertransverse fusion of the low back, Trans. Southern Surg. Ass. **74:**193, 1963.
13. King, D.: Internal fixation for lumbosacral fusion, Amer. J. Surg. **66:**357, 1944.
14. McElvenny, R. T.: To stalk a centaur, Amer. J. Orthop. **5:**264, 316, 332, 1963.
15. Mixter, W. J., and Barr, J. S.: Rupture of the intervertebral disc with involvement of the spinal canal, New Eng. J. Med. **211:**210, 1934.
16. Norton, P. L., and Brown, T.: The immobilizing efficiency of back braces: their effect on the posture and motion of the lumbosacral spine, J. Bone Joint Surg. **39-A:**111, 1957.
17. Raney, F. L., Jr., and Adams, J. E.: Anterior lumbar-disc excision and interbody fusion used as a salvage procedure (abstr.), J. Bone Joint Surg. **45-A:**667, 1963.
18. Sacks, S.: Anterior interbody fusion of the lumbar spine, J. Bone Joint Surg. **47-B:**211, 1965.
19. Shanewise, R. P.: Anterior intervertebral lumbar spine fusions, Western J. Surg. **71:**212, 1963.
20. Smith, A. DeF.: Discussion, J. Bone Joint Surg. **30-A:**565, 578, 1948.
21. Stewart, D. Y.: The anterior disk excision and interbody fusion approach to the problem of degenerative disk disease of the lower lumbar spinal segments, New York J. Med. **61:** 3252, 1961.
22. Truchly, G., and Thompson, W. A.: Posterolateral fusion of the lumbosacral spine, J. Bone Joint Surg. **44-A:** 505, 1962.
23. Watkins, M. B.: Posterolateral fusion of lumbar and lumbosacral spine, J. Bone Joint Surg. **35-A:**1014, 1953.
24. Wiltberger, B. R.: The Dowel intervertebral-body fusion as used in lumbar-disc surgery, J. Bone Joint Surg. **39-A:**284, 1957.

9. Spondylolisthesis: classification and etiology

Leon L. Wiltse, M.D.

The author wishes to present a classification of spondylolisthesis which, it is hoped, will include all types of the disease. This classification will be based principally on etiology in so far as that is possible, and an attempt will be made to explain the sometimes elusive etiology of the various types.

The term "spondylolisthesis" was coined by Kilian[10] in 1854. It is derived from the Greek *spondylo,* meaning spine, and *listhesis,* meaning to slip or slide down a slippery path. The term "spondylolysis," applied when there is a defect in the pars interarticularis without any forward slipping, is formed by combining *spondylo* with *lysis,* which means to dissolve. Several other terms, such as spondyloschisis (*schisis* meaning cleavage, crack, or fissure) and rachischisis (*rachis* meaning spine or vertebra), have been used. *Schisis* emphasizes the idea of a crack or fissure and *lysis* emphasizes dissolution.

According to our studies, about 50% of the cases involving a defect in the pars interarticularis will not show appreciable slipping and therefore can be designated as cases of spondylolysis. However, in the younger patient this can usually be converted into spondylolisthesis by having the patient stand up with weights on his shoulders and then relax so as to let the lumbar spine slide forward on the first sacral vertebra. Fig. 9-1 shows 2 of our patients in whom a very slight slip is converted to definite spondylolisthesis. Since isthmic spondylolysis and isthmic spondylolisthesis are fundamentally the same disease, they will be treated the same in this paper and discussed under the same general term, "spondylolisthesis."

Spondylolisthesis—that is, slipping of all or part of one vertebra forward on another—may result from several causes. The type of most clinical importance is that in which the lesion is in the isthmus or pars interarticularis. However, there are several other conditions that permit this forward slip of one vertebra on another. The following is a classification we have used—one that we believe covers all of the different types. This discussion will be limited to spondylolisthesis of the lumbar spine, except to note that the disease does occur in the cervical spine.[3, 5, 7, 15]

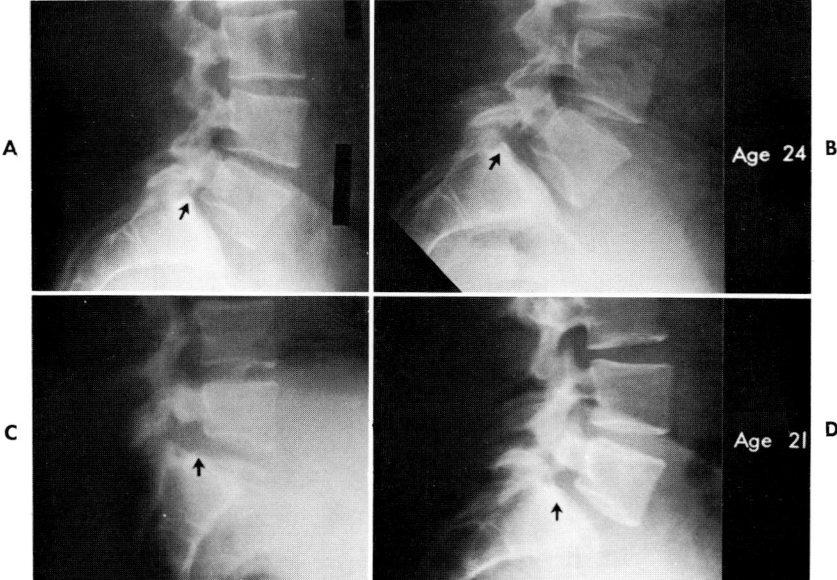

Fig. 9-1. A and **C,** In each of these roentgenograms the patient is supine on the x-ray table. **B** and **D,** Same two patients, now standing with 30 pounds of weight on the shoulders. Note the forward slip in each case. This will happen regularly in young patients. As a rule the younger the patient, the more pronounced the instability will be.

Mention will be made of this in the appropriate places in the classification. There have also been a few instances of pars defects in the thoracic spine, but to our knowledge the only cases of spondylolisthesis in the thoracic spine have been those due to fracture-dislocation secondary to severe trauma.

Classification

Type I. Isthmic. In this type the lesion is in the pars interarticularis. The following are the subtypes of isthmic spondylolisthesis:

- **A. Separation or dissolution of the pars.** There may or may not be forward slip. This is the commonest type in persons below the age of 50 and is the one we see most often in practice. It has been called "true" spondylolisthesis. However, other types may be just as "true."
- **B. Acute fracture.** This is rather rare and results from severe trauma. Dislocation may accompany it. Healing will usually follow if the dislocation is reduced and the spine immobilized.
- **C. Spondylolisthesis acquisita.** This is the type that occurs at the uppermost or lowermost vertebra of a spinal fusion, due to the extra stress on the area.[1, 8] There is another type of acquired spondylolisthesis, which is actually iatrogenic and which we are seeing occasionally now. This one is due to removal of the supporting structures by extensive surgery. In some cases of intractable back pain several operations are done. A few patients have had very radical laminectomies, some even with the removal of part of the pedicle. A very few of these have shown some slipping forward. (See Fig. 9-2.)

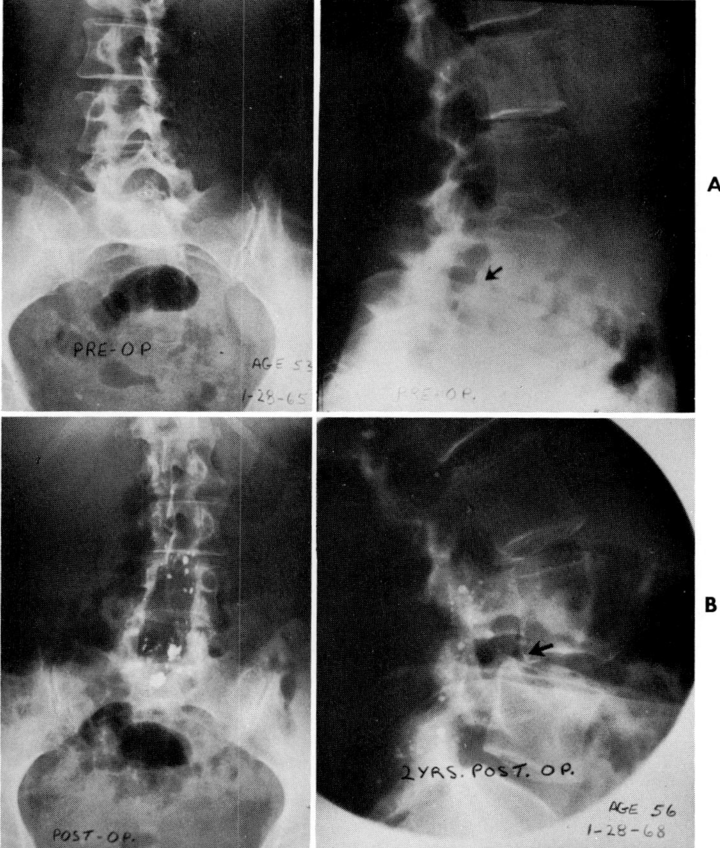

Fig. 9-2. A, Films taken previous to operation in a 56-year-old white female. Note that L4 shows a normal relationship with L5. **B,** Three years later, after two extensive laminectomies; note the wide laminectomy defect in the lower left anteroposterior view and the slip forward of L4 on L5 in the lower right roentgenogram. (Courtesy Dr. J. Gordon Bateman, Long Beach, Calif.)

D. Elongation of the pars without separation. This type is fundamentally the same as subtype A above, but the pars elongates instead of coming apart.

Type II. Congenital. In this type, failure of the supporting structures, from congenital weakness or insufficiency, allows the vertebra above to slip forward on the one below. There is no pars defect and there is no spondylolisthesis at birth.

Type III. Degenerative. This type is due to the giving way both at the facets and at the annulus also.

Type IV. Pedicular. In this type there is either a loss of continuity or an elongation of the pedicles.

Type V. Pathological. This type is caused by severe pathology and is mentioned only for completeness. It is due to destruction of the supporting structures from tuberculosis, cancer, or other disease. Massive fracture-dislocation or dislocation from severe trauma falls into this group.

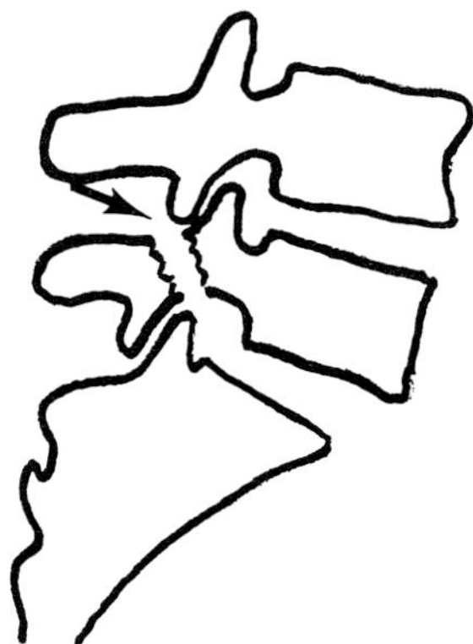

Fig. 9-3. Schematic drawing of isthmic spondylolisthesis with a defect (at arrow) in the pars interarticularis.

Etiology of the various types of spondylolisthesis

Type I. Isthmic

Subtype A. Separation: "true" spondylolisthesis (Fig. 9-3)

The etiology of this particular type has been the subject of extensive study. There has been a good deal of speculation, and numerous theories have been advanced as to its origin. Most of the articles on spondylolisthesis refer to this type. Although I have a bibliography listing 832 articles on this subject, I have no delusion that my list is complete.

The defect is in the part of the lamina between the articular facets: the pars interarticularis, in other words. To demonstrate this lesion, we normally take a large anteroposterior roentgenogram, a large lateral, a spot lateral, oblique views, and a Ferguson view of the lumbosacral area. The 45-degree lateral obliques are the best views to demonstrate this lesion, but the 30-degree caudocephalad view often gives good confirmatory evidence. If there is still doubt, 30-degree and 60-degree lateral obliques will often confirm the presence of this lesion. Also, a patient's standing with weights on the shoulders may cause the pars to separate more, and a lateral film may demonstrate the lesion. This is especially true in young people. Planigrams have been of limited value.

Factors to be considered in determining etiology

Before I present my concept of etiology of this condition, let us review some of the peculiarities of this disease.

1. It occurs only in man. I corresponded with all of the veterinary schools in the United States and in many other parts of the world. There is no record of defective pars interarticularis in any animal below man.

2. Man alone has true upright stance. Defects in the pars interarticularis have been found in the skeletons of prehistoric man; he, too, had upright stance. Defects do not occur in other primates. Schultz reviewed 4,000 primate skeletons without

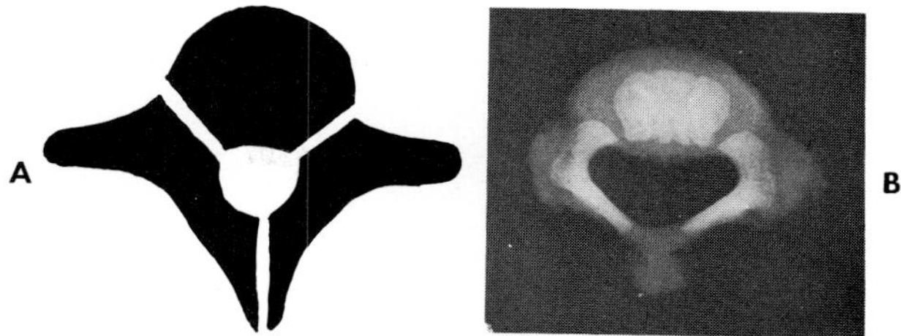

Fig. 9-4. A, Three primary ossification centers of vertebrae. **B,** Cephalocaudal roentgenogram of L5 in a newborn infant. Note that there is no line of fusion near the pars.

finding one pars interarticularis defect. Rosenberg[18] has collected evidence which indicates that in the human being those who have never stood up will not have pars defects. He has taken roentgenograms of 125 patients in an institution, none of whom had ever stood up. In these he found not a single pars defect. The chances of this occurring by sheer coincidence are quite remote.

3. Man alone has true lumbar lordosis. While some animals stand on their hind legs part of the time, they do not have true lumbar lordosis.

4. Man alone has bipedal gait. The bipedal gait may produce certain torsorial stresses not present in other animals.

5. There is no evidence that the defect is present at birth.[2, 20] The incidence of this disease increases until adulthood[20, 21, 29] but does not increase thereafter in the white race. The commonest age of onset is between 5 and 6 years. In the 36 families I studied,[28] no defects were found in members below the age of 5 years; yet the incidence was 40% in members of these families who were above the age of 10. Defects do occur rarely below the age of 5. Dr. Bernard Klieger[11] has a patient in whom spondylolisthesis of L5 with a high degree of slip was discovered at age 6 weeks. The child has been watched for years now and definitely has a pars defect. This is the youngest such patient that I am aware of. The child had never stood up, of course, when this defect was discovered, and this fact may seem to conflict with the findings of Rosenberg[18] concerning patients who had never stood. The defect could be due to birth trauma or other injury that babies sometimes receive.

6. The vertebrae ossify from three primary centers: one for the vertebral body and one for each lateral mass. There is never any sign of division or defect in these lateral masses at birth. (See Fig. 9-4.)

7. Fractures in the pars interarticularis are uncommon. Except in rare instances, known fractures of the pars interarticularis resulting from severe trauma have healed.[28]

8. Fractures in other parts of the spinal arch show evidence of attempted healing, but this is not seen in the typical defect in the pars interarticularis. Stress fractures in other areas of the body usually produce abundant callus.[21]

9. What slipping is going to occur ordinarily occurs before the age of 20. Only

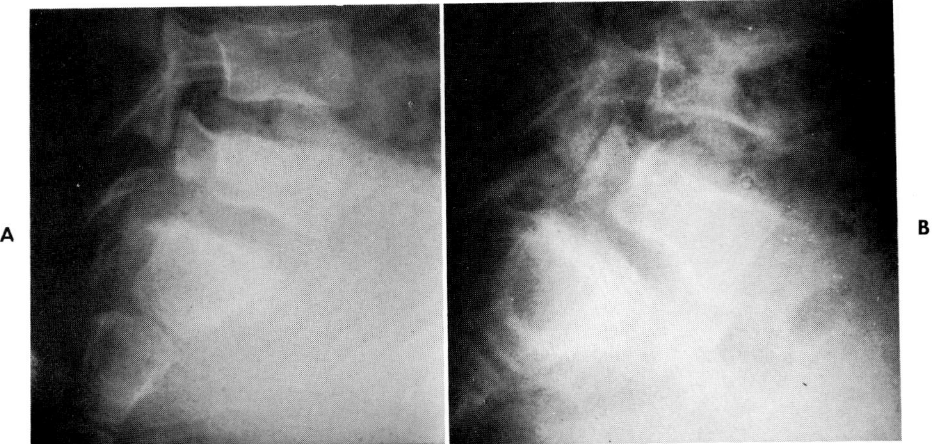

Fig. 9-5. A, Lateral roentgenogram of a boy at age 9 shows minimal slipping. **B,** Same child, age 13. Note rather severe slipping. There had been no known trauma in the interim.

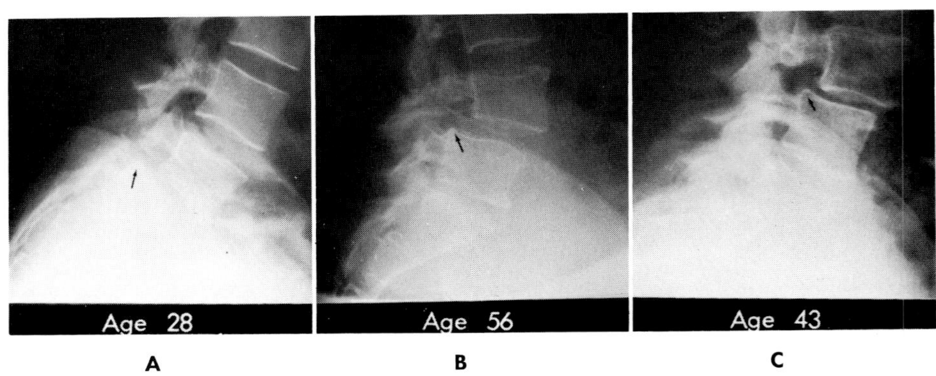

Fig. 9-6. Patients with different levels of isthmic spondylolisthesis. **A,** Pars defect with slip at L5. **B,** Pars defect with slip at L4. **C,** Pars defect with slip at L3.

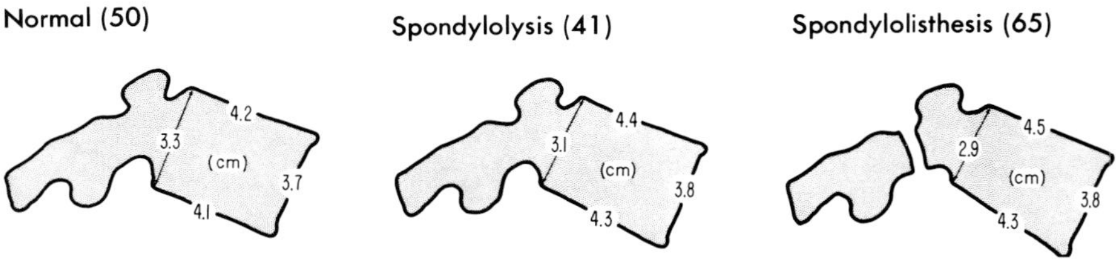

Fig. 9-7. Comparative average measurements of fifth lumbar vertebrae. It is this author's belief that the increased pressure on the posterior border of L5 due to the instability of not having intact pars causes the height of the posterior part of the body to become less. (From Wiltse, L. L.: J. Bone Joint Surg. **44-A:**539, 1962.)

rarely does slipping increase after 20 unless there has been surgical intervention. The period of most rapid slipping is between the ages of 10 and 15.[12] (See Fig. 9-5.)

10. Unilateral defects occur in the presence of an otherwise normal appearing lumbar vertebra. Assuming that dissolution does not occur, it is difficult to see how stress and strain alone could cause wide separations on one side only of a brittle bony ring.

11. Defects in the pars interarticularis are not always found in those parts of the spine in which there is the most stress and strain (Fig. 9-6). In Stewart's study, approximately 10% of the defects were found in the first three lumbar vertebrae.[21] Among Alaskan natives he found that the incidence of pars defects at the various levels was as follows: L5, 67%; L4, 25%; L3, 6%; L2, 1+%; L1, 2%. Roche and Rowe in 1952 reported the following incidence in Americans of all ethnic backgrounds: L5, 85%; L4, 9%; L3, 3−%; L2, 2+%.

12. In some cases the defects are much narrower than the amount of forward slipping of the body, suggesting an attempted healing or possibly that the pars interarticularis lengthened before coming apart, as taffy candy might do when pulled. (See Fig. 9-17.) In others, there is no slipping in the presence of a very wide defect, suggesting that resorption has progressed far beyond what was necessary to permit separation.

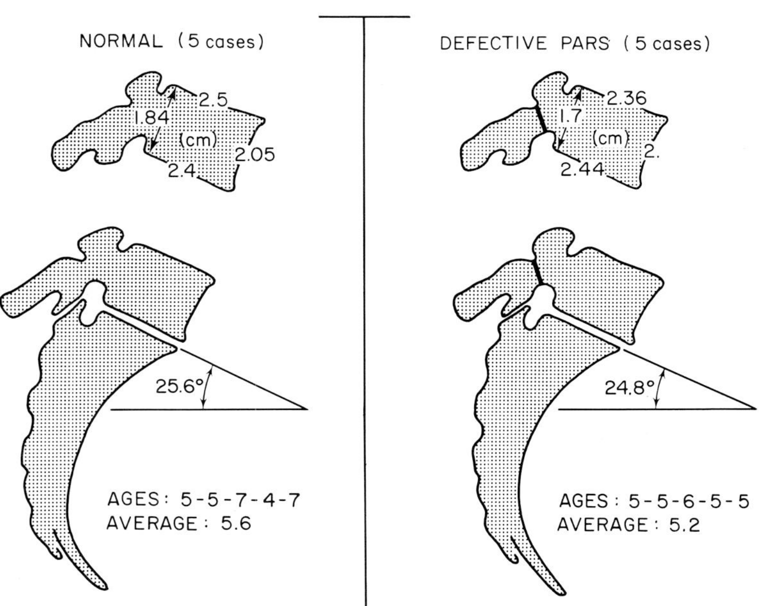

Fig. 9-8. Comparative average measurements of fifth lumbar vertebra and angle of inclination of top of sacrum in young children. The changes in the shape of the body seen in older groups are secondary and are due to instability; they have nothing to do with the development of the defect in the first place. (From Wiltse, L. L.: J. Bone Joint Surg. **44-A:**539, 1962.)

13. The trapezoid body of the fifth lumbar vertebra, so often seen in the adult with spondylolisthesis, is not present in the young child at the age when the defect appears (Fig. 9-7).

14. The pinching off appearance seen on roentgenogram between the superior facet of the sacrum and the inferior facet of the fourth lumbar vertebra, which has been blamed for cutting through the pars, is not present in the young child at the age when the defect appears.

15. The slightly increased lumbar lordosis seen in the adult is not present in the child with spondylolisthesis at the age when the defect appears (Fig. 9-8). Actually, the sacrum often assumes a vertical position with the pelvis in flexion in the presence of high-grade slip (Fig. 9-9).

16. There are well-documented cases of young children and adolescents with negative roentgenograms in whom full-blown spondylolisthesis has later developed.[4] (See Fig. 9-10.)

17. The overall incidence of the defect in Americans will be in the neighbor-

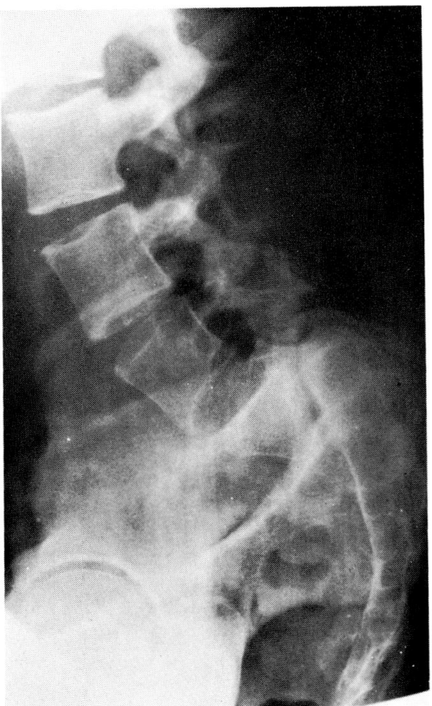

Fig. 9-9. Note that the sacrum is completely vertical, a situation characteristic of children with severe slip. In this author's opinion it appears to be the result of an effort to keep L5 in place. It may also be an effort to relieve the spasm in the hamstrings. (From Phalen, G. S., and Dickson, J. A.: J. Bone Joint Surg. **43-A:**506, 1961.)

hood of 5%. No absolutely accurate studies are available. Roche and Rowe,[17] from a study of 4,200 adult skeletons, found a smaller incidence (4.2%) but their material may have been weighted with Negro skeletons, in which the incidence is low. They found in their studies that the incidence in the white male was 6.4%, Negro male 2.8%, white female 2.3%, and Negro female 1.1%. Hasbe[9] found the incidence in Japanese to be 5.5% in 125 skeletons studied. Stewart[21] found Eskimos to have by far the highest incidence, as high as 50% in isolated communities north of the Yukon.

18. According to our studies[29] of 1,134 consecutive roentgenograms of the spine, spina bifida is thirteen times more frequent when it is associated with a defect in the pars interarticularis than in a normal spine. The wide open sacrum is four times as frequent in the presence of pars defects.

19. There is a definitely increased incidence of the severe degrees of scoliosis of the lumbar and lower thoracic spine in association with defects of the pars interarticularis in the lumbar area as compared to normal.[29] We found in reviewing 1,134 roentgenograms of the lumbar and lower thoracic spine from our office files that in 1,009 normal spines compared with 125 spines with defects of the pars interarticularis the mild and moderate degrees of scoliosis were practically equal, but severe scoliosis was four times as frequent in the spines having pars defects as it was in the normal ones.

20. There is a definite familial incidence of defective pars, according to our studies.[28, 29]

21. The vertebral segment showing a defective pars varies in a single family. Several vertebrae may be affected in the same individual. In a pair of identical twins with spondylolisthesis, the twenty-fourth segment was involved in one and the twenty-fifth segment in the other (Fig. 9-11). In the twin with the twenty-fourth segment involved, the twenty-fifth segment was fused to the sacrum; in the other twin the twenty-fifth segment was free. That we might be sure of the segment, our roentgenograms included the entire spine from the atlas to the sacrum. Friberg[6] reported an infant who, even though she had never walked, had defects at several levels. These observations suggest that there may be, in a given individual, several vertebrae with dysplasia in the pars interarticularis. Usually only the one subjected to the greatest stress or afflicted with the greatest dysplasia develops the defect. Again one might question how we explain the occasional case such as Friberg's, the patient who had defects at 11 months of age and had never walked, in the light of Rosenberg's work, where no defects were found in persons who had never stood up.[18] In such cases there may have been a very severe degree of dysplasia in the pars. Also there could have been injuries—as in the battered child syndrome, etc. Fig. 9-12 shows a family with different segments involved.

22. Transitional vertebrae, being rather stable, are virtually immune to the defect.[20]

23. There are many cases in which the pars has elongated very severely, permitting a high-grade slip, but without pars separation. Persons in these cases often

have brothers and sisters with typical pars defects, which would indicate that this condition of elongated pars is the same disease as is present in those with typical pars defects. (See Figs. 9-13 and 9-14.) The author knows of several other families showing this phenomenon.

24. We are seeing cases of teen-age boys with several pars fractures up and down the lumbar spine. Often several of these heal, but usually one or two levels remain unhealed. (See Fig. 9-15.)

25. We have shown by tetracycline uptake studies that the bone in the pars is similar to normal bone. The following study was done in a young white male adult with spondylolisthesis in whom spine fusion was to be done; it was anticipated that the loose element of the fifth lumbar vertebra would be removed at surgery. One gram of tetracycline was injected intravenously twenty-four hours before surgery. At surgery we carefully removed the loose element, damaging it as little as possible. Some soft tissue was left on the stump of the pars on each side. This material was

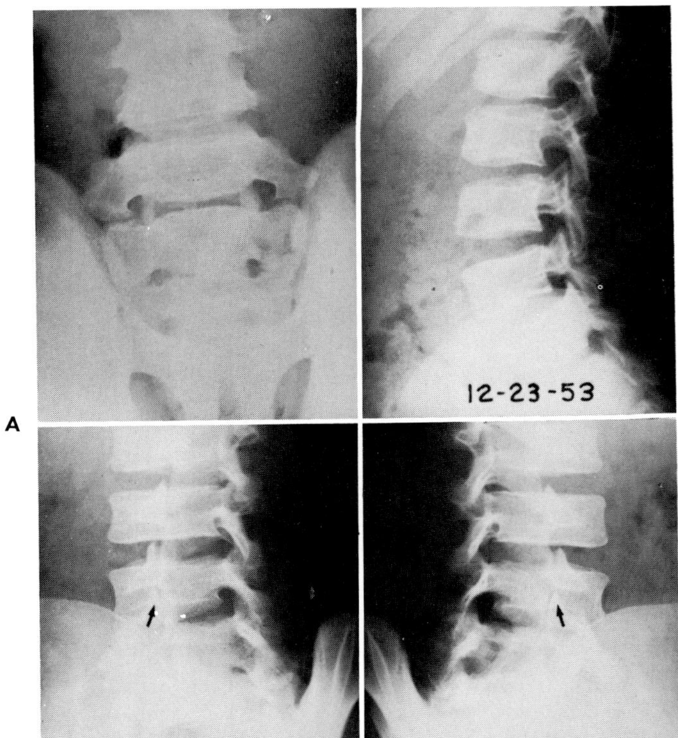

Fig. 9-10. A, W. M. at age 11. He was hurt in a football pileup. Roentgenograms are negative for pars defects. **B,** Because of continued pain in the low back, repeat roentgenograms were taken five months later. Note pars defect at L5 but no slip. **C,** Nine years later, definite slip can be seen. (Courtesy Dr. Homer Pheasant, Los Angeles, Calif.)

studied under the ultraviolet microscope, with the spinous process as a normal control area for comparison. It was noted that the bone tissue at the line of defect in the pars interarticularis was cortical bone and had the same uptake of tetracycline as the spinous process, which we believed to be normal bone. Dr. Marshall Urist of the University of California, Los Angeles, kindly assisted in this work. It would

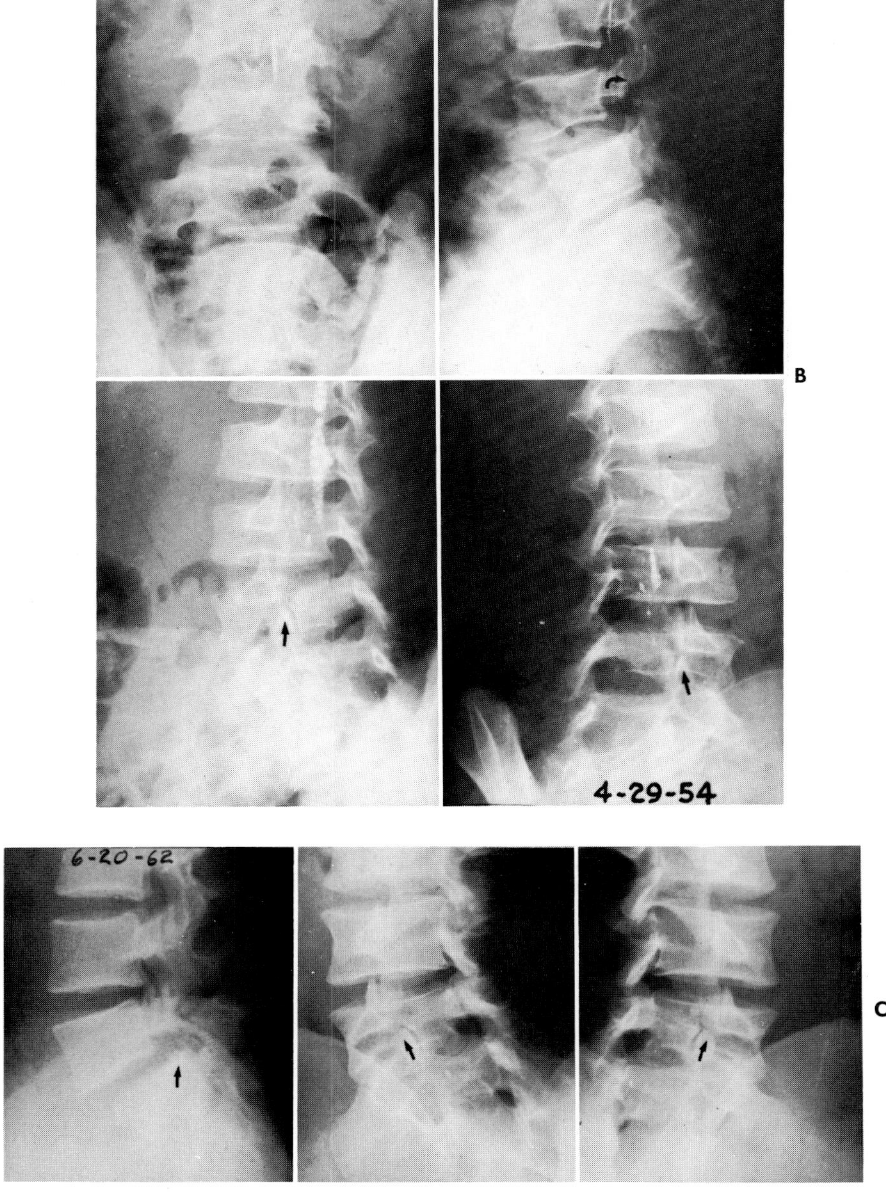

Fig. 9-10 cont'd. For legend see opposite page.

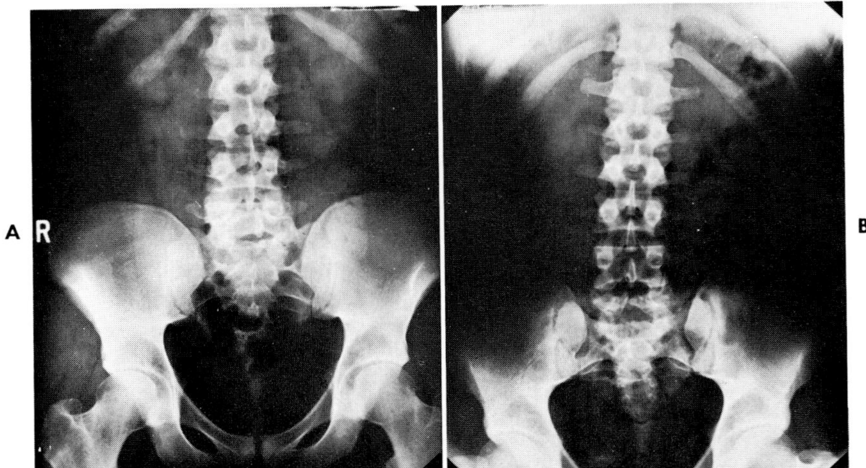

Fig. 9-11. Anteroposterior roentgenograms of identical twin boys, 18 years old. In one twin, **A,** there are five free lumbar segments, with defects in the pars interarticularis of the fifth lumbar vertebra or the lowest segment. In the other twin, **B,** there are six free lumbar vertebrae, with defects in the lowest mobile segment. In both boys complete roentgenograms from C1 down to the sacrum were made, to identify the segment. Spina bifida of the twenty-fifth segment was present in both. An interesting point to be made here is that segmentation of the spine seems not to be genetically controlled but spina bifida is. (Courtesy Dr. J. Gordon Bateman, Long Beach, Calif.; reprinted from Wiltse, L. L.: J. Bone Joint Surg. **44-A:**554, 1962.)

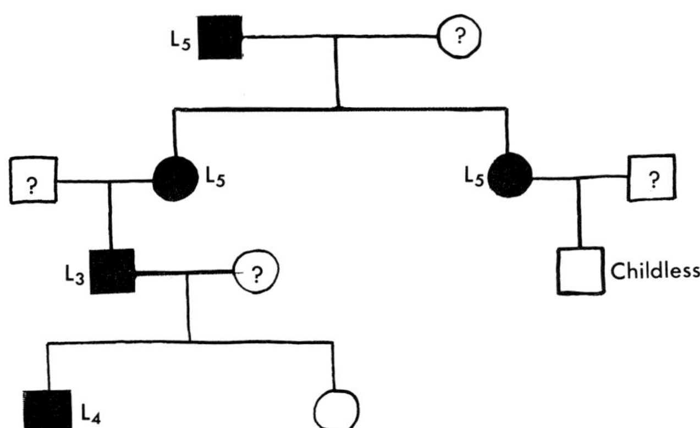

Fig. 9-12. Four generations of one family. Note that defect occurs at different levels in the same family. (Courtesy Dr. J. B. Josephsen, San Jose, Calif.)

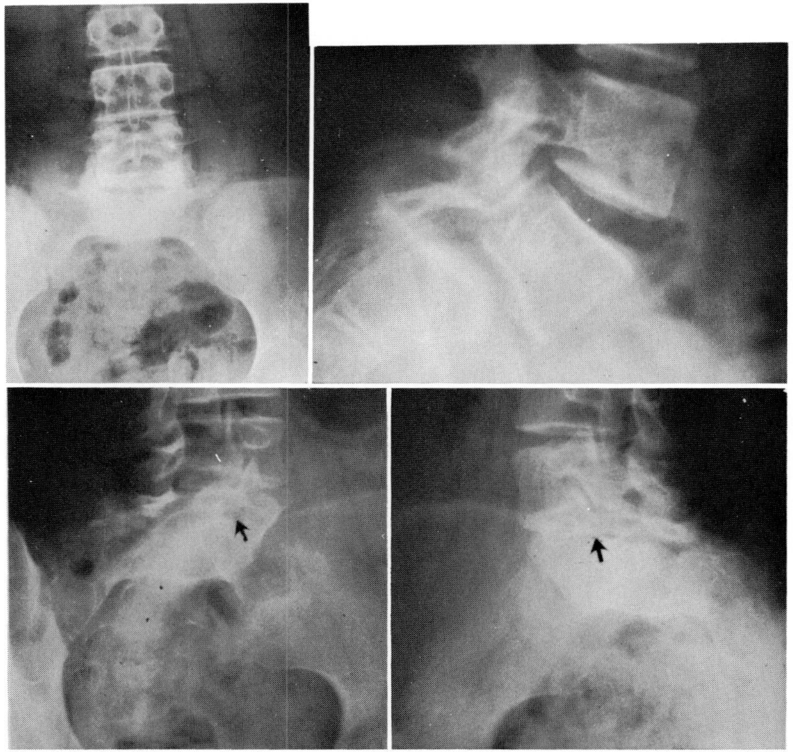

Fig. 9-13. Note 30% slip but no pars defect. Fig. 9-14 portrays the family in which this patient is the proband. (Courtesy Dr. Louis Valli, Los Angeles, Calif.)

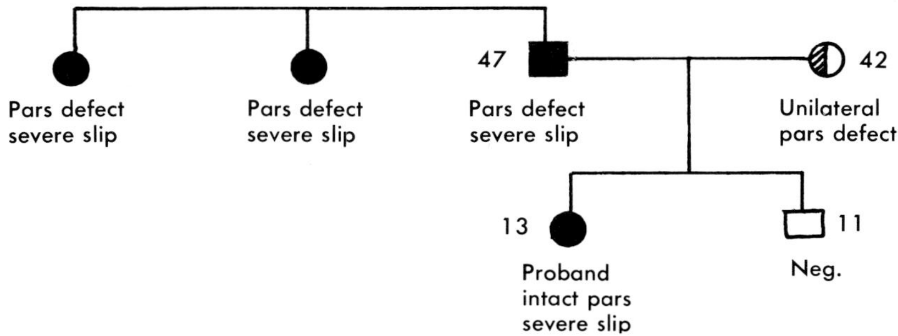

Fig. 9-14. The 13-year-old girl in the second generation is the proband. She had elongated but intact pars. Other positive members had typical pars defects. (Courtesy Dr. Louis Valli, Los Angeles, Calif.)

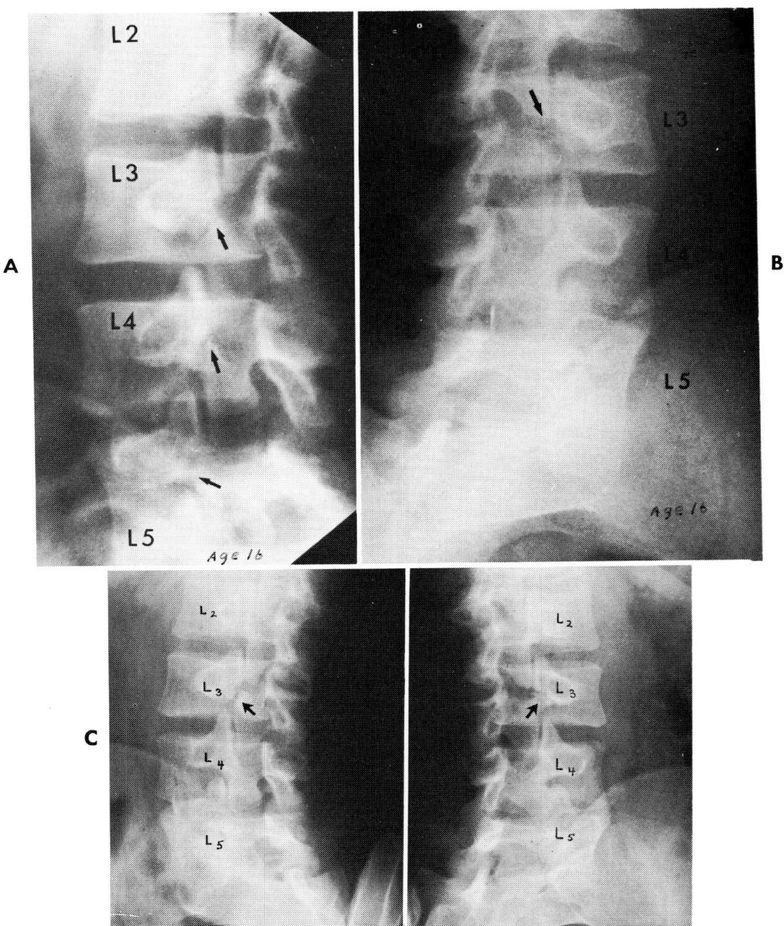

Fig. 9-15. A, W. M., age 16, was hurt in a scuffle in front of a theater and beaten up by some sailors. Note pars defects of L3, L4, and L5 (at arrows). **B,** Defect of L3 is indicated. **C,** The pars of L4 and L5 have healed. Both pars of L3 remain defective (arrows). (Courtesy Dr. Irwin Markovitz, Canoga Park, Calif.)

appear from this study that the defective pars interarticularis is not a portion of bone of low vitality, as has been suspected, but is functioning as other bone does and contributing to the body's pool of bone metabolism.[25, 29] This would not preclude the possibility that there are differences in the structure of the bone in this area, which would affect its reparative ability. This ability is an extremely complex one and is as yet not well understood. We have all seen similar fractures in different individuals vary widely in rate of healing; and we have seen fractures go on to nonunion when, by all the usual criteria, they should have healed. The study described above does not measure this factor.

Author's concept of the etiology of isthmic spondylolisthesis subtype A

Considering all the facts known about this type of spondylolisthesis, I believe that the defect in the pars is due to the following factors:

1. A hereditary defect or dysplasia, probably in the cartilage model of the arch of the affected vertebra and usually of several vertebrae in this same individual
2. The particular stresses and strains upon the pars interarticularis in the lower lumbar spine due to the erect stance and to the lumbar curve

As a result of the physical force of strain or tension, combined with the factor of dysplasia, the reparative process that bone normally is undergoing all the time progresses more toward bone resorption than toward bone formation. Microfractures occur during play or from injury. In most children these heal during rest, but in the person destined to get a pars defect these progress to dissolution. In some the factor of dysplasia is so pronounced on one side that a defect will occur unilaterally at a point where strain must be relatively slight. In others defects occur in the upper lumbar spine where, also, the element of strain must be less. If separation occurs in spite of the relatively small amount of the strain, the hereditary dysplasia in the pars interarticularis must be especially pronounced.

It would seem, then, that the lesion represents a stress fracture in a very special situation in that it occurs in a slender isthmus of cortical bone which, when a person is standing upright, is continually under at least some tension or torsional stress and in which the reparative abilities are poorer than average.

Type I. Isthmic

Subtype B. Acute fracture of the pars with or without forward slip of the vertebral body

This subtype includes only fractures through the pars, other kinds of fracture-dislocation not being included. These usually heal if immobilized.

The question arises when one sees a pars defect after acute injury as to whether this defect in the pars represents a recent fracture or not. Rarely do we have roentgenograms that were taken before the accident. If we did have a negative roentgenogram that had been taken before the accident, it could be the best evidence that we were dealing with an acute fracture. In such cases the spine should be immobilized in a cast from knees to nipple line. Healing would probably occur.

Often we have a situation where there has been an acute injury and the pars has the appearance of an acute fracture but we cannot be absolutely sure. This poses something of a problem. One is reluctant to subject a patient to eight weeks of recumbency just on a hunch that this lesion is acute; yet if he is allowed to be up and around, healing will probably not take place. An ordinary corset or brace does not actually limit motion at the lumbosacral joint. As a practical matter, we can assume that these are not acute fractures and be right most of the time.

We are now seeing quite a few high school football players who have had back pain for some time and who keep right on playing. When roentgenograms are finally taken, there may be several pars fractures up and down the spine. On follow-up we find that some of these line fractures heal, but so far in no case where we have seen multiple line fractures in the pars have all of the defects healed. These must certainly be acute or at least relatively recent fractures. I feel, but have no proof, that if these boys were kept recumbent in a body spica these might all heal. (See Fig. 9-15.)

Type I. Isthmic
Subtype C. Spondylolisthesis acquisita

It is felt that acquired spondylolisthesis results from the increased strain and stress on the pars at the upper or rarely at the lower end of a fused segment of spine.[1, 8, 24] Injury to the pars at the time of the fusion operation may play a part. (See Fig. 9-16.) Most cases seem to occur in patients fused for spondylolisthesis, so the basic underlying predisposition which affects several vertebrae must be a factor in its occurrence. Sullivan and Bickell[23] reported a series of three such cases.

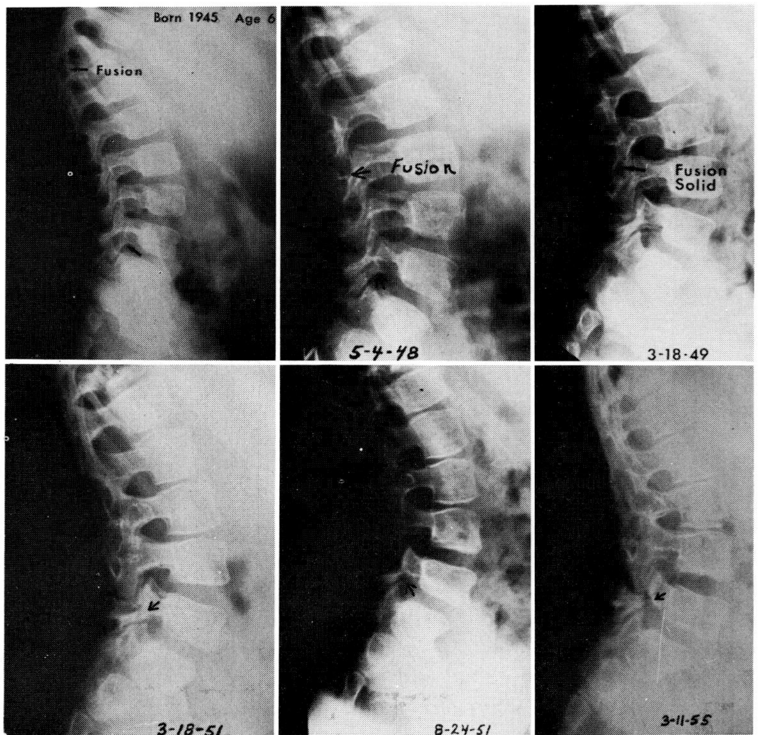

Fig. 9-16. This child had a spinal fusion as noted. Instead of the pars breaking at the top of the spinal fusion it came apart at the lower end, in this case through the pars of L5. However, the defect showed up between the ages of 5 and 6—the usual age for the defect to show up in the pars. The question might be raised as to whether this is a case of spondylolisthesis acquisita or as to whether the child would have developed a defect without the fusion above. (Courtesy Dr. Earl Feiwell, Long Beach, Calif.)

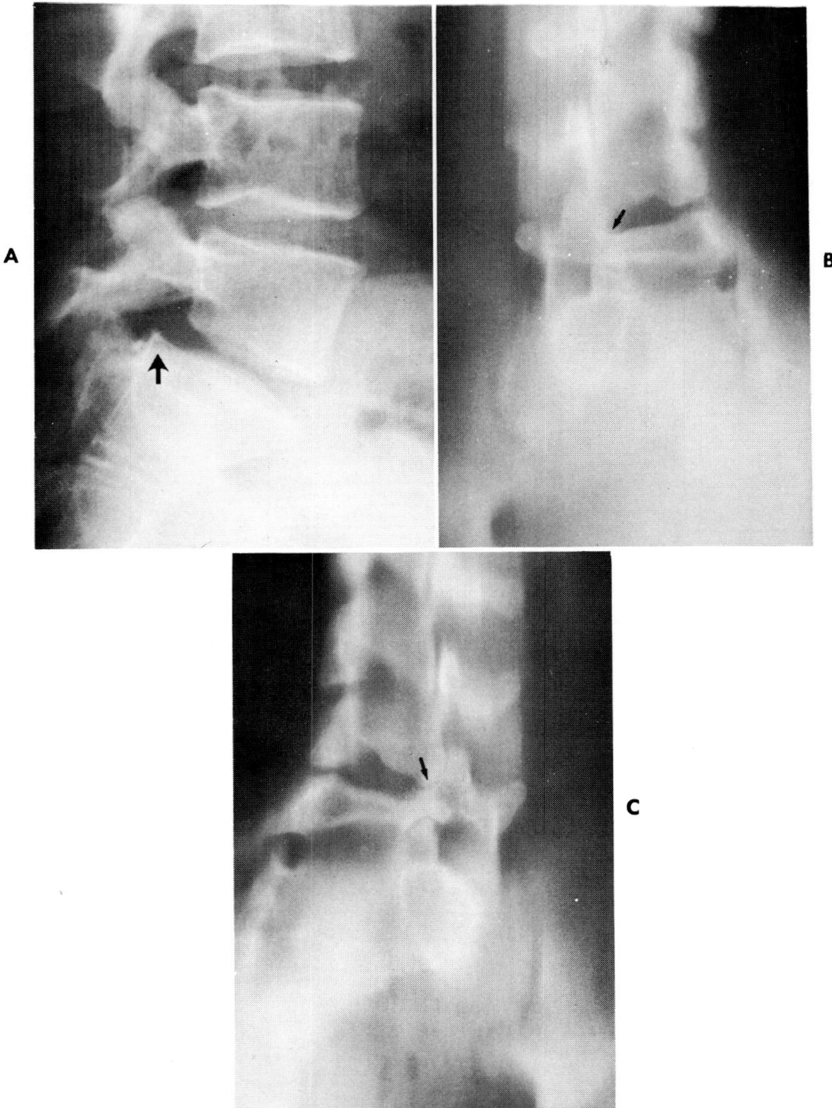

Fig. 9-17. A, Note moderate slip. **B** and **C,** Note elongated but nearly intact pars. A very fine line can be seen in the middle of the pars, suggesting that it has made a valiant effort to heal and has virtually succeeded but has elongated in the process. (Courtesy Dr. Edward Gillman, Long Beach, Calif.)

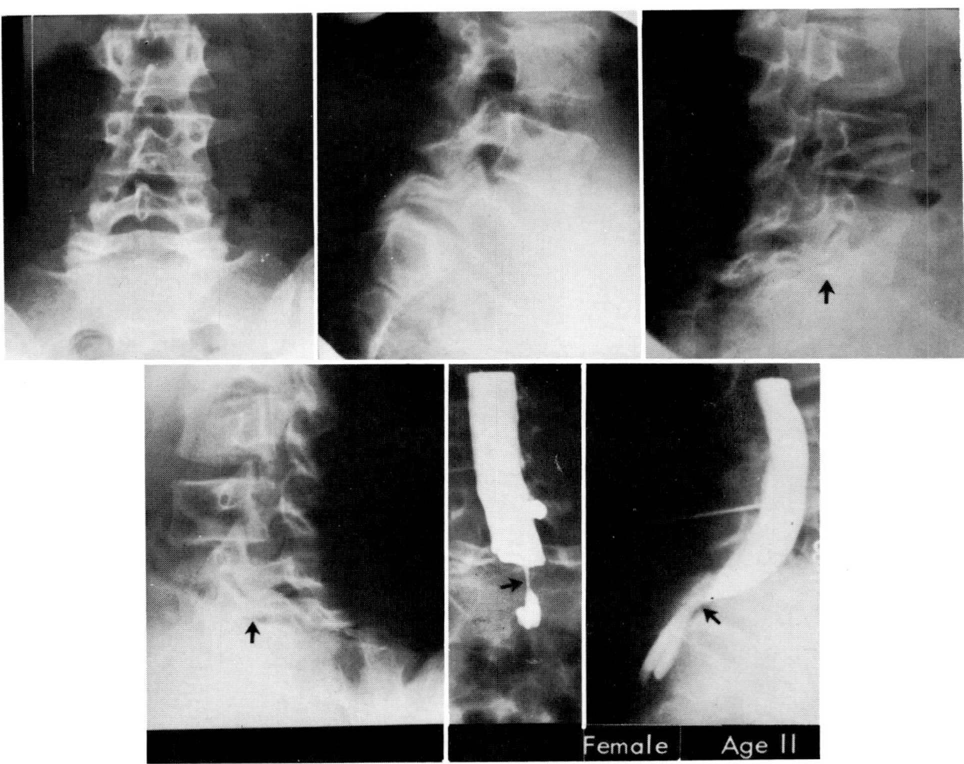

Fig. 9-18. Note that this child had intact pars. This was proved at surgery. She had tight hamstrings and "spastic" gait. See Fig. 9-19 showing this child's family tree. (Courtesy Dr. John Howard, Los Angeles, Calif.)

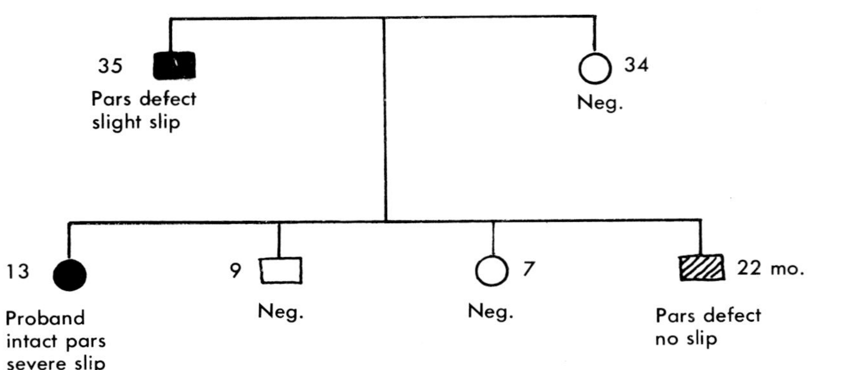

Fig. 9-19. Proband had severe slip with intact pars. Her father and brother had typical pars defects with spondylolisthesis.

In two of their three cases the lesion healed when the patient was immobilized in a cast.

Type I. Isthmic

Subtype D. Elongation of the pars without separation (Fig. 9-17)

This classification includes a large group of cases—from those showing a minor degree of slip to others with a very high-grade slip but all with an intact pars. In the cases showing a high grade of slip there is often the syndrome of tight hamstrings and peculiar "spastic" gait.[16] There may be inadequacy of the supporting structures in the lumbosacral region. Often there is deficient development of the top of the sacrum. Wide spina bifida is often present in L5 or S1 and S2. Often several vertebrae in the lumbosacral area show spina bifida, but the pars interarticularis is intact. This group has been labeled "congenital" by Newman.[14] The interesting thing is that several of our patients who show these congenital defects and fall into this category have parents and siblings with typical pars defects. This would indicate that the two types are the same basic disease but with different manifestations. (See Figs. 9-18 and 9-19.)

We have, then, cases in which there is typical spondylolisthesis due to separation in the pars interarticularis in the same families with another group having these congenital defects in the supporting structures with elongated but intact pars.

Type II. Congenital

Probably no child is born with spondylolisthesis. In a few cases there are congenital abnormalities of the spine that permit forward slip of one vertebra upon

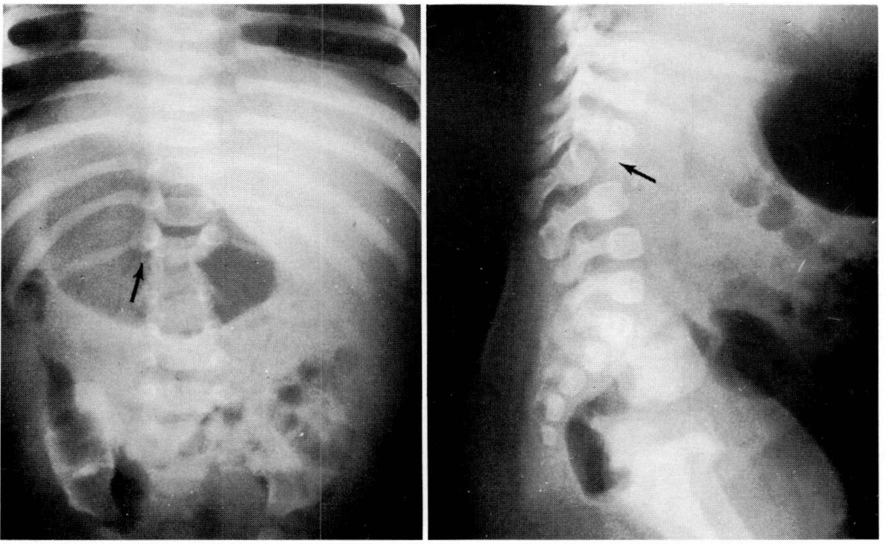

Fig. 9-20. A 6-week-old child with severe slip of L1 on L2. We have watched this child for two years. There has been no evidence of sensory or motor disturbance. (Courtesy Dr. Robert Shlens, Los Angeles, Calif.)

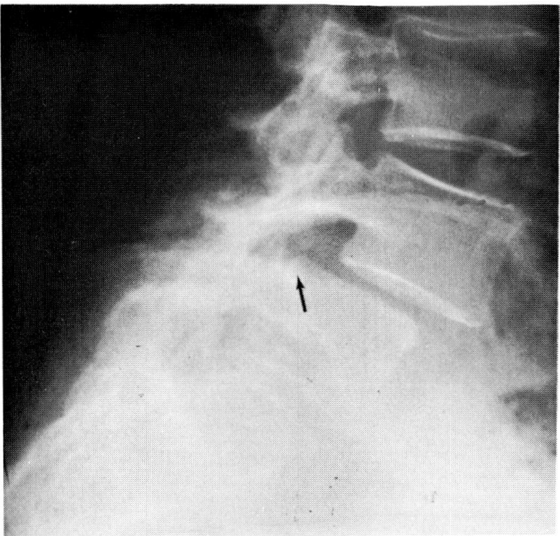

Fig. 9-21. Severe slip due to degenerative spondylolisthesis in a white female, age 67. Degenerative spondylolisthesis cases seldom slip more than 25%. There is degenerative disease, with giving way at both the annulus and the facets.

another. We have seen a few such cases in the upper lumbar area (Fig. 9-20). We have chosen to call these congenital because the congenital abnormalities are so striking, even though there is probably no slip at birth. This is a rare type of lesion.

Type III. Degenerative (Fig. 9-21)

The patients showing this type of slip are very numerous. In these cases there is degeneration of both the disc and the facets. The facets often show severe degeneration, having a somewhat similar appearance, as seen at operation, to a knee with advanced degenerative arthritis. Often the capsule of the facet joint is full of fluid. With both the disc and the facets degenerated, there is little to stop the body of the upper vertebra from slipping forward on the one below. The normal annulus fibrosus permits little anteroposterior slip, but the degenerated annulus does. As the cartilage erodes on the facets, the ligaments loosen and permit the inferior facets of the upper vertebra to slip forward between the superior facets of the one below. These seldom slip more than 25% but have been noted to slip 33%.

The L4, L5 space is most commonly affected, with the L5 and L3 spaces following in that order. Rosenberg[18] has observed that, when this occurs at L4, the L5 vertebra is more stable than average, thus causing more of the motion to occur at the L4 space, so that it is the one affected. Often there is a block-shaped body of L5, and a higher percentage than average show sacralization of L5. There is no pars defect.

The incidence increases as age increases, and our figures indicate that this is actually the most common type of spondylolisthesis in the very aged.

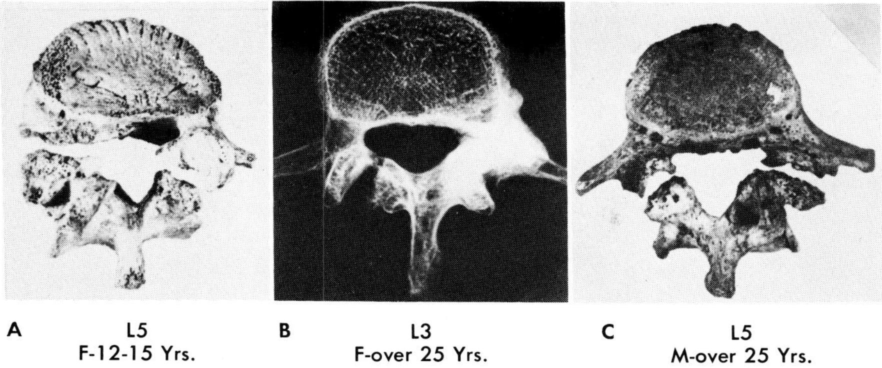

Fig. 9-22. **A,** Fifth lumbar vertebra with a defect through the pedicle on the left and through the pars on the right. **B,** Roentgenogram of third lumbar vertebra. The defect through the right pedicle is partly united. Note the marked repair reaction in the pedicle as contrasted to the lack of such reaction about the defect through the left pars interarticularis. **C,** Fifth lumbar vertebra with defects through the pedicles, both sides. In this specimen the defects are behind the transverse processes, not in front of them as in **A.** In addition, there is a defect through the pars interarticularis on the left so that the superior articular process on this side is a separate piece of bone (not shown). (From Stewart, T. D.: J. Bone Joint Surg. **35-A:**937, 1953.)

The fact that the incidence is so much higher in women would suggest that hormonal factors are important in its development. It never occurs before the age of 40 and usually not before age 50. Osteoporosis would not seem to be a factor in its etiology, since the defect is more common in the Negro female and Negroes are less affected by osteoporosis than are Caucasians.[19]

Type IV. Pedicular

This type is caused by fracture or elongation of the pedicles. This is a rare type in the lumbar area and is of little importance. When fractures of the pedicles do occur, they attempt to heal[21, 22] and may heal in a normal or slightly elongated position. Occasionally, bone diseases such as Paget's disease may cause stretching of the pedicle at one level and thus fulfill the criteria for spondylolisthesis. Stewart[21] observed fractures of the pedicles in some of his Eskimo skeletons. (See Fig. 9-22.) Strangely, most fractures of the pedicle seem to be unilateral with a unilateral pars defect on the other side.

Type V. Pathological

This type is caused by severe pathology. It is mentioned only for completeness. In this group I have chosen to place spondylolisthesis caused by destructive disease such as tuberculosis or cancer. Charcot's disease will rarely permit one vertebra to slip forward on the one below. Severe fracture-dislocation or dislocation alone from major trauma is included here. The etiology is usually quite clear and needs no discussion.

Reverse spondylolisthesis

Although reverse or retrograde spondylolisthesis was not mentioned in the classification, it is mentioned here in the discussion because it bears the name. However, it hardly fulfills the requirements to be called spondylolisthesis, since by definition *listhesis* means to slip or slide down an incline. These cases would seem to slide up an incline.

The appearance of posterior slip of one vertebral body on the one below is seen in the following situations:

1. The body of L5 may be thick, as compared with a thinner body of S1. Or the body of L5 may be kidney shaped,[26] thus giving it the appearance of being slipped back without its actually being so. (See Fig. 9-23.)

Note in Fig. 9-24, *C,* that one might be led to believe that there was a posterior slip of L5 on S1; but if one measures the bodies of these two vertebrae, it will be noted that the anteroposterior diameter of L5 is greater than that of S1.[27] This could be due either to an actual increase in the size of the body of L5 or to a kidney-

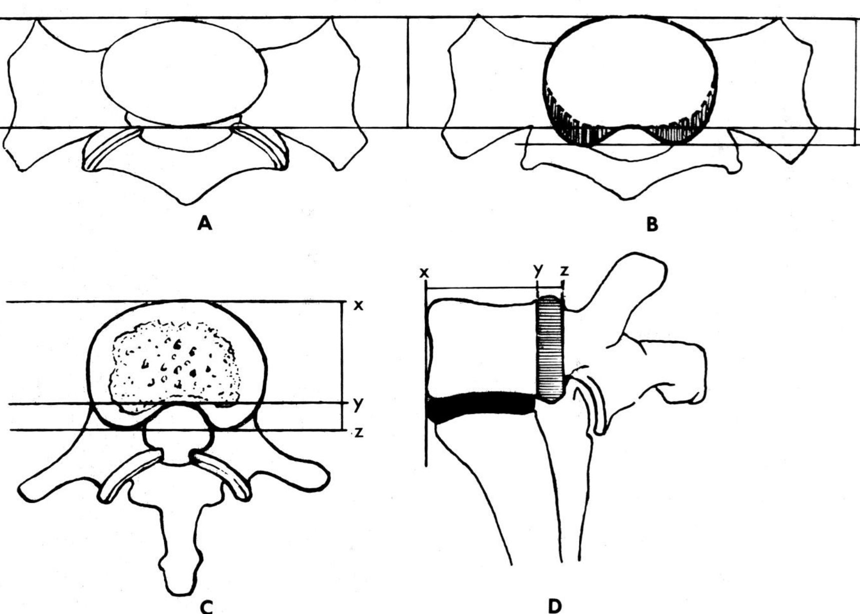

Fig. 9-23. A, Note that the body of S1 is oval. **B,** The body of L5 is kidney shaped on its posterior surface. **C** and **D,** Note that the anteroposterior diameter of L5 is the same as that of S1 only in the "hilum" or central portion.

The two poles of the kidney-shaped L5 may lie behind the posterior margin of the sacrum in a lateral x-ray film, thereby giving an illusion of retro-displacement unless both the anterior and posterior margins of the vertebrae are viewed and compared. If the anteroposterior diameters of the two vertebrae are measured and that of L5 is found to be greater, there may be an illusion of retro-displacement without true retro-displacement being present. This, then, would be a case of pseudo retro-spondylolisthesis. (From Willis, T. A.: J. Bone Joint Surg. **17:** 347, 1935.)

shaped body of L5 such that the corners of the body cast a shadow on the roentgenogram, which is posterior to that of the body of S1. This is not true retrograde spondylolisthesis and might be called pseudo retro-spondylolisthesis.

2. Narrowing and degeneration of the disc may occur, but with the facets holding and acting as a fulcrum (Fig. 9-24, *A* and *B*). These represent true posterior

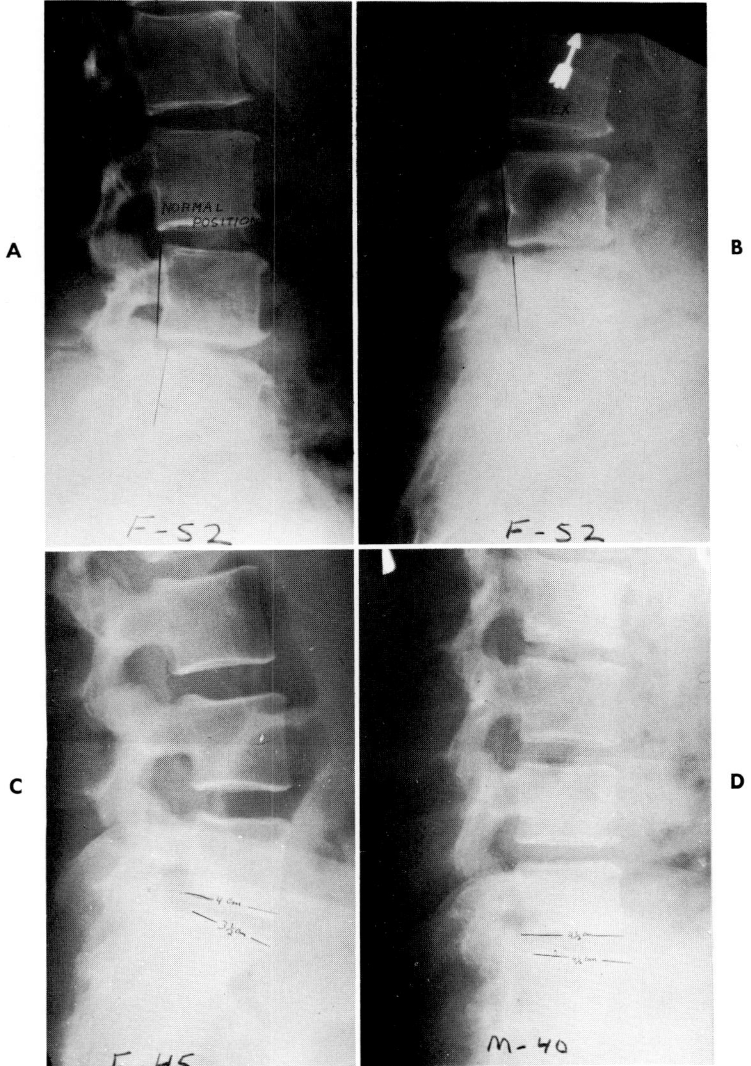

Fig. 9-24. A, True retro-spondylolisthesis. **B,** Same patient as at left, with spine flexed so the posterior slip disappears. **C,** In this case the anteroposterior diameter of L5 is greater than that of S1. This represents a case of pseudo retro-spondylolisthesis as described by Willis. **D,** A case of true retro-spondylolisthesis of L5 on S1. Note that the anteroposterior diameters of the bodies are equal but that L5 is slipped back on S1.

slip—a pathological process. It is true retro-spondylolisthesis. The facets remain relatively normal but the inferior facets of the vertebra above do slide down on the superior facets of the one below. The ligaments of the facets stretch, but the cartilage at the facets remains relatively normal.

3. Posterior slip may exist only during hyperextension. This is seen in early degeneration of a disc and is the so-called "primary instability."[13]

Occasionally, this is the first visible roentgenographic sign of disc degeneration. It is likely that in all cases of retro- or reverse spondylolisthesis this sign is present initially.

• • •

In the cervical vertebrae we often see cases of degenerative spondylolisthesis and we occasionally see the pedicular type due to fracture or nonunion of the pedicles.[7] True isthmic spondylolisthesis in the upper five cervical segments is extremely rare and possibly does not occur, since in the cervical spine the part between the articular facets is very short except in C6 and C7 where there is a reasonably well developed pars interarticularis. I have one patient in whom I think I can definitely say that there is a fracture of the pars of C6. If fractures do occur in this short pars, and they may, they probably heal and this is why we do not see them more often.

Summary

The various types of spondylolisthesis in the lumbar spine have been presented and the etiology of each discussed. Spondylolisthesis of the cervical spine was mentioned briefly and it was noted that at least three types do occur in the cervical spine.

To my knowledge there is no case reported of spondylolisthesis of the thoracic spine except those of fracture-dislocation from severe trauma. Pars defects do occur in the thoracic spine.

The common type of isthmic spondylolisthesis where the defect is in the pars interarticularis is believed to be a stress fracture through a segment of bone that has diminished ability to repair itself. This diminished ability is hereditary.

Retrograde spondylolisthesis is discussed briefly because it bears the name, but this is probably a misnomer. It would seem better to simply call it "posterior displacement."

References

1. Anderson, C. E.: Spondyloschisis following spine fusion, J. Bone Joint Surg. **38-A:**1142, 1956.
2. Batts, M., Jr.: The etiology of spondylolisthesis, J. Bone Joint Surg. **21:**879, 1939.
3. Cornish, B. L.: Traumatic spondylolisthesis of the axis, J. Bone Joint Surg. **50-B:**31, 1968.
4. Cozen, L.: The developmental origin of spondylolisthesis; two case reports, J. Bone Joint Surg. **43-A:**180, 1961.
5. Durbin, F. C.: Spondylolisthesis of the cervical spine, J. Bone Joint Surg. **38-B:**734, 1956.
6. Friberg, S.: Studies on spondylolisthesis, Acta Chir. Scand **82**(supp. 55)**:**1, 1939.

7. Hadley, L. A.: Congenital absence of the pedicle from cervical vertebrae; report of three cases, Amer. J. Roentgen. **55:**193, 1956.
8. Harris, R. I., and others: Acquired spondylolisthesis as a sequel to spinal fusion, J. Bone Joint Surg. **45-A:**1159, 1963.
9. Hasbe, K.: Die Wirbelsaule der Japaner, Z. Morph. Anthrop. **15:**259, 1913.
10. Kilian, H. F.: Schilderungen neuer Beckenformen und ihres Verhalten im leben Bassermann und Mathy, Mannheim, 1854 (cited by Brocher)
11. Klieger, B.: Personal communication.
12. Laurent, L. E., and Einola, S.: Spondylolisthesis in children and adolescents, Acta Orthop. Scand. **31:**45, 1961.
13. Morgan, F. P., and King, T.: Primary instability of the lumbar vertebrae as a common cause of low back pain, J. Bone Joint Surg. **39-B:**6, 1957.
14. Newman, P. H.: The etiology of spondylolisthesis, J. Bone Joint Surg. **45-B:**36, 1963.
15. Perlman, R., and Hawes, L. E.: Cervical spondylolisthesis, J. Bone Joint Surg. **33-A:** 1012, 1951.
16. Phalen, G. S., and Dickson, J. A.: Spondylolisthesis and tight hamstrings, J. Bone Joint Surg. **43-A:**505, 1961.
17. Roche, M. B., and Rowe, G. G.: The incidence of separate neural arch and coincident bone variations, Anat. Rec. **109:**233, 1951.
18. Rosenberg, N.:. Personal communication, 1966.
19. Rosenberg, N.: Articular spondylolisthesis. Paper read at the meeting of the American Orthopaedic Association, Castle Harbour Hotel, Bermuda, May 28, 1962.
20. Rowe, G. G., and Roche, M. B.: The lumbar neural arch: roentgenographic study of ossification, J. Bone Joint Surg. **32-A:**554, 1957.
21. Stewart, T. D.: The age incidence of neural arch defects in Alaskan natives, considered from the standpoint of etiology, J. Bone Joint Surg. **35-A:**937, 1953.
22. Stewart, T. D.: Examination of the possibility that certain skeletal characteristics predispose to defects in the lumbar neural arches, Clin. Orthop. **8:**44, 1956.
23. Sullivan, C. R., and Bickell, W. H.: The problem of traumatic spondylolisthesis; a report of three cases, Amer. J. Surg. **100:**698, 1960.
24. Unander-Scharin, L.: A case of spondylolisthesis lumbalis acquisita, Acta Orthop. Scand. **19:**536, 1950.
25. Urist, M.: Personal communication.
26. Willis, T. A.: The separate neural arch, J. Bone Joint Surg. **13:**709, 1931.
27. Willis, T. A.: Lumbosacral retrodisplacement, Amer. J. Roentgen. **90:**1263, 1963.
28. Wiltse, L. L.: Etiology of spondylolisthesis, Clin. Orthop. **10:**48, 1957.
29. Wiltse, L. L.: The etiology of spondylolisthesis, J. Bone Joint Surg. **44-A:**539, 1962.

10. Osteoporosis and fractures of the spine

George E. Spencer, Jr., M.D.

Back pain in the elderly patient is a symptom complex which we must all be concerned with and be competent to treat, because of the increasing population of geriatric patients. It is estimated that approximately 20% of elderly people develop osteoporosis.[9] Osteoporosis with compression fractures of the dorsolumbar spine is the pathological condition with which we must now concern ourselves.

The fractures are the problem that brings the patient to us. These are not major fractures and often they are not diagnosed or treated. Many of these patients are living in extended care facilities or nursing homes and may not come to anyone's attention for indefinite periods of time. They may have multiple compression fractures when first seen.

The characteristic of osteoporosis is that it is a generalized disease of bone with a decrease in bone mass.[1] Bone is a very active living tissue that is being both formed and resorbed, thereby depending on the balance between the two activities to determine its state when we examine the skeleton. When there is an increase in resorption, the net effect of the balance is on the loss side and a catabolic state exists. The bone mass decreases without loss of volume and this weakens the bone. The serum calcium and phosphorus levels remain normal in this disease process. The serum alkaline phosphatase may be normal or slightly low.

Osteoporosis involves the spine and pelvis and areas of cancellous bone more persistently than cortical bone. We see this in the many hip and spine fractures we treat in these patients. It is interesting to observe that fracture healing is usually unaffected in this disease and that a fracture is an excellent stimulus to bone formation.[9]

The causes of osteoporosis have been well outlined by Albright and Reifenstein.*

- I. Defect in osteoblasts
  - A. Loss of stress and strain
    - 1. Atrophy of disuse

*From Albright, F., and Reifenstein, E., Jr.: The parathyroid glands and metabolic bone disease, Baltimore, 1948, The Williams & Wilkins Co.

B. Lack of estrogen
   1. Postmenopausal state
   2. Congenital hypoestrinism: ovarian agenesis
C. Congenital osteoblastic defect
   1. Osteogenesis imperfecta

II. Defect in matrix
   A. Loss of androgen
      1. Eunuchoidism
      2. ? Senile osteoporosis
   B. Loss of protein
      1. Malnutrition
      2. Hypovitaminosis C
      3. Cushing's syndrome
      4. "Alarm reaction"

III. Defect unknown
   A. Acromegaly
   B. Idiopathic osteoporosis

This still remains an excellent functional plan for grouping the various causes of osteoporosis, even though there are discrepancies. We are all familiar with disuse osteoporosis as we see it with cast immobilization of the skeleton. In this type, there is a loss of stress, with a reduction in bone formation and a resultant catabolic

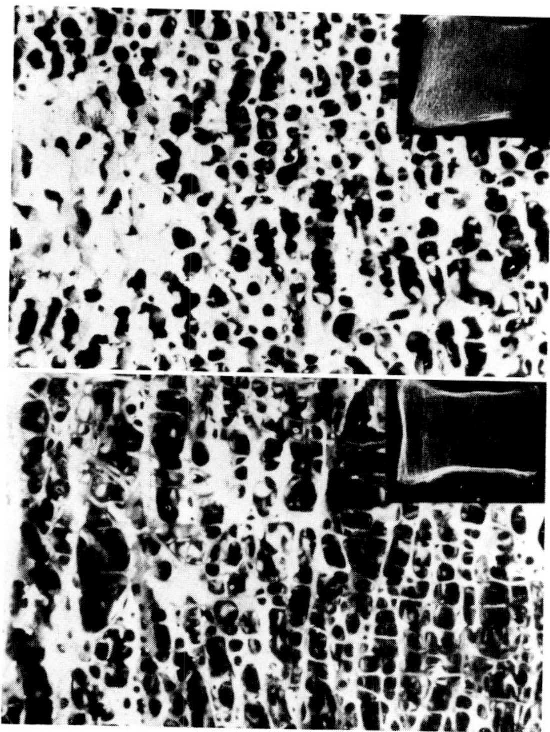

Fig. 10-1. Normal bone above and osteoporotic bone below. Note the diminution of mass and the thin trabecular pattern.

state. This kind of osteoporosis is reversible when stress is again increased.[10] The other causes of osteoporosis result in a catabolic state because of the increase in bone resorption and the imbalance that results.[3, 4, 7]

The gross pathology of osteoporosis is seen in Fig. 10-1. Normal bone above is contrasted with osteoporotic bone below. The trabeculae are thin, as are the end-plates. It is stated that x-ray evidence of osteoporosis begins to be visible only when 40% of the bone mass is lost.[6] It is therefore a rather inaccurate means of determining loss of bone mass. When such evidence is seen, the loss is fairly far advanced.

One of the physical characteristics seen in persons with osteoporosis is their loss of height. Some patients lose four or five inches in height in a year or two. This occurs because of multiple compression fractures with anterior wedging of the vertebrae. As individuals shorten, they also increase the anteroposterior diameter of the chest, with expansion and shortening of the waist. Their body configuration changes quite markedly and their clothes fit poorly. They have back pain with the wedging and micro-fractures that are occurring until they no longer compress. After they stabilize for a few months, their pain improves gradually.

These compression fractures may result from normal trauma or from such minimal trauma that the patient is unable to recall the incident. Very frequently, the patient's x-ray films will not show any fractures at the initial examination when they become symptomatic. However, if one repeats x-ray examination a few weeks later, the fracture and wedging are visible and most probably secondary to settling from resultant micro-fractures. Usually, multiple vertebrae are involved.

The treatment recommended is not fully agreed upon, and various medications are being recommended or condemned as their results unveil themselves with time and careful observation.

When one sees a patient with an acute symptomatic fracture or fractures of the vertebrae, a short period of bed rest on a firm bed is recommended. The patient is urged to be active while in bed but not to sit up. Prone lying is encouraged if he can tolerate it. We recommend that the patient remain down seven to ten days and then we ambulate men in a Taylor back brace and the women in a full-length dorsolumbar corset with steel stays. A Taylor back brace can also be used, of course, on women if they will tolerate it. We recommend that they apply and remove their supports while in bed and encourage them to be active in order to lessen the superimposed effects of disuse osteoporosis. The patients are advised to wear their supports a minimum of three months and then gradually discontinue them. If their pain continues or if they prefer to wear the support, we encourage them to do so with the hope that we can prevent or lessen future fractures of the vertebrae. Gentle exercises of the extension type only are recommended for the younger patients after six weeks but, if they cause symptoms or are difficult, they are not encouraged.

Hormonal therapy has been used on patients for a long period of time, and in the female patient estrogens are recommended. The dosage for one of the medications used, ethinyl estradiol, is 50 μg. It is found that, when androgens are added, the estrogens are more efficient. One has to be careful of the side effects of using androgens in females. Methyltestosterone, 10 mg. per day, is used as the androgen. A drug such as Halotestin, 2 mg., is also very effective. Many companies make medications such as Deladumone and Formatrix, which are the combined medications and can be used for hormone therapy in males and in females. In the male patient, it is recommended that methyltestosterone be used daily but one must be certain that there is no evidence of neoplasm in the prostate gland or any medical problem that could be accentuated by using male hormones. Anabolic hormones such as Dianabol and Norandrolone are also used. They have fewer side effects but are not as strong in their anabolic effect. It has been found that these medications function to lessen the catabolic reaction in the bone or the increased bone resorption. These actually function as anticatabolic medications.[5]

The dietary needs of the patient are thought, because of the recommendations of Nordin,[8] to be an adequate- or high-calcium diet. It has been found that a patient given a high-calcium diet can be placed into a positive calcium balance. However, his bone turnover as measured by bone kinetics does not show any change. The patient should take at least 800 mg. of calcium per day.

During the past five years, it has been recommended that a fluoride be used to treat osteoporosis. We have treated patients with sodium fluoride, 22 to 66 mg. per day. This is thought to be a fairly strong therapeutic dose. The use of fluoride is thought to be effective because it should strengthen the molecule so that bone resorption will be inhibited. However, it is known that patients and animals with chronic fluoride poisoning from prolonged fluoride intoxication may readily sustain fractures.

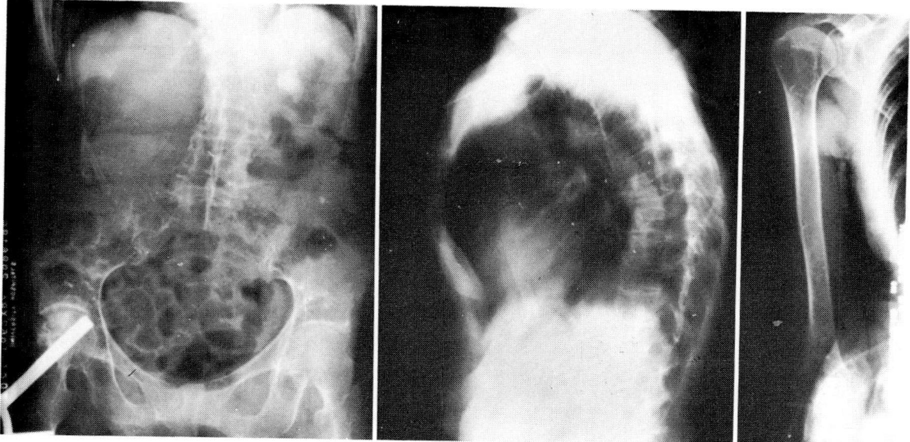

Fig. 10-2. A 69-year-old white female with advanced osteoporosis. Note the multiple compression fractures, increased anteroposterior diameter of the chest, and healed fracture of the right hip.

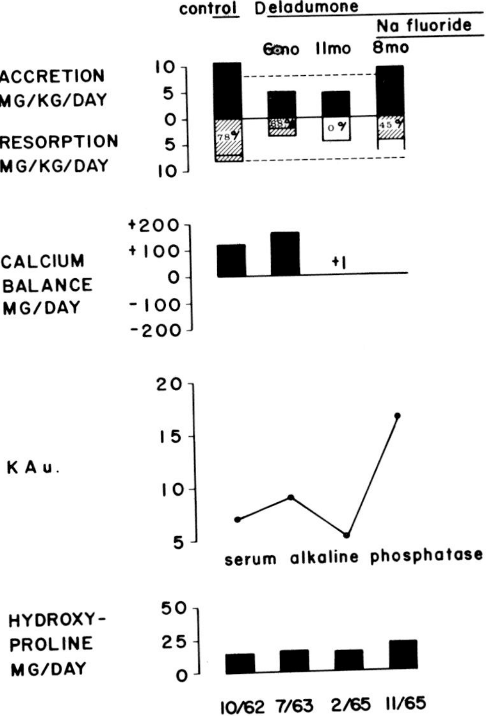

Fig. 10-3. Kinetic and balance data of patient in Fig. 10-2.

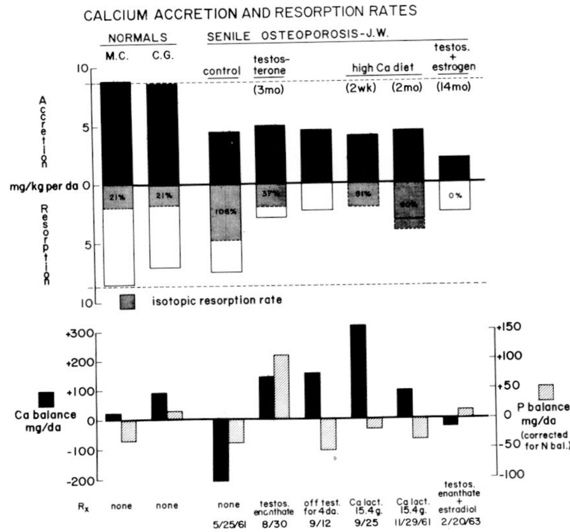

Fig. 10-4. Kinetic and balance data for J. W. show a favorable response to testosterone. The positive state is not maintained and the disease is only arrested, not reversed.

High-phosphorus diets have been tested during the past eight months. The patients that are on this dietary regimen are symptomatically improved. However, they have not been studied long enough for us to come to any definite evaluation of results. A fairly typical patient with osteoporosis is shown in Fig. 10-2. Note that the humerus definitely shows osteoporosis. There are multiple compression fractures in the thoracic spine and there is an increased anteroposterior diameter of the chest. A healed hip fracture, with the internal fixation device in place, can be seen. Fig. 10-3 shows the data of a kinetic and balance study of this patient. The accretion and resorption rates have been determined, using calcium 47 as recommended by Bauer[2] and Lafferty.[5] The patient's control period shows that her accretion rate was within a normal range and her resorption rate was slightly less so that she was in a state of positive calcium balance during this time. The patient's alkaline phosphatase was also normal and the hydroxyproline levels were within normal ranges. It is felt that hydroxyproline levels are a good measure of bone collagen formation. It is noticed that the patient responded to Deladumone by slowing down her bone formation and resorption and then had an increase in the accretion rate while on sodium fluoride therapy. There was also an elevation of the patient's alkaline phosphatase. Because of these findings, it was felt that she was having a satisfactory response to her medication.

Fig. 10-4 shows the kinetic and balance study of a male patient with senile osteoporosis. His control period showed him to be in negative calcium and phosphorus balance and his resorption exceeded his accretion. Testosterone lowered his resorption rate and reversed his balance. This reversal was not maintained, however, and the patient returned to equilibrium. We therefore only arrested his disease and did not cure his problem.

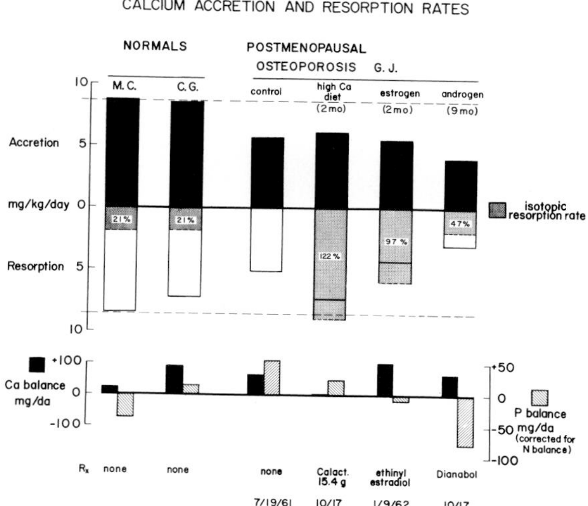

Fig. 10-5. Kinetic and balance data of a white female 64 years of age.

Fig. 10-5 shows a patient with postmenopausal osteoporosis and her response to a high-calcium diet, estrogen, and androgen. Her bone turnover appeared to be slowed but the disease was only kept in an arrested state by her therapy.

Fig. 10-6 shows the lumbosacral spine radiographs of an elderly male with senile osteoporosis. He had been treated for eight months with a high-phosphorus

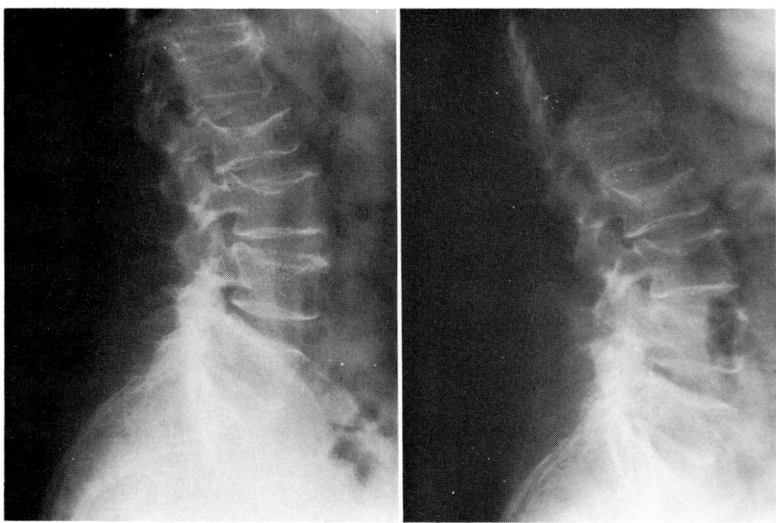

Fig. 10-6. This patient is being treated with a high-phosphorus diet. The x-ray film on the right shows no change after eight months of therapy.

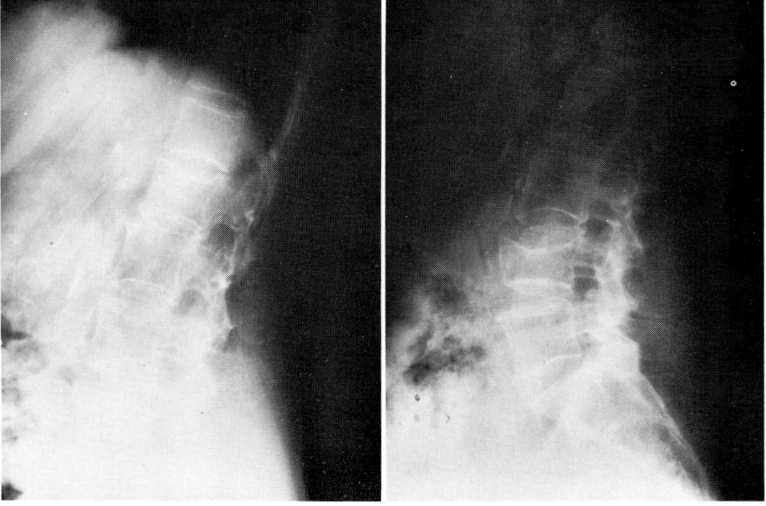

Fig. 10-7. This patient has received 22 mg. of sodium fluoride daily for twenty-six months. Note that there is no change in the x-ray appearance after twenty-six months.

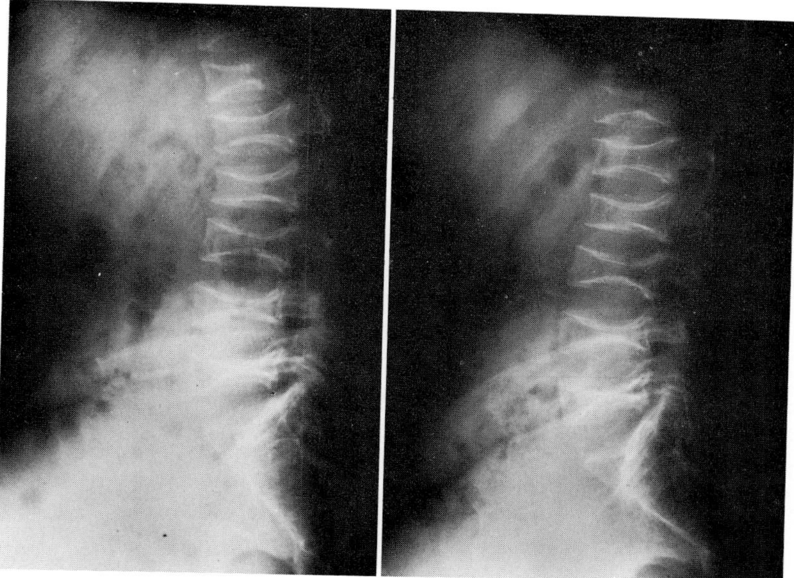

Fig. 10-8. A 30-year-old white male with idiopathic osteoporosis. There is no change after sodium fluoride therapy, 44 mg. daily. The x-ray film on the right was taken after twenty-four months of therapy.

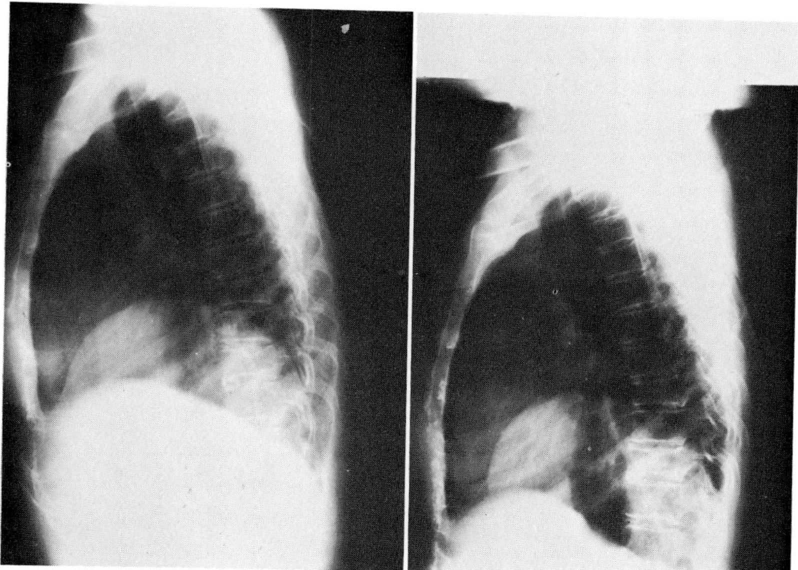

Fig. 10-9. A 59-year-old white female with fractures of one lumbar and two thoracic vertebrae. The x-ray film on the right was taken after three months of estrogen-androgen therapy and shows no change.

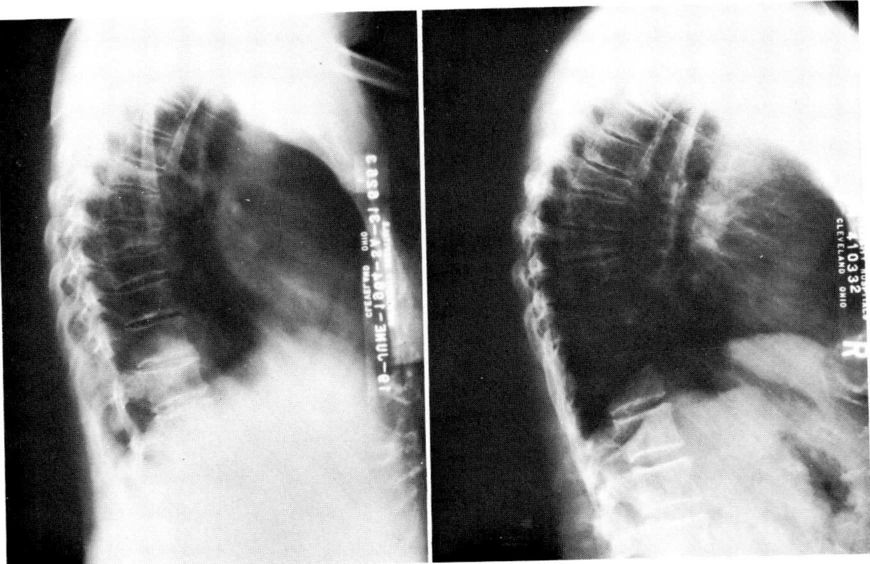

Fig. 10-10. A 61-year-old white female after three and a half years of 66 mg. of sodium fluoride daily. Note the change in the x-ray films, that on the right showing increased density.

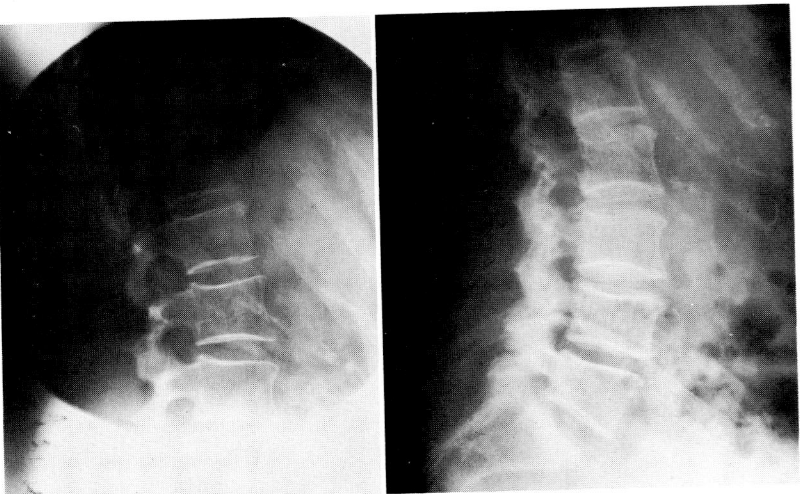

Fig. 10-11. A 61-year-old white female after three and a half years of 66 mg. of sodium fluoride daily. Note the change in x-ray appearance on the right, showing increased density.

intake. There was no change shown on his radiographs, but only a short period of time had elapsed and further observation will be needed to more fully evaluate this method.

Fig. 10-7 gives the radiographs of a patient with postmenopausal osteoporosis who was treated with 22 mg. of sodium fluoride daily for two and a half years. Her metabolic and kinetic studies show only an elevated alkaline phosphatase. The radiographs show no essential change after twenty-six months of treatment.

Fig. 10-8 shows the radiographs of a 30-year-old white male with idiopathic osteoporosis. He has been under treatment with sodium fluoride but has shown no improvement on his radiographs or his metabolic studies.

Fig. 10-9 shows the radiograph of an active, 59-year-old female who is an accountant. She sustained compression fractures of two thoracic and one lumbar vertebrae when she raised a window. She was treated with bed rest for one week, then ambulated in a dorsolumbar corset. She was also treated with hormones and, after three months, was placed on gentle extension exercises. She is gradually discontinuing her support.

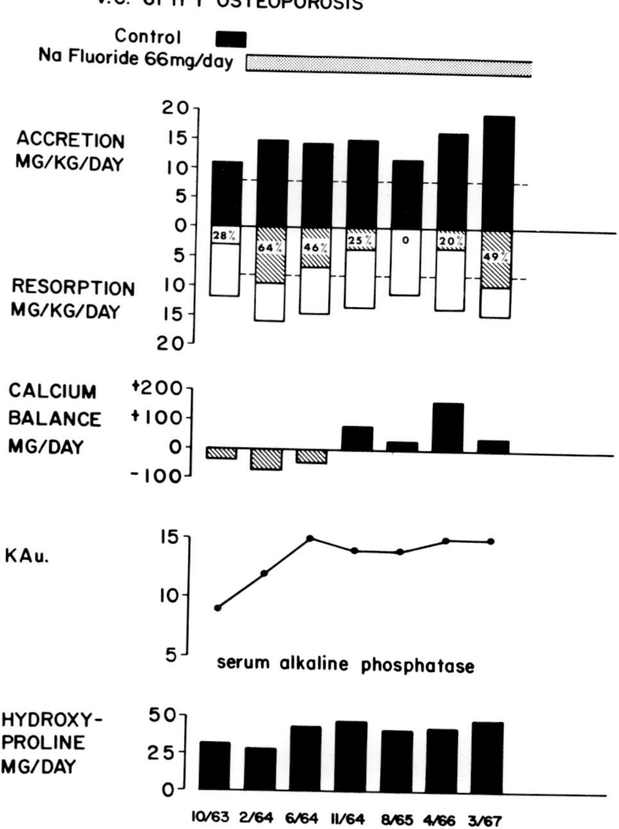

Fig. 10-12. Kinetic and balance data of patient shown in Figs. 10-10 and 10-11.

Figs. 10-10 and 10-11 show the radiographs of a 61-year-old white female with postmenopausal osteoporosis. She has been taking 66 mg. of sodium fluoride daily for three and a half years. The patient is very active and well otherwise. Her compression fractures came from minor trauma. There is a definite change in the patient's radiographs after three years of treatment: an increase in radiodensity and a thickening of the trabeculae. This is the only patient we have treated who has shown radiological change.

Fig. 10-12 shows this woman's metabolic and kinetic data. They are not remarkable except for the elevation of her serum alkaline phosphatase. Liver function tests were done repeatedly and there was no diminished function revealed by them. She was continued on her medication. In the summer of 1967, she was gardening in her yard and was working in a kneeling position. She sat back slowly on her hips and felt pain in her left hip. She did not concern herself seriously with this but did use crutches until she was checked two months later. Fig. 10-13 shows the radiograph taken in October, 1967. Note the partially impacted fracture of the left femoral neck. It is in slight varus. This is consistent with fractures seen to result from mild trauma in patients with osteoporosis. It was very discouraging to have this occur in the only patient who we thought was showing such a satisfactory response to treatment. Her fracture has healed but we have stopped her medication and she is now on hormone therapy.

In summary, it is recommended that patients with acute compression fractures and osteoporosis be given a few days of bed rest and then be ambulated with a

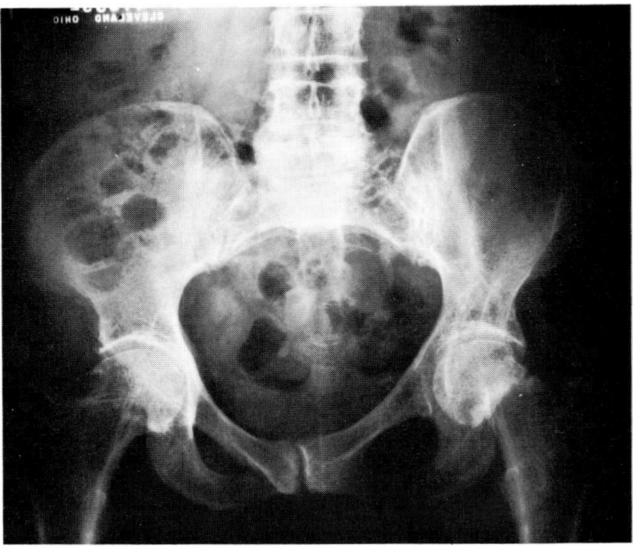

Fig. 10-13. X-ray film of patient shown in Figs. 10-10 to 10-12, following a spontaneous fracture of the left femoral neck after she had increased her bone density on sodium fluoride therapy.

back support. The diet should be high in protein and include 800 mg. of calcium daily. A pint of milk provides this. Hormones still remain the most satisfactory treatment and we know they at least arrest the disease even though they will not cure it. Prophylactic treatment to prevent osteoporosis will be the best treatment when it can be accomplished.

References

1. Arnold, J. S.: Quantitation of mineralization of bone as an organ and tissue in osteoporosis, Clin. Orthop. **17:**167, 1960.
2. Bauer, G. C. H., Carlsson, A., and Lindquist, B.: Bone salt metabolism in humans studied by means of radiocalcium, Acta Med. Scand. **158:**143, 1957.
3. Fraser, R., Harrison, M., and Ibberston, K.: The rate of calcium turnover in bone, Quart. J. Med. **29:**85, 1960.
4. Heaney, R. P., and Whedon, G. D.: Radiocalcium studies of bone formation in human metabolic bone disease, J. Clin. Endocr. **18:**1246, 1958.
5. Lafferty, F. W., Spencer, G. E., Jr., and Pearson, O. H.: Effects of androgens, estrogens and high calcium intakes on bone formation and resorption in osteoporosis, Amer. J. Med. **36:**514, 1964.
6. Macnab, I.: Sound Slide 31, American Academy of Orthopaedic Surgeons.
7. Nordin, B. E. C.: Investigation of bone metabolism with calcium^{47}; a preliminary report, Proc. Roy. Soc. Med. **52:**351, 1959.
8. Nordin, B. E. C: Pathogenesis of osteoporosis, Lancet **1:**1011, 1961.
9. Urist, M. F.: Observations bearing on the problem of osteoporosis. In Rodahl, K., Nicholson, J. T., and Brown, E. M., Jr., editors: Bone as a tissue, New York, 1960, McGraw-Hill Book Co.
10. Whedon, G. D.: Osteoporosis: atrophy of disuse. In Rodahl, K., Nicholson, J. T., and Brown, E. M., Jr., editors: Bone as a tissue, New York, 1960, McGraw-Hill Book Co.

11. Pulmonary function in scoliosis

Scott R. Inkley, M.D.

Any discussion of the problems of cardiorespiratory changes in scoliosis requires a brief review of some basic concepts of pulmonary physiology, a discipline that has developed in the last few years and may not be familiar to those who finished their medical school education twenty or so years ago. An attempt to discuss these points in the short time allowed must, of necessity, be superficial. Therefore, admittedly guilty of oversimplifying, I will attempt to outline several aspects of lung function and some of the ways in which scoliosis may interfere with the normal physiology of the lung.

If we think of the lung for a moment, we recall that it is a highly complicated organ having a thin-walled membrane and a large surface area with blood on one side and air on the other. Any malfunction of either the heart or the lung (in airway, thoracic wall, diaphragm, lung covering, or stretchability of the lung itself) may interfere with the performance of this exchange system.

Approaching the air pump or "bellows" function first, we can divide the abnormalities that develop in the lung and its encasing structures into two broad categories as seen in Fig. 11-1, where the overall size of the bar reflects total lung capacity (TLC); the stippled area, vital capacity (VC); and the dark area, residual volume (RV). Residual volume is the air left in the lung after a forced expiration. In the left-hand bar, the normal relationship of residual volume and vital capacity is depicted, and the two other bars represent obstructive and restrictive types of malfunction. Restrictive abnormalities embrace all the nervous, muscular, or structural (scoliosis) changes, abnormalities of pleura or pleural space, and intrinsic disease of the lung parenchyma that leads to reduction in total lung capacity and vital capacity. Obstructive lesions result in obstruction to flow of air and are characterized by the three well-known clinical entities—asthma, emphysema, and chronic bronchitis. As seen in this illustration, residual volume remains at normal or slightly reduced levels in restrictive disease and increases significantly in obstructive disease. However, on comparing residual volume to total lung capacity (RV/TLC) in a patient with a restrictive disease, one might be misled into thinking that there was obstructive disease present if the ratio of RV/TLC were considered as the prime feature of obstructive disease. This ratio, therefore, must be examined

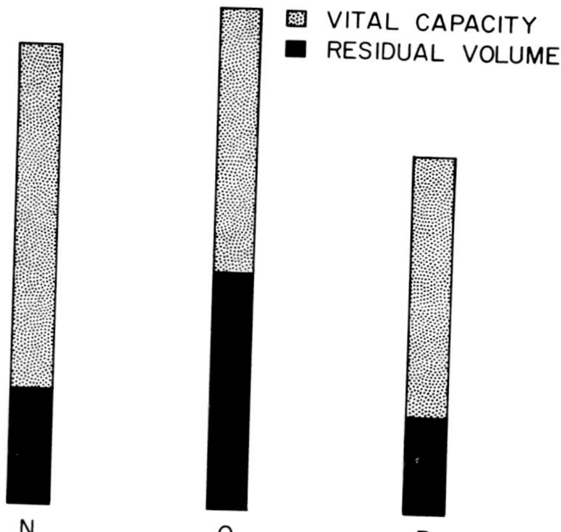

Fig. 11-1. Total lung capacity is indicated by the total bar, residual volume by the dark area, and vital capacity by the stippled area: **N,** normal lung; **O,** obstructive abnormality; and **R,** restrictive abnormality.

in the light of VC and TLC as compared to the predicted value for that individual patient. Patients with restrictive diseases such as scoliosis usually show little or no evidence of airway obstruction at all but, just as other patients, may have obstructive airway disease in addition to their restrictive disease, as seen in Fig. 11-2. In any group of patients with scoliosis, the characteristic feature therefore is a restrictive type of disease with normal to slightly reduced RV and a major reduction in VC over the predicted value for sex, height, and age. Timed VC and maximum breathing capacity may be close to normal.

Abnormalities of the blood-circulating system may also be divided into two broad groups: (1) pump abnormalities such as congenital or acquired defects in the heart and (2) abnormalities of the pulmonary vascular bed. Generally speaking, the total vascular bed is either normal or decreased, as noted in Fig. 11-3. A decrease can be related to congenital abnormalities such as absence of pulmonary arteries or to acquired lesions such as pulmonary embolism or pulmonary artery thrombosis. Reduction of the pulmonary vascular bed to a point where cardiac output in response to exercise is limited certainly results in failure of the gas exchange system.

Perhaps the most difficult concept to achieve and the commonest abnormality to occur in clinical situations has to do with the distribution of both blood and gas, or air, in the proper ratio. Blood must be distributed to those areas of the lung which are being ventilated and air must be distributed to those areas of the lung which are being perfused. This relationship is known as the ventilation/perfusion relationship, or as the $\dot{V}/\dot{Q}$ ratio where $\dot{V}$ = ventilation per minute and $\dot{Q}$ = perfusion per minute in whatever portion of the lung is under consideration.

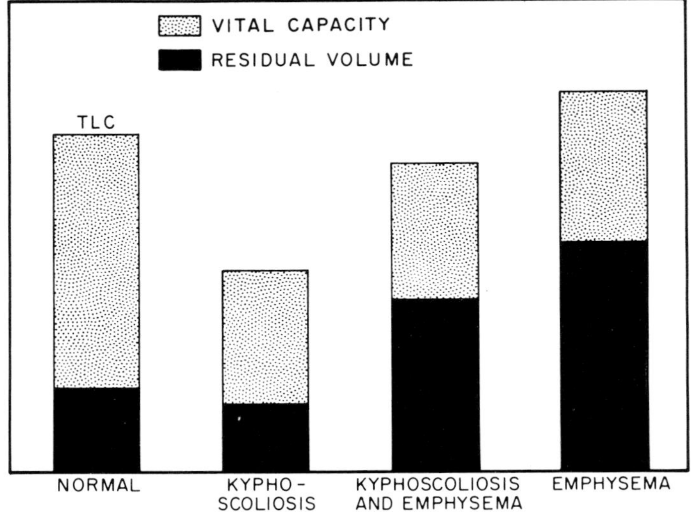

Fig. 11-2. Variations in distribution of residual volume and vital capacity in the normal person and in restrictive, combined restrictive and obstructive, and obstructive disease are shown.

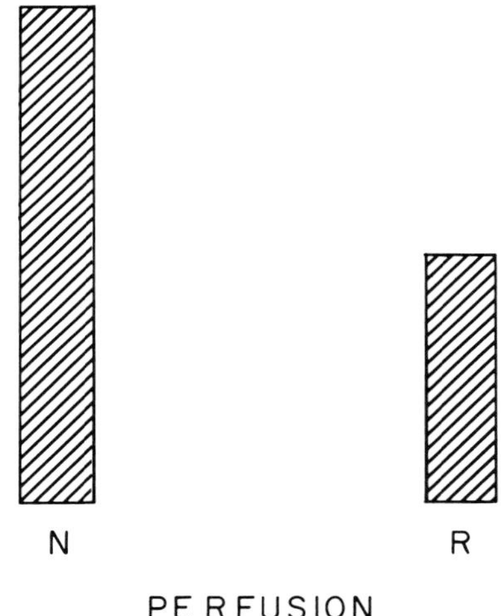

Fig. 11-3. Perfusion, as indicated by the bars, may be normal or be restricted as would occur in a reduced pulmonary capillary bed.

In the normal upright lung, a discrepancy exists in $\dot{V}/\dot{Q}$ in which the apices, which are poorly perfused, are still ventilated. Therefore the ratio of ventilation to perfusion is heavily weighted in favor of ventilation in the upper lung and is heavily weighted in favor of perfusion in the lower part. Fig. 11-4, *N*, shows blood flowing to the lower two-thirds of the upright lung, and the overall size of the bar is the ventilated lung.

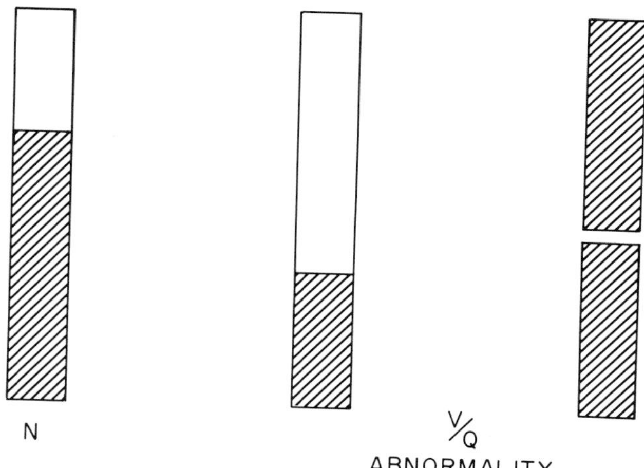

Fig. 11-4. The bar on the left indicates the normal relationship of perfusion and ventilation in the upright normal lung. Total lung capacity is represented by the whole bar and the perfused portion by the hatched area. In V/Q abnormality total prefusion may be reduced; or, as noted in the bar on the right, the perfused portion of the lung may not be ventilated, producing a "physiological shunt."

In the second part of Fig. 11-4, perfusion is markedly reduced in relation to ventilation, as one might expect to see in pulmonary embolism.

The third illustration represents the commonest clinical condition to account for anoxia, and one of great practical importance so far as patient management is concerned. As the diagram indicates, perfusion is occurring in unventilated portions of the lung and leading to what is, in effect, a shunt of blood from the right to the left side of the heart. Typical examples of this would be pneumonia or atelectatic areas behind an obstructed airway. The average overall relationship between ventilation and perfusion is on the order of 4 to 5, or 0.8. When this overall ratio falls, anoxia begins to develop.

Evaluation of both the ventilation/perfusion relationship and ventilation itself depends on a laboratory measurement that has become widely available within the last seven or eight years. This is the determination of partial pressures of oxygen and carbon dioxide by the electrode technique,[5] which has made the procedure one that can be readily carried on in a clinical setting. Partial pressure of gas is directly related to the percentage of the whole which that particular gas constitutes. Partial pressure of a gas in a liquid medium such as arterial blood reflects the partial pressure of the gas, in the gas to which the liquid has been exposed—in this instance, alveolar air.

Fig. 11-5 represents partial pressures of oxygen, nitrogen, carbon dioxide, and water vapor in three different locations: (1) room air saturated with water at 37° C., (2) average perfused alveoli, and (3) arterial blood. There are slight differences between alveolar partial pressures and arterial partial pressures, brought about primarily by venous admixture after blood leaves the pulmonary capillary.

Arterial partial pressures reflect, therefore, the mean alveolar pressure. So far as oxygen is concerned, this is a more sensitive indicator than arterial hemoglobin oxygen saturation because of the hemoglobin dissociation curve which permits relatively high saturations with low partial pressures of oxygen, as illustrated in Fig. 11-6.

By means of arterial pCO_2 values, it is possible to determine the adequacy of alveolar ventilation. Because of highly sensitive central nervous system receptors,

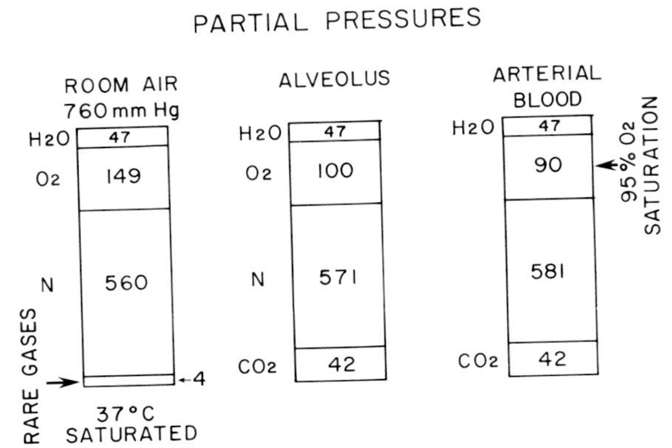

PARTIAL PRESSURES

ROOM AIR
760 mm Hg
H2O 47
O2 149
N 560
RARE GASES 4
37°C
SATURATED

ALVEOLUS
H2O 47
O2 100
N 571
CO2 42

ARTERIAL
BLOOD
H2O 47
90
95% O2
SATURATION
581
CO2 42

Fig. 11-5. The bars indicate the partial pressures of various gases as found in room air, alveoli, and arterial blood.

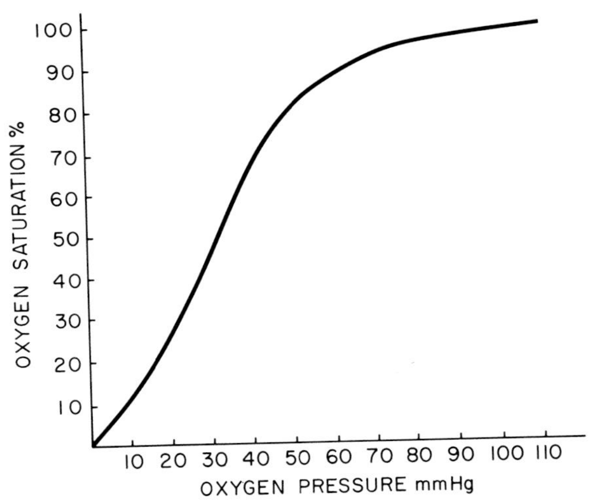

Fig. 11-6. Hemoglobin dissociation curve showing relationship between partial pressure of oxygen and percentage saturation of hemoglobin with oxygen.

partial pressures of carbon dioxide are kept within a very narrow range, with ventilation increasing or decreasing as this value rises and falls. In theory, alveolar ventilation is a term used to indicate the amount of air which is exhaled per minute that has actually come in contact with the pulmonary capillary bed. In the normal individual, this will usually be tidal volume minus predictable anatomical dead space times respiratory rate per minute. In patients with diffuse obstructive disease, such as emphysema, where large areas of lung may be ventilated but have no capillary bed (Fig. 11-4), dead space may be significantly increased and alveolar ventilation be much smaller than would be predicted on the basis of tidal volume and respiratory rate. Suffice it to say: alveolar ventilation should reflect carbon dioxide production by the body and should rise and fall enough to maintain a state of equilibrium so far as partial pressures of carbon dioxide are concerned. It can therefore be said also (1) that when partial pressures of arterial carbon dioxide rise, hypoventilation exists and (2) that in the presence of alveolar hypoventilation, partial pressures of oxygen always fall. Ventilation/perfusion abnormalities, however, are often associated with normal or low values for pCO_2 and are characterized by low values for pO_2.

Most of the patients we have seen who have scoliosis uncomplicated by severe muscle or central nervous system disease, below the age of 35, exhibit little or no evidence of hypoventilation or clinically detectable ventilation/perfusion abnormalities. This has not been the experience of all authors presenting studies of this entity, however.[6] Several have reported unusual ventilation/perfusion changes in patients who have no significant clinical change in blood gases.[2, 4] This change has been characterized by increased perfusion in the apices of the lung, over what would normally be anticipated. The reasons for this are far from clear but are associated with an actual increase in the diffusion of carbon monoxide into the blood by the single breath method of Foerster.[3a]

Exactly what happens to these individuals as they grow older is not clear. It is, however, apparent that the incapacitating and often fatal development of cor pulmonale, with which the internist is concerned in the fourth to sixth decades, is related to inadequate alveolar ventilation. In these patients high arterial levels of pCO_2, low pH, and low pO_2 characterize the picture of kyphoscoliotic heart disease. Bergofsky and co-workers in their comprehensive review of this problem outlined possible pathways for termination of this disease.[1]

A number of studies have shown that low partial pressures of oxygen, coupled with high partial pressures of carbon dioxide and low pH, may be associated with increased pulmonary vascular resistance (Fig. 11-7). Long-standing[3] hypoventilation or increased work of breathing, therefore, either with or without the added complication of infection and the development of severe ventilation/perfusion problems with decrease in oxygen supply to the myocardium, may lead to chronic pulmonary artery hypertension and right-sided heart failure. Reversal of this picture depends on improvement of ventilation and careful addition of small amounts of oxygen administered with the danger of the so-called "paradoxical oxygen effect"

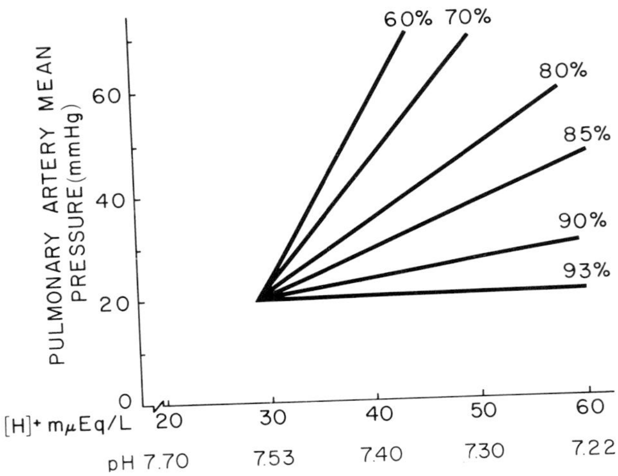

Fig. 11-7. This graph demonstrates the effect of lowering pH and oxygen saturation on pulmonary artery pressure. The isopleths refer to oxygen saturation. (From Ferrer, M. I.: Bull. N. Y. Acad. Med. **41**:942, 1965.)

in mind. The old concept of pulmonary hypertension secondary to torsion of vessels due to chest deformity is no longer accepted.

In any evaluation of changes that scoliosis produces on the cardiorespiratory system, a question of great interest is naturally related to the effect of either surgical or nonsurgical correction of the back deformity. Does correction improve or worsen the ventilatory parameters of these patients? And, even further, does such correction ultimately prevent the end-stage picture of cor pulmonale? The answer to the last question obviously lies years in the future and will be available only after careful evaluation of patient populations, such as ours, has been carried out. The immediate effects of corrective procedures on ventilatory function are also difficult to assess, as has been pointed out in a paper recently presented to the Scoliosis Research Society and presently in press.[4a]

Ventilatory changes by and large indicate a slight improvement after surgery in the group that was studied. However, when correction is made for changes in height of the patient, the improvement is not striking. Further evaluation of these results will depend also on long-term follow-up of this patient population. One problem that comes up in relation to overall use of pulmonary function techniques is the question of identification of patients who should not be subjected to surgery. To set an arbitrary cutoff value for lung function studies would be not only difficult but probably unreliable. We have operated on patients who had very severe respiratory malfunction, with minimum complication. On the other hand, some patients with modest abnormalities may have rather marked difficulties, particularly in the presence of postoperative infection or atelectasis. I think the greatest value, from a clinical point of view, of the preoperative evaluation is that it can be used to identify those patients who may be expected to present the most hazardous postoperative course, and therefore will need the most watchful surveillance on the part of those who participate in their management. It is in these individuals that team evaluation and follow-up after surgery may be most helpful and, conceivably, life-saving.

Obviously any pulmonary infection such as bronchitis or the recent onset of acute upper respiratory infection should be dealt with preoperatively and, if necessary, cause cancellation of surgery. Any patient who presents a problem of postoperative secretions should be managed with a deep tracheal suctioning and postural drainage with clapping. If this is ineffective, he should be given a tracheotomy so that bronchial toilet can be assisted and artificial ventilation instituted if necessary. It is in these individuals that the abnormality of ventilation/perfusion is most striking. Presence of a normal or low arterial pCO_2 in these individuals, coupled with a low pO_2 even in the presence of administered oxygen, indicates ventilation/perfusion abnormality and the need for vigorous improvement of bronchial toilet and even for bronchoscopy if secretions appear to be a problem. Blood gas changes of low pO_2 and high pCO_2 are an indication for assisted ventilation. Arterial blood therefore should be the determining factor in such a patient if problems of this sort develop.

In summary, we see that scoliosis may produce a restrictive type of abnormality of ventilation. Chronically inadequate ventilation of the alveolar capillary bed may lead to pulmonary hypertension and kyphoscoliotic heart disease. Not all patients with scoliosis develop these severe changes. Surgical correction of the curvature does not produce major changes in the restrictive abnormality. The long-term effect of such correction must await further study. Preoperative evaluation of ventilation is important in order to identify those patients who will need intensive postoperative follow-up. Ideal arrangements should include a team approach to the management of such patients.

References

1. Bergofsky, E. H., Fishman, A. P., and Turing, G. M.: Cardiorespiratory failure in kyphoscoliosis, Medicine **38:**263, 1959.
2. Dollery, C. T., Gillam, P. M. S., Hugh-Jones, P., and Zorab, P. A.: Regional lung function in scoliosis, Thorax **20:**175, 1965.
3. Ferrer, M. I.: Disturbances in the circulation in patients with cor pulmonale, Bull. N. Y. Acad. Med. **41:**942, 1965.

3a. Foerster, R. E., Fowler, W. S., Bates, D. V., and Van Lingen, B.: The absorption of carbon monoxide by the lungs during breath holding, J. Clin. Invest. **33:**1135, 1954.

4. Loken, M. K., and Westgate, H. D.: Evaluation of pulmonary function using xenon^{133} and the scintillation camera, J. Roentgen. Nucl. Med. **100:**835, 1967.

4a. Makley, J. T., Herndon, C. H., Inkley, S. R., Doershuk, C., Matthews, L. W., Post, R. H., and Littell, A. S.: Pulmonary function in paralytic and non-paralytic scoliosis before and after treatment, J. Bone Joint Surg. **50-A:** 1379, 1968.

5. Severinghaus, J. W., and Bradley, A. F.: Electrodes for blood pO_2 and pCO_2 determination, J. Appl. Physiol. **13:**515, 1958.
6. Westgate, H. D.: Pulmonary function in scoliosis, Proceedings of American Thoracic Society, May 22, 1967.

12. Nonoperative treatment of scoliosis

Walter P. Blount, M.D.

During the time of Hippocrates, about 400 B.C., crude mechanical therapy was tried in an effort to straighten crooked backs that were called scolioses. Two thousand years later, the uncomfortable, inefficient cuirasses that armorers fashioned from metal were equally unsuccessful in preventing or correcting these deformities. Not until Hessing designed a corset about three hundred years later was there anything approaching adequate support. At the turn of this century there were literally hundreds of different scoliosis braces.

At about that time the more efficient plaster jacket was applied effectively in several German and Swiss clinics. The head was included to maintain adequate distraction much as in the modern localizer cast. Good correction of the scoliosis was obtained but frequently lost because the support was removed too soon.

Early in this century the Klapp system of exercises was recognized in Europe as effective while the children were under treatment in the hospital. Modifications of several European techniques were used by many orthopaedic surgeons in this country. Exercises were prescribed and the patient was "watched" while the deformity became progressively worse. The futile nonoperative management of scoliosis was condemned by most responsible orthopaedic surgeons.

This treatment was so unsatisfactory that after 1914 many American orthopaedists followed Hibbs' lead and fused the crooked spines after partial correction. The results achieved by most orthopaedic surgeons were so bad that the operative approach prevailed in only a few clinics.

By 1940 so much had been learned from the early operative failures that spine fusion finally succeeded, and the results have continued to improve since.

The first Milwaukee brace was presented in 1945 as a means of correcting and holding the scoliotic spine after a fusion operation. Until 1957 Dr. Schmidt and I said repeatedly that it should be used only rarely in the nonoperative treatment. Not until the Milwaukee brace had proved its value was nonoperative treatment worthy of consideration as an alternative to surgery.

As the brace was simplified and used more frequently, we gradually came to realize its value without operation in preventing spinal curves from becoming worse. It was used occasionally in paralytic scolioses and in some adolescent

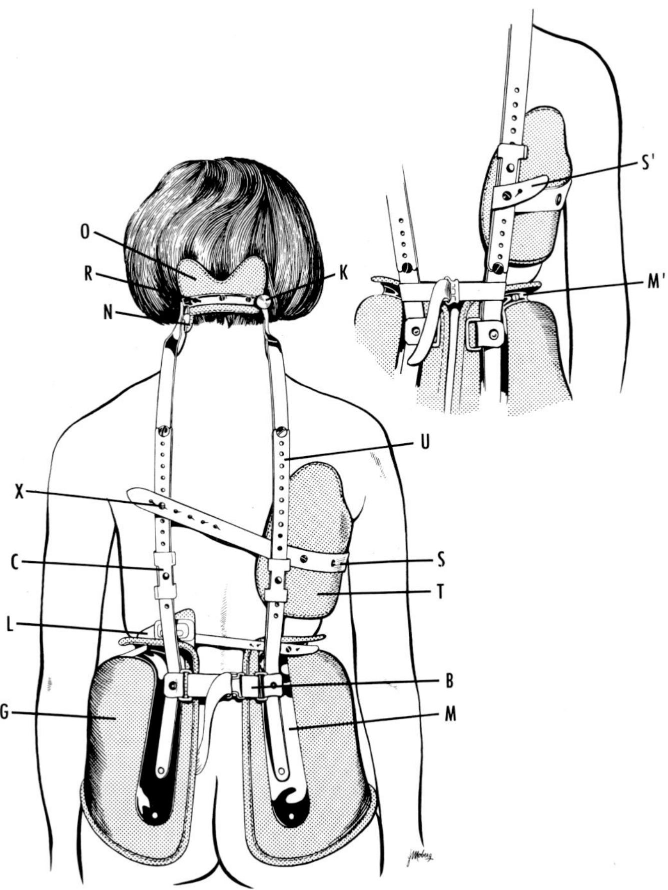

Fig. 12-1. Standard Milwaukee brace shows the detail of the occipital pad, **O,** which is notched to avoid pressure on the occipital protuberance; the neck ring, **R,** is hinged in front and fastened behind to a knurled nut, **K;** the neck pad, **N,** is to cushion the holding force against the neck as the patient is shifted to the left by the thoracic pad, **T;** the posterior uprights, **U,** are twisted 90 degrees at the cephalad ends and attached to the lateral sides of the neck ring. The twist makes them slightly flexible in two directions. The strap, **B,** which tightens the pelvic girdle, **G,** is fastened by a buckle; a framework of Monel metal, **M,** reinforces the girdle. It must be formed into half of a narrow cylinder in the waistline where the cowhide of the girdle is molded deeply. The lumbar pad, **L,** may be slipped under the girdle or between the leather and the Monel metal as correction is obtained. The pad is floated on a nylon strap that is secured at both ends by truss studs. A similar stud, **X,** secures the strap for the thoracic pad. The pad is effective at first in reducing the rib hump. Later, to avoid exaggeration of thoracic lordosis, the strap may be curled around the nearest bar (**S′,** insert) and held with the truss stud. As the girdle is tightened, the nylon belt may be shifted to the posterior bars. Note the detail of the narrowly molded Monel metal, **M′,** at the waist. (From Blount, W. P., and Bolinske, J.: Phys. Ther. **47:**919, 1967. Reprinted with permission from Physical Therapy, journal of the American Physical Therapy Association.)

idiopathic curves that were acceptable and near the completion of growth. As early as 1954 the brace proved in a few growing children that it was successful in improving curves that would previously have required fusion.[1] There was obviously something "different" about this brace[9]—the first in the history of medicine to actuate the permanent improvement of spinal curvatures.[6]

Except for Spitzy's active device that made the child stand tall because there was a sharp button under the chin and another under the occiput, all of the previous braces had relied on passive correction with elastic straps, balloons, and mechanical levers. They were usually worn only during the day. They failed to bring about any lasting correction and rarely prevented the curve from getting worse.

The Milwaukee brace afforded comfortable, passive support by distraction and the holding force of lateral pads.[4] At the same time it was fitted loosely about the torso. Active improvement of the deformity was readily accomplished by cooperative patients.[7] As the curve straightened, the holding pads were advanced and the brace elongated, often excessively. We learned that if the occipital support fitted snugly, the chin pad should be lowered until the chin could be raised 3 or 4 cm. from the pad.

The child participated in all activities except body contact games. The brace prevented the deformity from increasing. The torso could move only in the direction of correction. As the spine shifted into an improved position, the brace took up slack.

Most deformities reached the maximum correction in three months but some continued to improve for several years. Much depended upon the skill with which the brace was employed and the vigor and frequency with which the patient reduced the deformity by the active corrective force of his daily activity and specific exercises in the brace.[5] The success of the treatment varied also with the age of the patient and the flexibility of the spine.

The value of this program was recognized in many clinics in several countries. The combined efforts of orthropaedic surgeons and orthotists with varied backgrounds led to significant improvements in the brace. At first it was supplied with only a single thoracic pad (Fig. 12-1). The correction of lumbar curves was not attempted. Later a lumbar pad was perfected (Figs. 12-1 and 12-2). Its holding force against the second and third spinous processes was remarkably effective. This force was largely passive but the patients were taught to shift away from the lumbar pad actively.

Correction of a right thoracic curve frequently elevated the left shoulder and made the left first and second ribs and scapula protrude. This was particularly noticeable with the double thoracic curve that Moe[8] has described. Unsightly bulging of the trapezius resulted. A ring flange (Figs. 12-2 and 12-3) was perfected to overcome this component of the deformity. With the aid of two or three basic pads, moderate deformity has been improved effectively by nonoperative means in a variety of curve patterns.

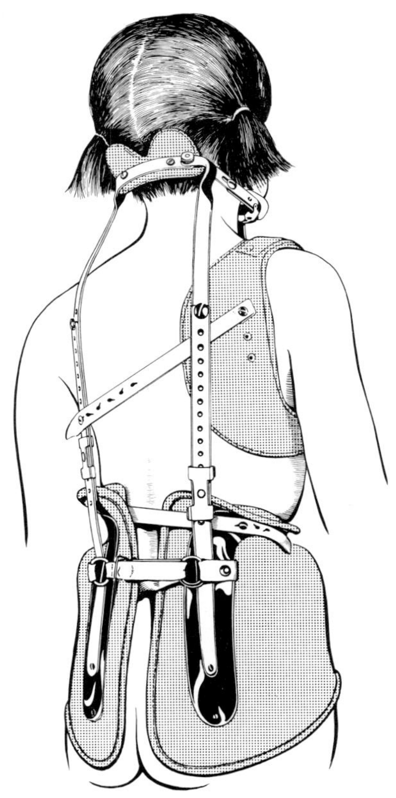

Fig. 12-2. A Milwaukee brace similar to that in Fig. 12-1, except that a ring flange has been used instead of a thoracic pad at the right shoulder to counteract the tendency of the lumbar pad to increase the right thoracic curve and elevate the right shoulder. This pad tends to increase the left upper thoracic curve. It provides some holding force against the seventh and eighth ribs on the right side. In recumbency the flange exerts a passive corrective force on the rib hump. The function of the ring flange may be changed by adjusting the attachment of the strap to the flange. As the screw is lowered, there is more lateral holding force against the ribs and less depression of the shoulder. The truss stud on the left may be raised until the strap is horizontal and there is no effect of holding down the right shoulder. The truss stud may even be raised higher to assist in the elevation of a depressed shoulder. Note that the notched occipital pad fits the contour of the back of the head and neck snugly and furnishes efficient distraction. The chin support may be lower than was originally thought to be expedient. As compared with Fig. 12-1, the back, but not the sides of the pelvic girdle, is higher and closely molded. This modification may be used without any lumbar pad when correction of the left lumbar curve is not important. Here there is a thin lumbar pad under the leather of the girdle. As the lumbar curve improves, the girdle is made more comfortable by shifting the thin pad to lie between the Monel metal and the leather of the girdle. This arrangement is almost as effective as the first. For a moderate lumbar curve, the pad in Fig. 12-1 is usually preferable.

Similar treatment of round back proved even more gratifying. True Scheuermann's disease or extremely poor posture without vertebral osteochondrosis was equally well managed by the combination of the Milwaukee brace and exercises.

For the support of the round back a single broad kyphosis pad was used posteriorly, just below the apex of the curve. The pelvic girdle furnished the holding force against the symphysis pubis and lower abdomen. The neck ring

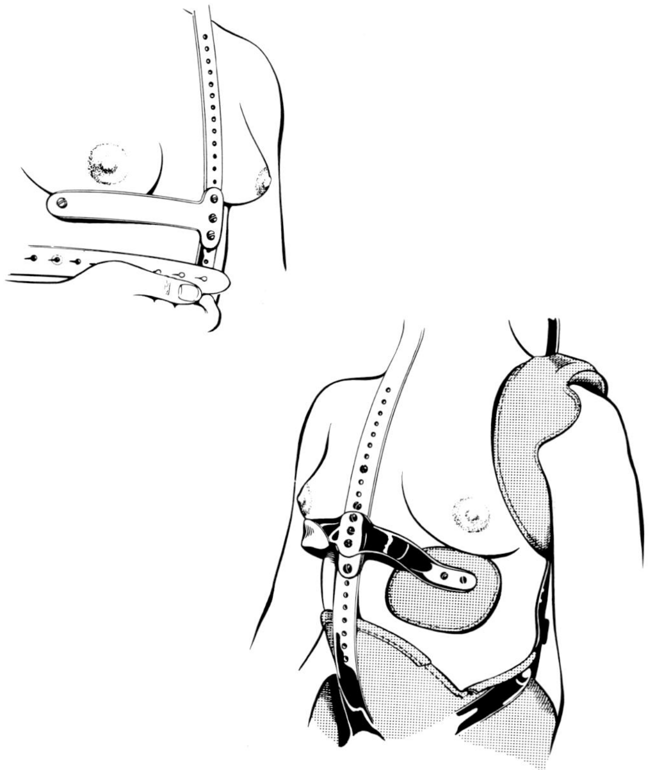

Fig. 12-3. The ring flange is seen from the front as used in correcting a left upper thoracic curve with bulging of the first two ribs under the trapezius muscle. Broadening the ring in front provides a comfortable check to keep the shoulder from drooping forward. Even without an anterior strap, the ring flange restricts shoulder motion. In the daytime it may be replaced by a thoracic pad (Fig. 12-1) in many situations. Sometimes, with a prominent rib hump, both pads may be worn at night. When the patient arches his back like a kitten, the ribs impinge on the pads and the spine rotates to fill out the thoracic valley on the opposite side. This effective exercise is possible only if the posterior bars are far enough from the torso. The inset (upper left) shows the conventional outrigger, terminating in a truss stud for attachment of the strap of the thoracic pad. In the larger figure, illustration at lower right, this outrigger has been combined with one on the opposite side. The small oval pad is most effective in the passive correction of a deformed and protruding anterior costal margin. It should not be used to restrain the normal bulging of the rib cage away from the thoracic pad.

contributed to the third holding force. To prevent undue pressure on the throat for the first few weeks, a sternal pad was held by an adjustable screw with the cephalad margin just above the level of the clavicles.

The patient could shift away from the pads as he wished. In addition, the pelvic tilt was maintained by the brace while the patient performed hyperextension exercises against resistance several times a day. The correction of deformity was rapid in the immature patient. As the treatment progressed and the posture changed, the superstructure was modified to maintain the head and neck in the corrected position.

I have published the results obtained in patients with moderate scolioses and round backs from various causes.[2, 3] Flexible spines corrected well with the Milwaukee brace. Rib humps were reduced, but frequently at the cost of increasing the thoracic lordosis. This tendency was successfully combatted if the child was sufficiently immature and if he persevered with energetic breathing exercises. If treatment was started when the child was young enough to actually grow straight, and if he continued with the brace and exercises full time until his spine was mature by all roentgenological criteria, the correction was maintained after the brace was discontinued.[1, 3] Several years' delay in closure of the vertebral apophyses in the mid-thoracic region sometimes required the prolonged use of the Milwaukee brace at night only.

A girl with a skeletal age of 15 with open vertebral apophyses will obtain compensation promptly.[1] A rib hump will diminish to a gratifying degree and the curvature will be reduced substantially in the brace. The curve does not become worse if the treatment is efficient.

Even though the brace is worn long enough, a girl of this skeletal age will usually lose most of the correction in the first few months after the brace is removed. She is too old to grow straight. She will remain compensated and the rib hump will be diminished. The curves are no worse and the parents are usually well satisfied. This outcome is particularly desirable when two major curves are about equal and 45 degrees or less.

In considering the indications for brace treatment we must include most adolescent patients with idiopathic curves of moderate severity and all young children, no matter what the etiology or the magnitude of the deformity.[3] It is surprising to the uninitiated to see what correction can be obtained with the skillful use of the brace in a 3- or 4-year-old child. We have started brace treatment with patients under 1 year of age but there are many practical objections and it is usually well to rely upon other corrective means such as the Denis Browne splint, plaster bed, or localizer cast until a year or two later.

Congenital curves may be improved by the brace. This is particularly true of cervicothoracic scolioses.[8] Compensatory curves are reduced and the appearance improved. Progression of a congenital curve may be retarded in a brace. Later, if it cannot be controlled, the curve may be fused short and the Milwaukee brace continued until the child is mature. The characteristically short stature associated with congenital scolioses makes the postponement of extensive fusion most desirable.

The spinal deformities associated with Marfan's and Morquio's diseases, cleidocranial dysostosis, and above all, infantile idiopathic scoliosis should be managed successfully with Milwaukee braces if these are applied early enough.

The method is not easier than operative fusion. It takes longer. It requires more patience and an attention to detail that may bore the older orthopaedist who treats scoliosis only occasionally. It is the eager, young orthopaedic surgeon who readily acquires the necessary knowledge and obtains the successful results. It is discouraging to hear professors of orthopaedics condemn the method without knowing anything about it.

There is no reason why one cannot start the nonoperative treatment and then, if the result is not acceptable, fuse the spine. One may plan the treatment of a young child with the hope of improving the scoliosis as much as possible and then holding this position until the child is of a suitable age for surgery.[6]

Cooperation of the parents and the patient is imperative. If their enthusiasm falters, there is no recourse but to fuse the spine. One cannot stop in the middle of the nonoperative treatment. If the brace is removed too soon, correction will be lost even though the child was young enough at the start of treatment and wore the brace faithfully for several years.

One may wean the patient somewhat earlier and more rapidly if the major curve is reduced to 10 degrees or less. If a young child corrects or overcorrects the curve, he need wear the brace only at night. It is well to continue with this program because it is difficult to get a patient to resume wearing the brace after it has been completely abandoned. Even though a young patient has stayed straight when out of the brace for several years, he may relapse during a rapid growth spurt and require further aggressive treatment. Keep him wearing the brace at night and occasionally during the day.

Long-continued pressure on the mandible may cause a bite deformity and flattening of the jaw. This complication has been overemphasized. If the occiput pad fits snugly and if the chin support is not raised too high, many patients with good dentition at the start of treatment will go through the entire course of therapy without significant changes in their bites. Prophylactic treatment with a retainer or a positioner at night may be desirable, however. Before the start of brace treatment all patients should be examined by an orthodontist, and a cephalometric roentgenogram, a photograph, and a bite mold should be made. These records and the cooperation of the orthodontist may be urgently needed later.

Summary

If treatment with the Milwaukee brace and exercises is started early enough, gratifying results will be obtained in scoliosis and round back deformities of moderate severity. The correction will be maintained if the treatment is continued until the patient is mature by all radiological criteria and he is then weaned gradually.

Fewer patients will require operations. Above all, one must condemn observational therapy: just "watching" the deformity progress until surgery is justified.

References

1. Blount, W. P.: Operative und nicht-operative Behandlung der Skoliose. Verhandlungen der Deutschen Orthopädischen Gesellschaft, 50 Kongress, München, Sept. 19 to 22, 1962, Stuttgart, 1963, Ferdinand Enke Verlag.
2. Blount, W. P.: The Milwaukee brace in non-operative scoliosis treatment, Acta Orthop. Scand. **33:**399, 1963.
3. Blount, W. P.: The Milwaukee brace in the treatment of the young child with scoliosis, Arch. Orthop. Unfallchir. **56:**363, 1964.
4. Blount, W. P.: Nonoperative treatment of scoliosis with the Milwaukee brace, Manitoba Med. Rev. **45:**478, 1965.
5. Blount, W. P., and Bolinske, J.: Physical therapy in the nonoperative treatment of scoliosis, Phys. Ther. **47:**919, 1967.
6. James, J. I. P.: Scoliosis, Baltimore, 1967, The Williams & Wilkins Co.
7. MacEwen, G. D., and Shands, A. R.: The improving prognosis in scoliosis: a deforming childhood problem, Clin. Pediat. **6:**210, 1967.
8. Moe, J. H.: Personal communication, 1967.
9. Riseborough, E. J.: Treatment of scoliosis, New Eng. J. Med. **276:**1429, 1967.

13. Methods and technique of evaluating idiopathic scoliosis

John H. Moe, M.D.

Classification of types and patterns of idiopathic scoliosis

Idiopathic scoliosis varies considerably in age of onset, rate of progression, degree and pattern of curvature, amount of structural change, cosmetic deformity, clinical symptoms, effect on pulmonary function, morbidity, and mortality.

The age of onset is difficult to determine unless there were diagnostic x-ray films of the spine made during infancy and throughout growth. Early roentgenograms are seldom available when the child is brought in late for evaluation and treatment. It is astonishing what a severe curve can already be present—with prominent scapula and hip, waist asymmetry, and poor posture—when the parents first notice that something is wrong. Often, it is the dress fitter or the physical education instructor rather than the parent or doctor who is first aware of the deformity. In recent years the pediatrician has realized the importance of early evaluation of scoliosis, and early referral of spinal curvatures to the orthopaedic surgeon is becoming more common.

James described what he called infantile idiopathic scoliosis in 1951 and 1954. The curves were mostly left thoracic and thoracolumbar in infants below the age of 3. They were most common in boys and 83% were progressive. By the age of 10 years nearly all of them had exceeded 70 degrees. James noted that some of the infantile curves of 20 degrees or less disappeared spontaneously below the age of 3 years. These he termed "resolving infantile idiopathic curves."

In 1955 Scott and Morgan published their analysis of 28 infantile idiopathic curves. These represented 12.8% of 218 progressive idiopathic scolioses that were analyzed. These 28 curves all progressed to 80 degrees or more. Ninety-three percent were left thoracic curves but in their group the sex ratio was equal. In 7 additional infants, resolving idiopathic curves straightened spontaneously within an average of two and one-half years. In this group of 7, only 2 patients had curves of more than 20 degrees.

In 1959 James, Lloyd-Roberts, and Pilcher analyzed curves in 212 patients with infantile idiopathic scoliosis and found 135 (63%) of them progressive. Of these, 111 (81%) were thoracic curves. In this same group of 111 thoracic curves, 90 (81%) were left-sided; 65 (58%) were in boys; 5 (4%) were present at birth, and 73 (66%) appeared during the first year of life. The ability of those writers to analyze the prognosis throughout the growing years was handicapped by surgical and other treatment instituted; but they were able to record curve measurement before treatment was started in 47 children up to the age of 5 years, in 37 between the ages of 6 and 10, and in 23 between the age of 11 and maturity.

Of the 47 children measured between the ages of 0 and 5 years, 20 (42%) had curves that were less than 70 degrees, in 23 (49%) curves were between 70 and 100 degrees, and in 4 (8%) they were over 100 degrees.

Of the 37 children measured between the ages of 6 and 10 years, curves in 10 (27%) were under 70 degrees, in 13 (35%) they ranged from 70 to 100 degrees, and in 14 (37%) curves had progressed to more than 100 degrees.

Of curves in the 23 patients untreated and measured from age 11 to maturity, only 2 (8%) were less than 70 degrees, 9 (39%) were between 70 and 100 degrees, and 12 (52%) were over 100 degrees.

In 1965, Lloyd-Roberts and Pilcher analyzed the natural history of 100 infants with idiopathic scoliosis present during the first year of life. The diagnosis was based on (1) a clinically evident curvature that did not disappear when the infant was suspended by the arms and (2) a rib prominence. Anteroposterior x-ray films taken in arm suspension confirmed the diagnosis. Bending x-ray views were not taken routinely. In this group of 100 infants, 67 were boys. All curves were thoracic, ranging from 5 to 40 degrees (suspended). In 10 infants pelvic obliquity was seen, and 83 had head molding (plagiocephaly). With an average follow-up of three years, complete resolution to a straight spine occurred in 92. Seventy-eight fully resolved within the first year of observation. Several initially deteriorated and then resolved, one from an increase of 27 degrees. Three developed secondary structural curves before resolving. Three with secondary structural lumbar curves have remained benign up to age 13. Only 5 in the whole group developed a progressive curve of bad prognosis. There were no special features in these curves.

Eighty-three had skull molding, frontal and occipital; sternomastoid tumors were found in 3 of these. Rib cage molding was present in all. In 50 it was present without x-ray evidence of rotation. Pelvic obliquity was found in 10, associated with limited abduction on the convex side.

In the same issue of the British Journal of Bone and Joint Surgery is a short report by Walker analyzing a group of 49 patients with infantile idiopathic scoliosis routinely treated with a Denis Browne scoliosis tray. In 81.7% the curves resolved and in 18.3% there was progression. Walker's report indicates that this treatment gives the same or slightly poorer results than those found in the analysis of the natural course as reported by Lloyd-Roberts and Pilcher.

Infantile idiopathic scoliosis in its progressive or resolving forms continues to be far more common in Great Britain and on the European continent than in the

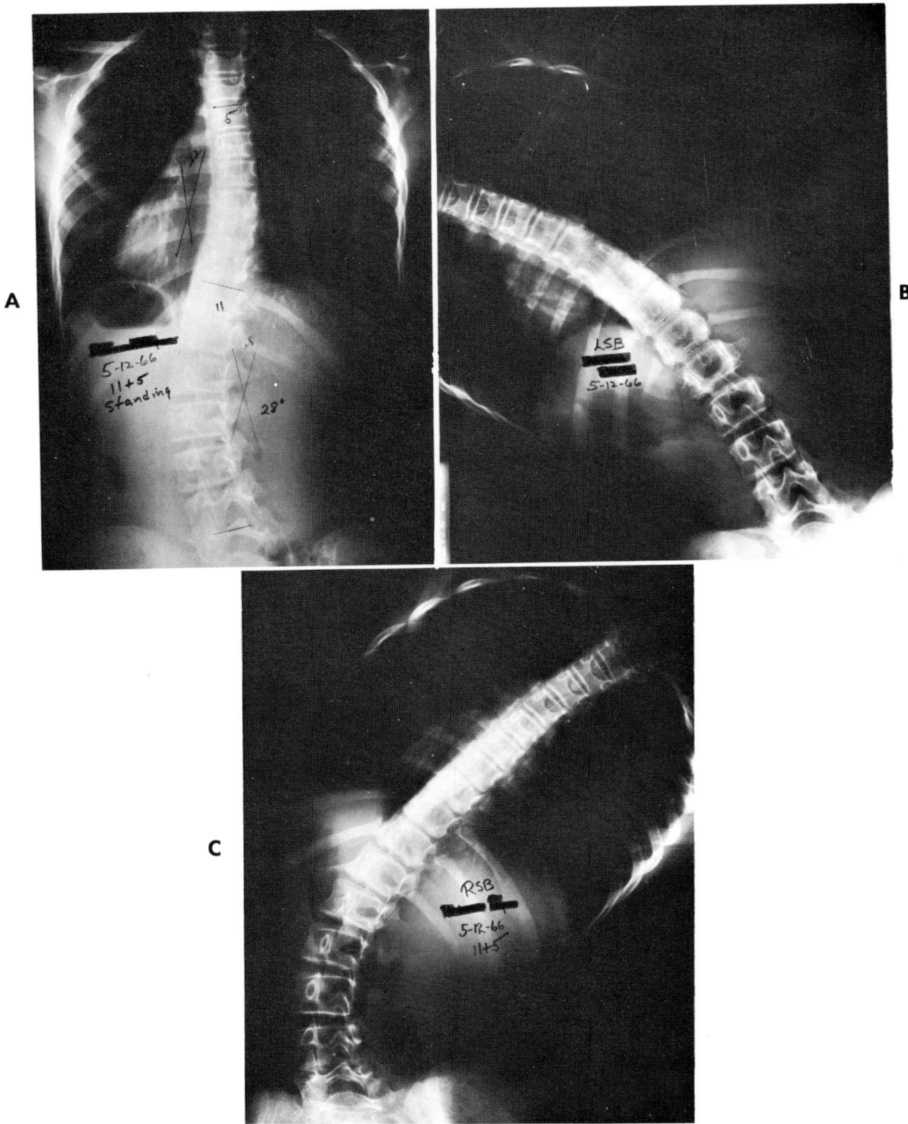

Fig. 13-1. D. R. **A,** Double primary curve, right thoracic, T5 to T11, 22 degrees, and left thoracolumbar, T11 to L4, 28 degrees. Note that L5 is also in the lumbar curve and has a slightly oblique "takeoff" from the sacrum. **B,** On left side bending the lumbar curve is completely flexible, including complete flexibility at the lumbosacral joint. The thoracolumbar curve overcorrects. **C,** On right side bending the thoracic curve is completely flexible except for borderline loss of normal flexibility at T7 to T10 region. Note lack of normal bending at L5 and at L4 to L5. This contributes to the formation and progression of the left lumbar curve.

United States and Canada. Its incidence in other parts of the world still remains to be investigated.

All juvenile and adolescent idiopathic scolioses begin as small flexible curves in previously straight spines. Presumably, this is true in the majority of the infantile variety, also, although a few have shown structural manifestations at birth.

Treatment of progressive infantile idiopathic scoliosis must be aggressive, for the problem magnifies as the curvature increases. When one is reasonably certain that spontaneous resolution is not going to materialize, the Denis Browne scoliosis splint (described in article by Walker[10]) will serve adequately in the infant. Risser localizer casts should be applied under intubation anesthesia if the curve is not easily controlled. With the new thermoplastic isoprene plastic used for the pelvic girdle, a Milwaukee brace can be fitted at an early age. Curves that have been neglected or are not controlled must have correction with a wedging turnbuckle cast and short fusion performed on the convex side of the central vertebrae of the curve. After this has matured, the Milwaukee brace will control the curve with greater efficiency. (See Fig. 13-23.)

The infantile idiopathic curve is likely to be detected and x-rayed while it is still small. The idiopathic curve that appears after the age of 3 is often unnoticed for some time. The exact age of transition from a straight spine to a laterally curved spine frequently remains in doubt. The "juvenile type" that occurs from age 3 to puberty is often not x-rayed until it is over 50 or 60 degrees and already has structural changes. When the curve is still small, side bending x-ray films may demonstrate complete flexibility. Later, they will show slight loss of flexibility, particularly within the apical area. The juvenile curves appearing after the age of 5 or 6 are like those of adolescence, occurring predominantly in girls, and most are initially right thoracic. (See Fig. 13-1.)

In the curves of adolescence it is likewise difficult to determine the exact time of onset. They are like the earlier curves in that the more growth remaining in the spine, the greater the potential for progression. Rapid growth spurts are likely to be associated with worsening of the scoliosis but not always.

Throughout the age range of the juvenile and the adolescent scolioses, curves will be found that do not progress for a number of years. Occasionally, curves will regress spontaneously without treatment.

The idiopathic curve of adolescence is most common in girls. Girls of the adolescent age are characteristically reticent to appear unclothed before their parents. The family physician is not likely to examine the girl's back and, as a result, early curves are unnoticed. Many a doctor is shocked when he suddenly discovers that his 12-year-old daughter has a severe curve that has just been noticed.

If we accept the thesis that idiopathic scoliosis develops as a flexible curve in a previously straight spine, we must also agree that there is extreme variability in the rate of progression and the severity of structural manifestations (Fig. 13-2). As in infantile idiopathic types, juvenile and adolescent curves may never become cosmetically deforming or assume significant structural changes. A few retain complete

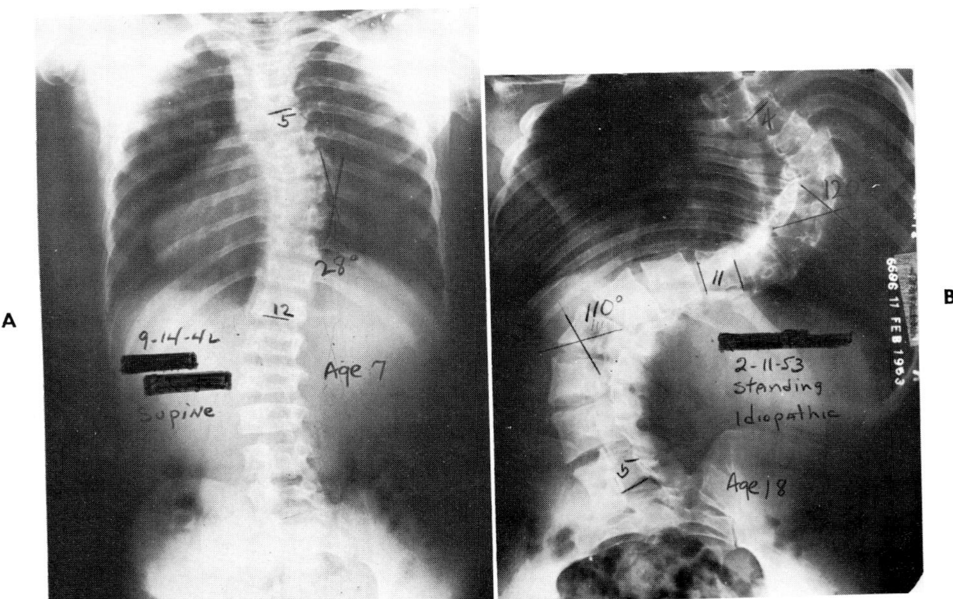

Fig. 13-2. A, Right thoracic curve is the larger but the left lumbar shows structural rotation. This may have been a right thoracic primary, with the left lumbar secondarily becoming structural, or the lumbar curve also may have been primary. To distinguish, early side bending x-ray films would be required. **B,** It is difficult to evaluate primary curves when they are of long duration and are severely structural. This patient would ordinarily be considered to have two primary curves. Were they so at their start?

flexibility throughout the growing years. Occasionally, one may show improvement during growth (Fig. 13-3). Some moderately deforming curves retain a high degree of flexibility into adult life.

Scolioses that retain flexibility and do not develop significant deformity have been called "postural curves" or "functional curves" in the past (Fig. 13-4). Both in juvenile and adolescent ages, small curves are discovered that are completely flexible on side bending x-ray study and that remain flexible, in the juvenile age particularly. This "postural" curve may show some variation in the degree of curvature on different occasions. Until structural fixation is demonstrated, these young persons need no treatment other than correction of bad postural habits. The severe idiopathic curve that was at first completely flexible and later assumed a structural change was a "postural" or "functional" curve that progressed.

A "functional" curve does occur when there is a leg length discrepancy. Such a curve has a lumbar or thoracolumbar pattern and is seen on the standing anteroposterior x-ray film, where the low pelvis is also noted on its convexity. The curve disappears on the sitting and supine films. It remains completely flexible and does not assume structural changes on x-ray view or on forward bending, unless it becomes a participant in a coincidental idiopathic structural scoliosis.

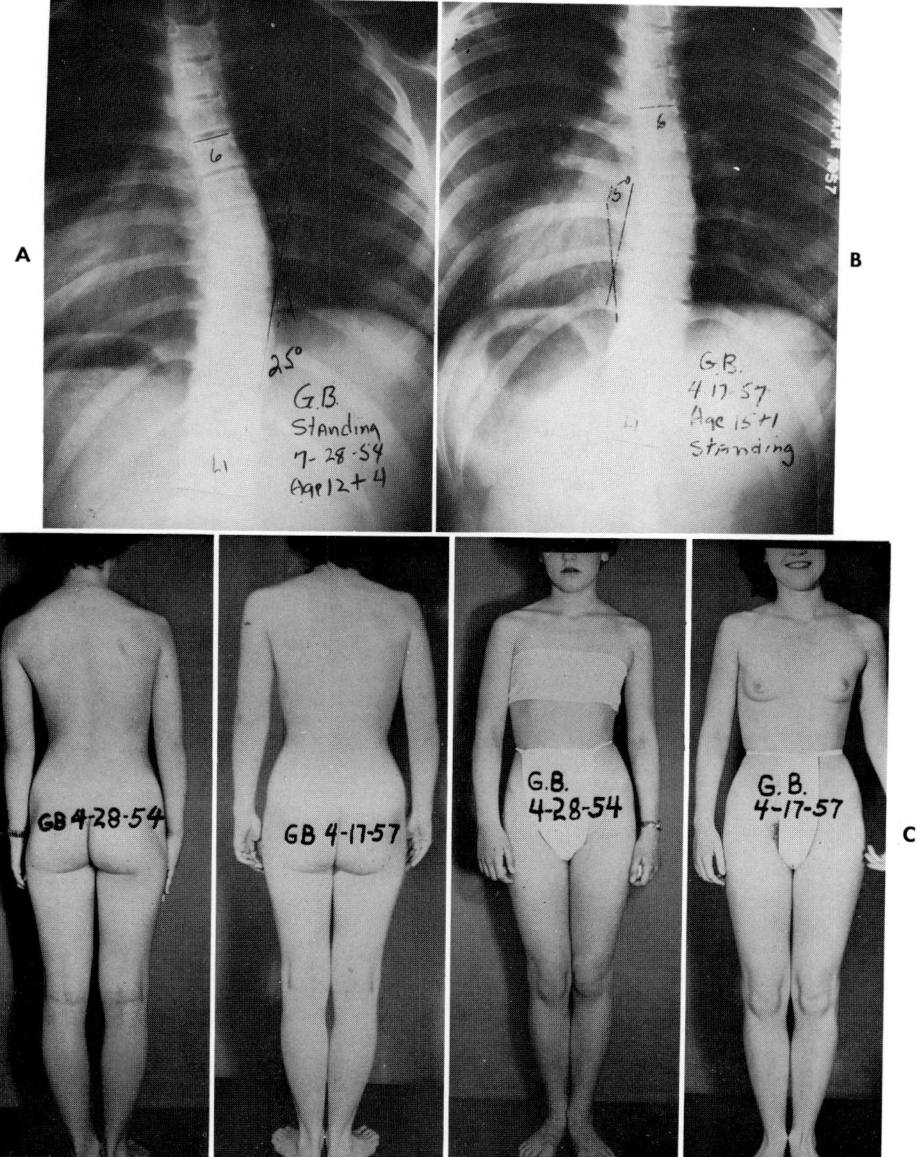

Fig. 13-3. A, X-ray film showing right thoracic curve, T6 to L1, 25 degrees at age 12 + 4. **B,** Three years later, the curve had spontaneously reduced to 15 degrees. There had been no treatment. **C,** Photographs of the patient, showing improvement in cosmetic appearance with regression of the curve.

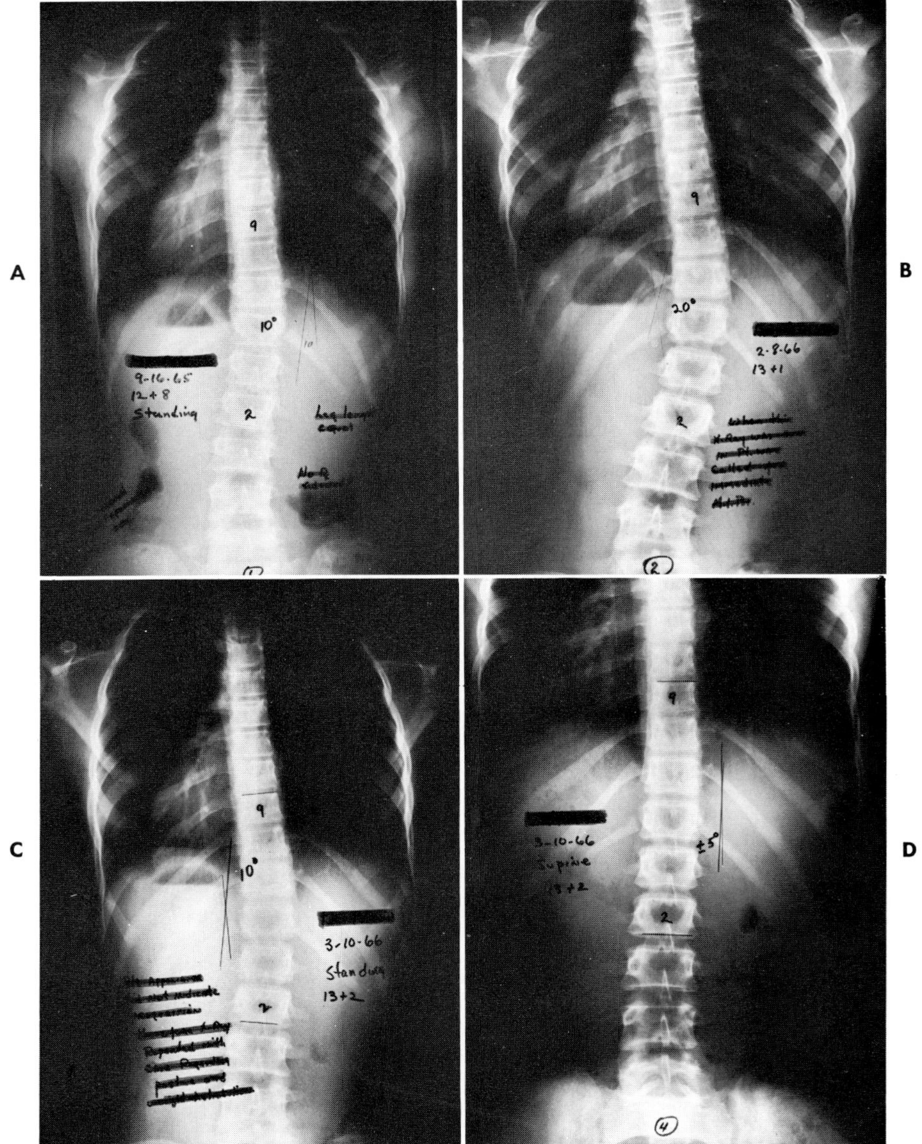

Fig. 13-4. L. P. **A,** At chronological age of 12 years 8 months, this patient had a minimal right thoracolumbar curve without rotation. The leg lengths were equal. The iliac apophyses showed beginning ossification anteriorly. Because of the minimal degree of curvature no treatment was advised; the parents were told to have another standing x-ray film made in three months and have this carefully reviewed. **B,** The parents waited five months and then reported to the orthopaedic surgeon for the x-ray examination requested. This showed an increase of the curve from 10 to 20 degrees. The patient was called in immediately for Milwaukee brace fitting. There now appeared to be a grade I rotation of the apical vertebrae. **C,** L. P. reported back one month later. Before the brace was ordered another standing x-ray film was taken with care to have equal weight distribution. This revealed no change in angulation from the original 10 degrees, standing. Side bending films were also taken, as well as a supine view. **D,** Supine view revealed almost complete straightening and no rotation.

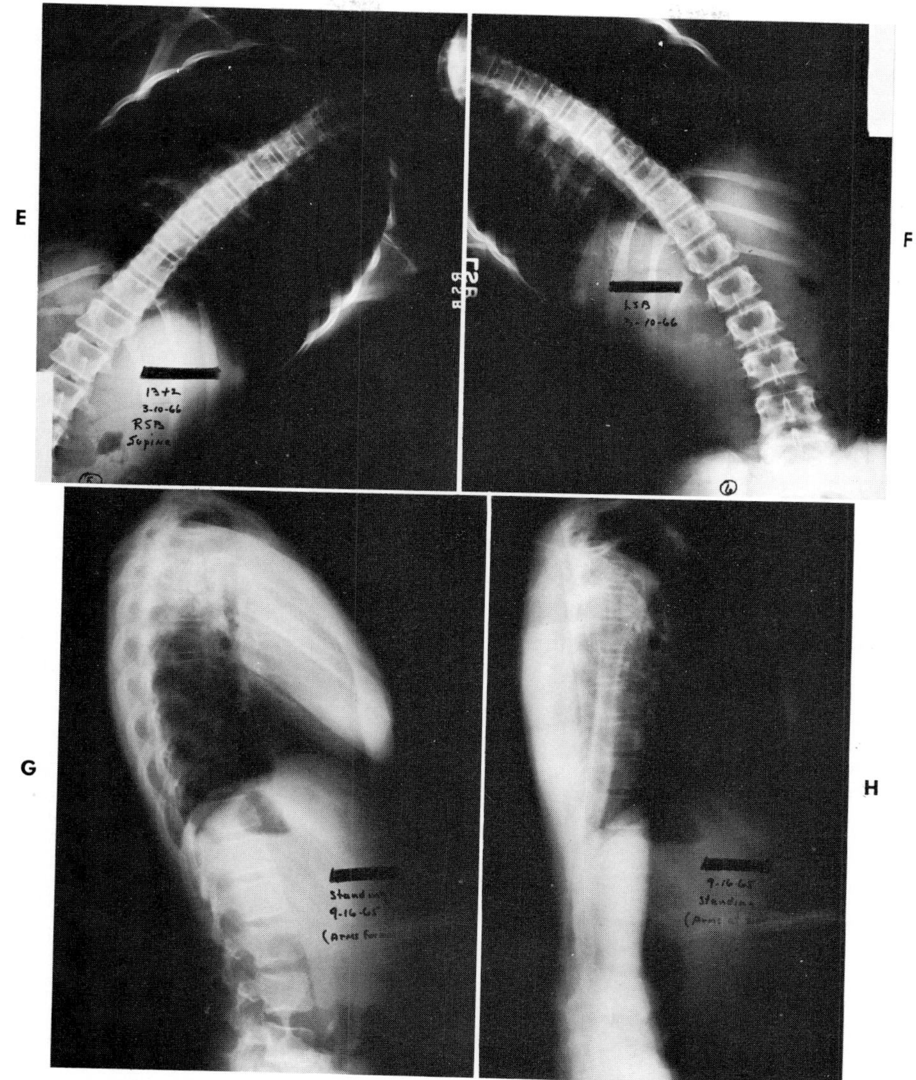

Fig. 13-4, cont'd. E, Right side bending x-ray film showed normal mobility. **F,** Left side bending x-ray views also showed normal mobility, and the brace order was canceled. This patient has shown no subsequent increase in curve angle or structural change. **G,** Of interest is a lateral spine x-ray film taken with the arms held forward resting on a bar. This revealed a normal physiological posterior thoracic curvature. Note the slight posterior protrusion of the rib cage. This is normal. **H,** X-ray film taken at the same time as that in **G** but with the arms held at the side and the patient in erect "military" position. There is a flattening of the normal posterior thoracic curve and even a slight reversal. The same will occur if the x-ray film is taken with the arms held directly overhead.

When this occurs, the short lower extremity with its low pelvis will increase the lumbar curve in the standing x-ray film; restoring a level pelvis will lessen the degree of curvature if it is flexible. On rare occasions the low pelvis is seen on the concave side of a lumbar curve. In this event it will play a helpful role in its treatment.

"Postural" curves are seen in patients who assume a relaxed slumping posture with weight unequally borne. When these curves are seen on the standing x-ray film, they may cause undue concern unless it is recognized that they represent only one frame of a motion picture. These are usually thoracolumbar curves. A curve localized within the thoracic spine is rarely postural. A curve that demonstrates even a small amount of loss of normal flexibility on side bending x-ray view is never to be diagnosed as a postural curve.

The importance of differentiating curve patterns in idiopathic scoliosis has not been emphasized in medical literature. Curves can best be designated by the level of the end vertebrae of each curve.

In 1950 Ponseti and Friedman provided a classification that has been used as a guideline in most subsequent writings. Some of their definitions need revision. Structural idiopathic curves seldom extend into the cervical spine although they often include the first thoracic vertebra. In the presence of cervical ribs, C7 to which the ribs are attached will often become a part of the thoracic curve. In other than this circumstance, idiopathic scoliosis very rarely develops a cervicothoracic curve pattern. Structural cervicothoracic curves do occur frequently in paralytic, congenital, high posttraumatic and postsurgical scolioses and in those of almost every other etiology.

In an x-ray film taken with the patient standing with both knees straight, a high pelvis on one side is due to an inequality of leg length or a difference in size of the innominate bones producing an inequality in height of the ilia. A high pelvis on the convex side of a lumbar curve is not detrimental, while a low one is.

Lumbosacral anomalies may interfere with mobility of the lower end of an idiopathic lumbar curve. (See Fig. 13-1.) Fixed obliquity occurs in some spines with lumbosacral spondylolysis or spondylolisthesis and may be the cause of a long thoracolumbar curve. These and other anomalies may cause an angulation between the L5 body and the sacrum and may contribute to the magnitude of an idiopathic lumbar curve. Spina bifida occulta does not appear to have an influence on spinal curvatures, although the incidence in idiopathic scoliosis is higher than normal.

Before classifying curve patterns, one must first clarify the meaning of the terms used in describing them.

Idiopathic scoliosis begins with a curve that we may call *primary,* and to balance the spine other curves develop secondarily for *compensation*. The primary curve may be single or two primary curves may develop simultaneously. When these two curves progress and develop structural changes similarly, they are called *double primary curves*. When an idiopathic right thoracic scoliosis has been present for a considerable period of growth and the compensatory curves have acquired structural qualities, it may be impossible to tell which of the structural curves was primary. When we recognize that curves are of major importance in magnitude and structural elements, they are called *major curves*. Such curves need not be primary. Structural changes are variable and include vertebral wedging, intervertebral disc wedging, joint distortion, rotational deformities, and soft tissue contractures.

The *secondary* or *compensatory* curves may remain completely flexible throughout vertebral growth or may lose flexibility and develop other structural characteristics best demonstrated by voluntary side bending x-ray films in the supine position.

The commonest idiopathic scolioses in the juvenile and adolescent age are the *right thoracic* with end vertebrae at T4 to T6 and at T11 to L2.

They begin as totally flexible curves of about 10 degrees and usually progress with loss of flexibility and the development of other structural changes. Such loss of flexibility is noted in the supine anteroposterior active side bending roentgenograms. In these earliest structural changes no asymmetry of the rib cage is noted on clinical forward bending examination. At first there is soft tissue contracture. As the curve increases, unequal pressure on the ring apophyses and on the cartilaginous growth plates develops. This may lead to inequality of the rate of growth on the convex and concave sides and ultimately produces vertebral wedging. (See Fig. 13-5.)

The right thoracic curve will progress more rapidly in both angulation and structural fixation than do the secondary curves above and below it. Ultimately, all three might become major curves. The less the structural fixation in the secondary curves, the less they need to be considered in the treatment program.

When the secondary lumbar curve has developed a high component of structural fixation, it is similar to the double primary curve (Fig. 13-2). Side bending x-ray films will demonstrate greater fixation in the right thoracic curve and confirm its primary nature. Such a structural lumbar curve often becomes a major curve that must be maximally corrected and fused along with the thoracic curve. When the secondary lumbar curve has retained a large flexible component, it will not require fusion. It will straighten sufficiently to establish balance with the corrected thoracic curve.

Most right thoracic primary curves have associated left high thoracic secondary curves, most often T1 to T5 or T1 to T6. When the right thoracic curves include T4 (or, as it does occasionally, T3), there is seldom any structural fixation in the half-hearted attempt to develop a high thoracic compensatory curve. On the other hand, the longer high left thoracic compensatory curves seldom remain completely flexible on side bending to the left. The structural fixation is seldom enough to require fusion in correction.

The clinical evaluation of the high thoracic curve is important. In this area curvatures of relatively small angulation, having a high degree of rotation and structural fixation, may produce a disfiguring asymmetry of the trapezius border of the lower neckline. The right thoracic curve pattern may have a left high

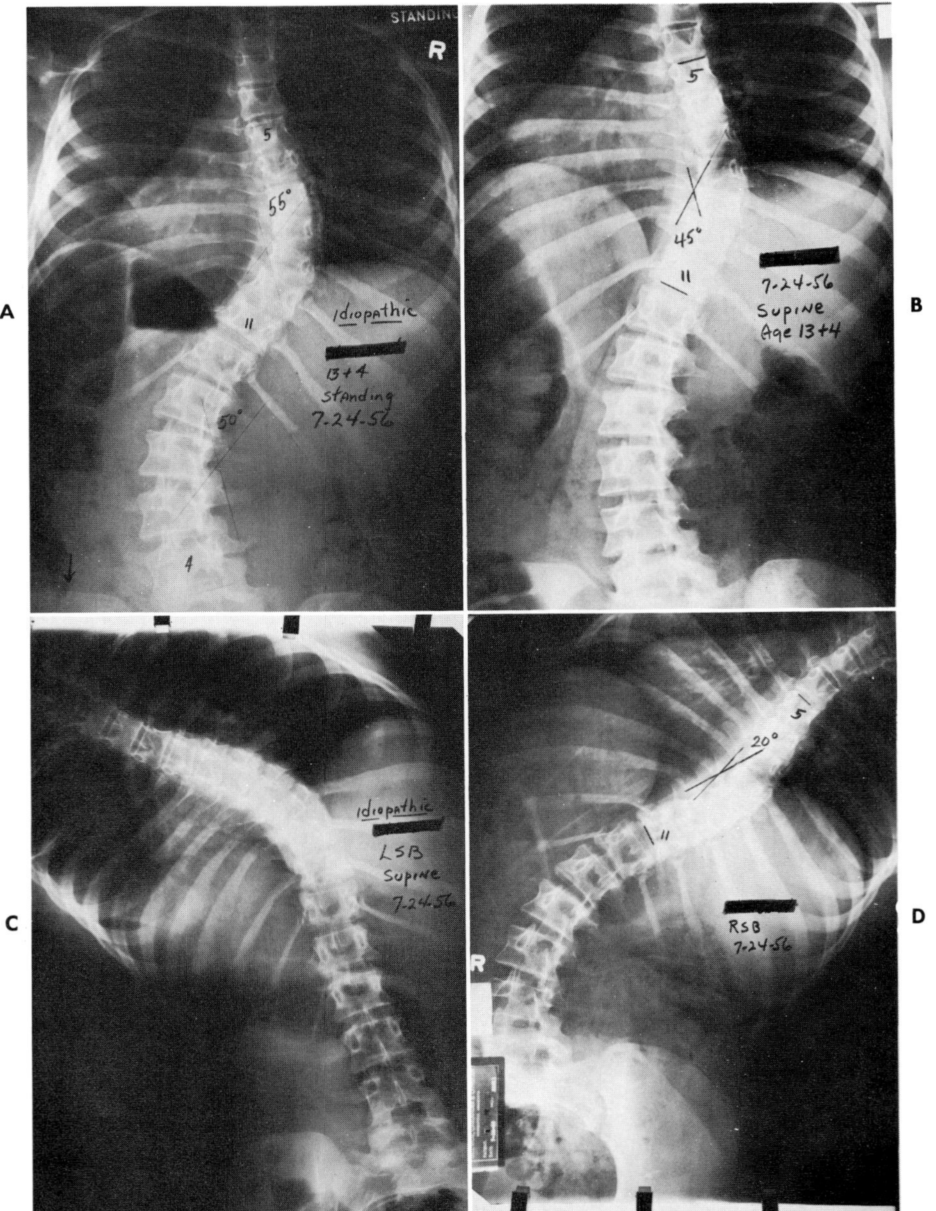

Fig. 13-5. For legend see opposite page.

thoracic secondary curve which demonstrates this structural deformity. In this event, correction and fusion of the right thoracic curve alone will accentuate the deformity produced by the uncorrected upper thoracic curve. Both curves need correction and fusion. (See Fig. 13-6.)

When the right lower and the left high thoracic curves develop and progress simultaneously, a *double thoracic major* pattern is established. In these, the degree

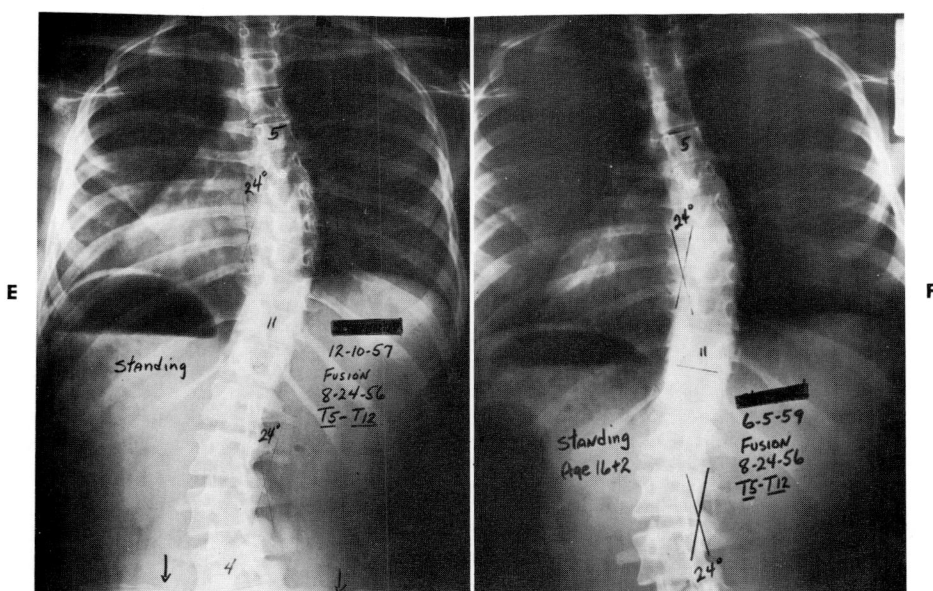

Fig. 13-5. A, Illustrative right thoracic idiopathic curve. Age 13 + 4. Iliac apophyses have appeared and have completed about half their excursion. The right thoracic curve is the major curve. The left lumbar curve is compensatory and flexible, although showing rotation on the standing film and clinically on forward bending. T5 to T11 are neutral in rotation. Fusion area will be either T5 to T11 or T5 to T12, preferably the latter to play safe. **B,** Supine view. There is correction of 10 degrees as compared with the standing x-ray appearance. **C,** On left bending, the compensatory curves show good flexibility. This means that if the major curve is corrected and fused, the compensation curves will straighten so as to balance the corrected major curve. **D,** On right side bending, voluntary, supine, the major curve straightens from 55 degrees standing to 20 degrees. Cast correction should aim at obtaining this amount of correction. In more structural and rigid curves, cast correction will usually exceed the correction shown on the bending film. **E,** Sixteen months after fusion, T5 to T12. Maximum correction was to 22 degrees. Minimal loss of correction during period of consolidation of the fusion. Full Risser localizer cast was worn for five months, then removed for x-ray films. These showed a substantial graft, so another full-length localizer cast was applied and the patient was allowed to be fully ambulatory. (She had not been allowed up the first five months.) At ten months after fusion, the full-length localizer cast was removed and a snug cast applied to the trunk under the arms. All external support was removed at eleven months after fusion, since the graft looked solid and mature. **F,** Three years after correction and fusion, there has been no loss. The flexible compensation curve has balanced the angle of the fused major curve. The patient presents an excellent cosmetic appearance.

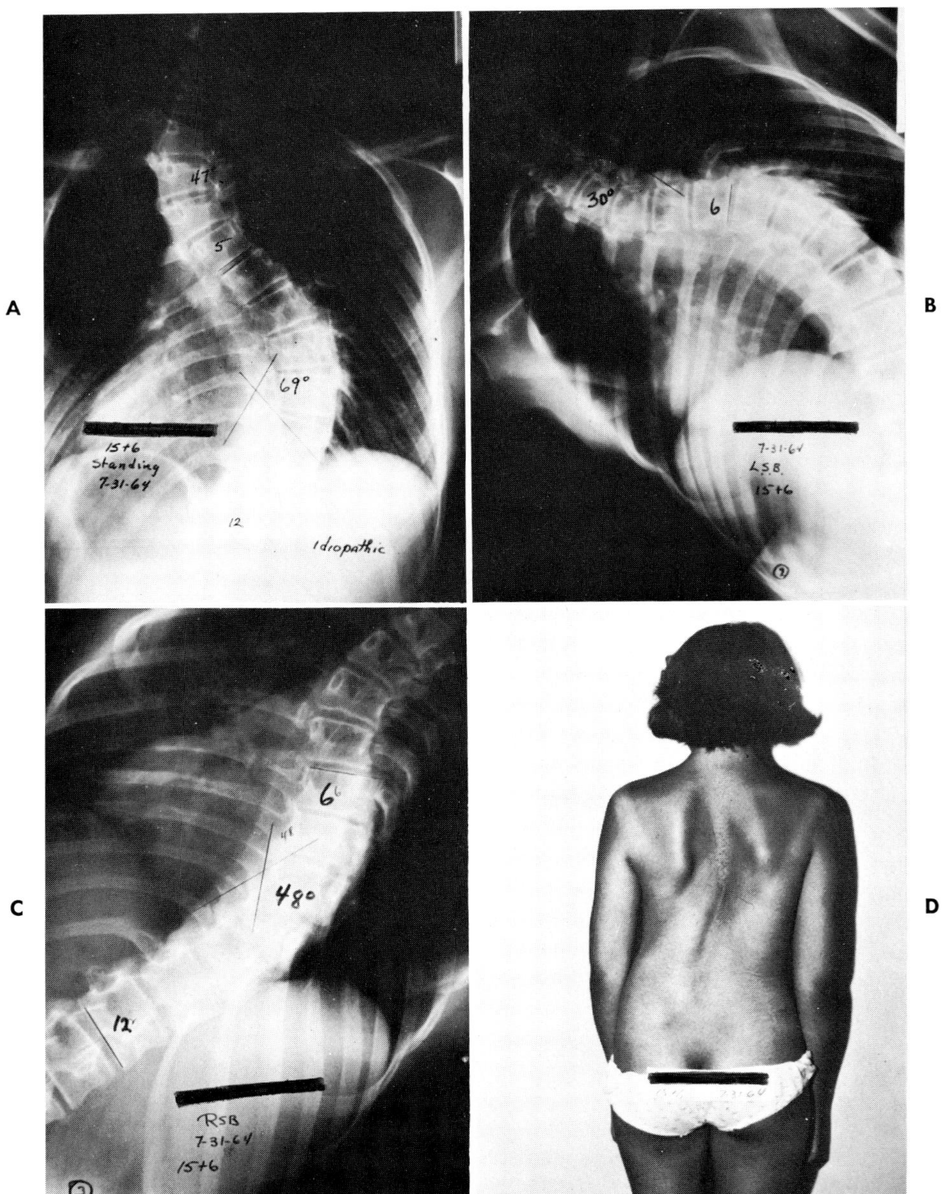

Fig. 13-6. C. V. O. **A,** Double thoracic major curve pattern. The left upper thoracic curve measures 47 degrees and the right lower thoracic 69 degrees (standing). **B,** Upper thoracic curve is 30 degrees structural on left bending (supine). **C,** Right bending curve has a 48-degree structural component on right side bending (supine). **D,** Preoperatively, there is little neck asymmetry. The magnitude of the right lower thoracic curve hides the disfigurement of the upper left thoracic curve.

of angulation and structural fixation tend to equalize. Sometimes, the high left thoracic curve is more structural. Two rib prominences accompany the two curves. In the true double thoracic primary curve pattern, the lumbar spine remains completely flexible. In this respect, the pattern differs from the right thoracic primary curve with a secondary high thoracic, which normally demonstrates a variable structural lumbar secondary curve.

The double thoracic primary curve can be assumed to be present when both thoracic curves are equally structural and the lumbar curve below is flexible, even when very early x-ray films are not available, for this is without question a distinct pattern. It is important clinically because it invariably calls for correction of both curves. In this pattern, the upper curve is of importance, for it is the harder to correct adequately, by nonoperative and operative correction alike.

The end vertebra of a thoracic curve may include the upper lumbar vertebrae so long as the apex of the curve lies within the thoracic spine. These are more appropriately called thoracic than thoracolumbar curves. The compensatory curve below does not tend to become highly structural. (See Fig. 13-7.)

The *double primary, combined thoracic and lumbar,* exists in two forms: the right thoracic–left thoracolumbar and the right thoracic–left lumbar. In these, both curves appear simultaneously and progress in a like manner.

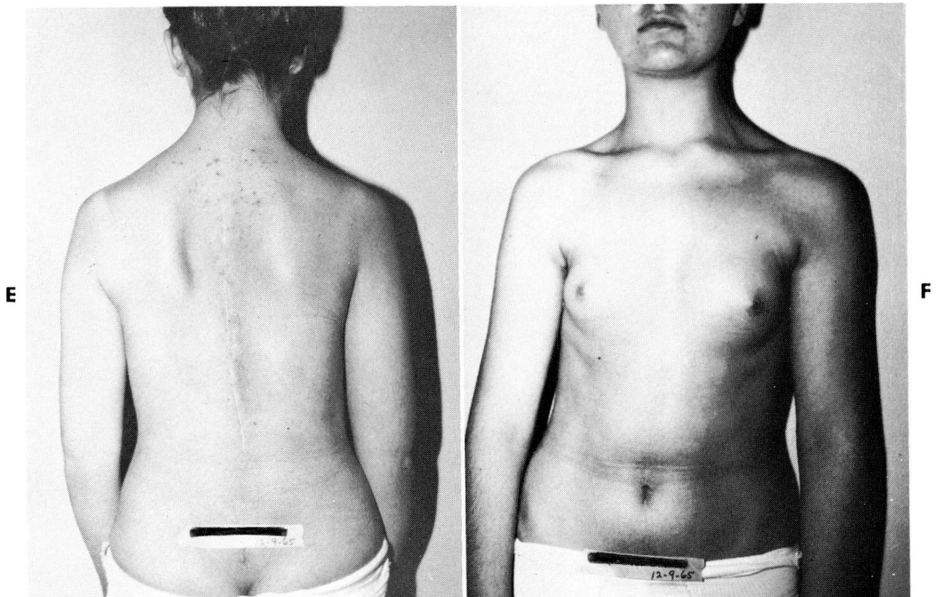

Fig. 13-6, cont'd. E, Right thoracic curve was corrected with Harrington instruments to 24 degrees. The upper hook was placed between T5 and T6 (into the convexity of the upper thoracic curve). The upper thoracic curve was not fused. The final result was poor because of trapezius neckline asymmetry due to the uncorrected upper thoracic curve. **F,** In the anterior view the neckline distortion is more evident.

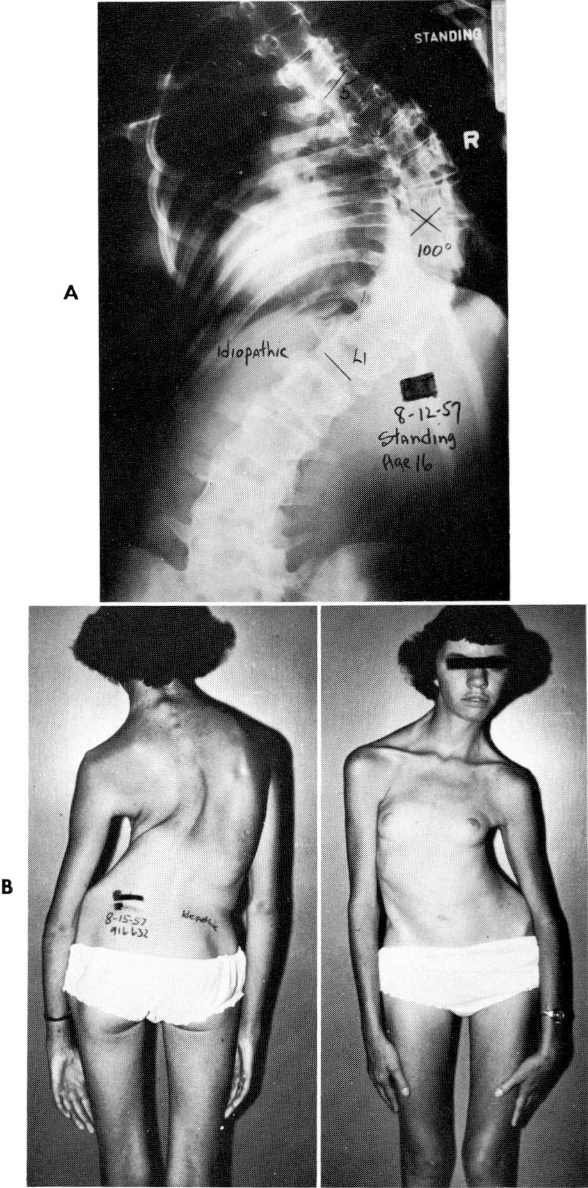

Fig. 13-7. A, Standing x-ray film of a severely structural idiopathic curve. This patient, age 16, had been informed by several orthopaedic surgeons that nothing could be done for her, because of the rigidity of her curve. **B,** Photographs of the 16-year-old patient, before correction and fusion. The right thoracic curve pattern is the most severely deforming.

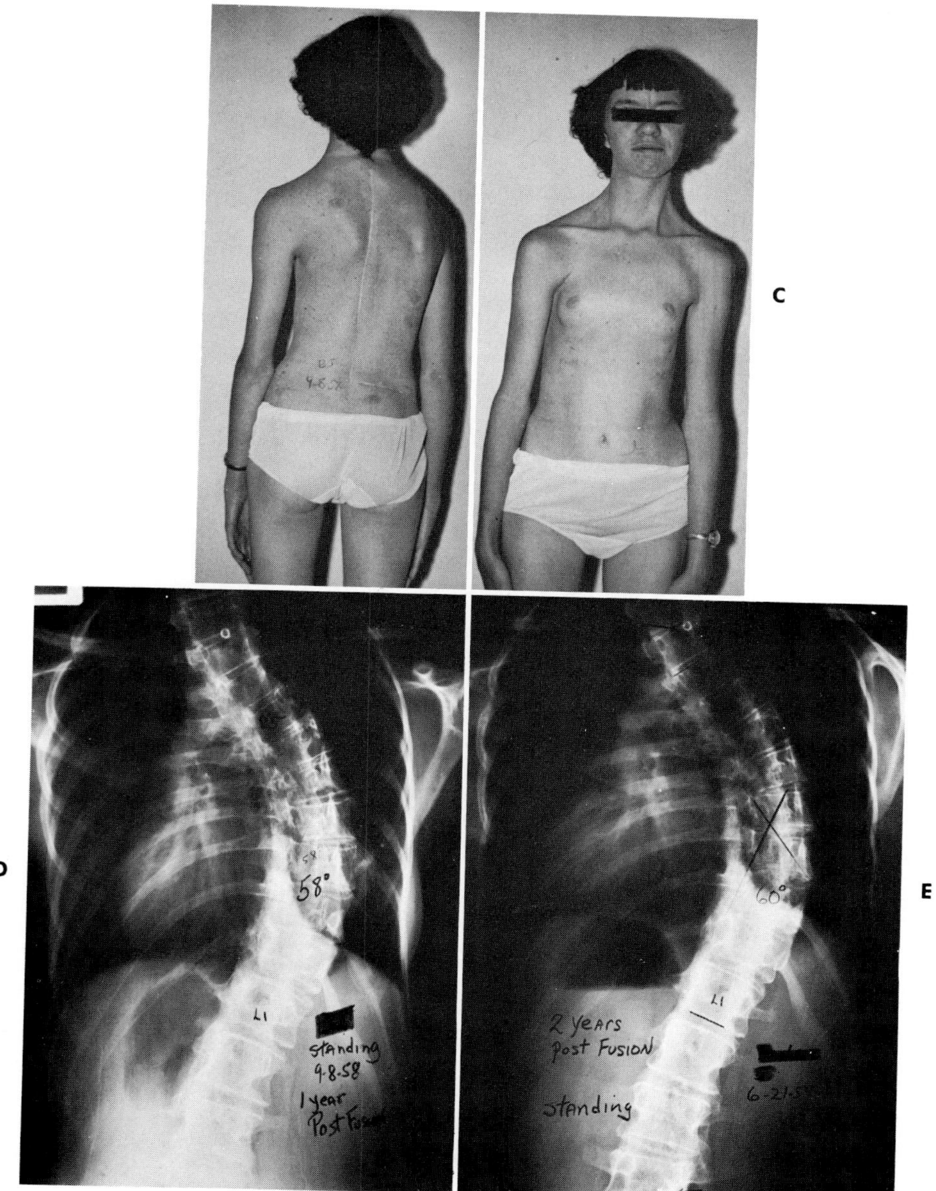

Fig. 13-7, cont'd. C, Photographs one year after correction and fusion. **D,** The 100-degree curve was reduced to 58 degrees by means of a Risser localizer cast without wedging. The measured curve was T5 to L1. T5 and L2 were neutral vertebrae. It was felt that the fusion should extend to L3, at least. The additional vertebra (L4) was included in the fusion area without any particular justification but was added on the basis of the adage "When in doubt, add a vertebra to the fusion area." Extensive fusions do less harm than do short fusions. **E,** Two years after the correction and fusion, the correction is fully maintained. The patient is compensated and pleased with the improvement.

The *right thoracic–left thoracolumbar* form consists of a relatively short thoracic curve, T3 or T4 to T8, T9, or T10, and a longer left thoracolumbar curve, T8 or T9 to L3 or L4 (Fig. 13-8). The thoracolumbar curve is always of greater angulation and is the most deforming. The thoracic curve is usually more structural and fixed on side bending x-ray films. To obtain maximum cosmetic improvement, both curves are usually corrected in maximal balance.

In the *combined thoracic and lumbar primary* pattern, the upper is purely thoracic and the lower purely lumbar. The transition between the two is usually T11 or T12. The lumbar curve ends at L4 or L5. It is in this combined pattern that the distinction between *primary* and *major* becomes more a matter of semantics than of practicality. (See Fig. 13-9.) In many patients with right thoracic primary curves, the lumbar secondary or compensatory curve has become highly structural and therefore both curves have become major. If these curves are added to the combined thoracic and lumbar primary pattern and to the combined thoracic and thoracolumbar pattern, the total pattern becomes quite common. James does place them into one group and indicates that they constitute a very frequent pattern.

The least common curve pattern found is the lumbar curve alone (Fig. 13-10). In these, only the lumbar curve is present, L1 to L5, and the thoracic spine is

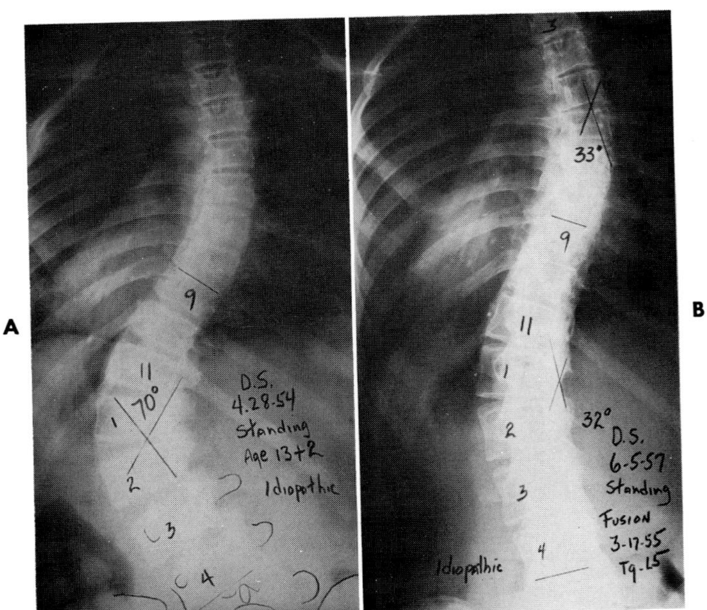

Fig. 13-8. A, A 70-degree left thoracolumbar idiopathic curve that was deforming. Such curves are worth correcting for cosmetic reasons. They are also productive of low back pain in adult life. **B,** The lower major curve, T9 to L4, was corrected to 32 degrees and T9 to L5 was fused. The upper curve was not fused. This is a combined right thoracic–left thoracolumbar curve pattern.

straight without a compensatory curve. Obviously, only the one curve needs treatment. Many are moderate curves having little cosmetic deformity. Correction and fusion may not be indicated if growth is complete. During growth, Milwaukee brace treatment is indicated (Fig. 13-11).

Evaluation of scoliosis by x-ray

The diagnosis, evaluation, and treatment of scoliosis requires a complete set of good x-ray films. While the number of views required will vary somewhat, the quality and size of the films will not. They must all be of excellent diagnostic quality with distinct visualization of the vertebral bodies, neither too dark nor too light. They must cover the entire curve and preferably the entire spine. In certain studies

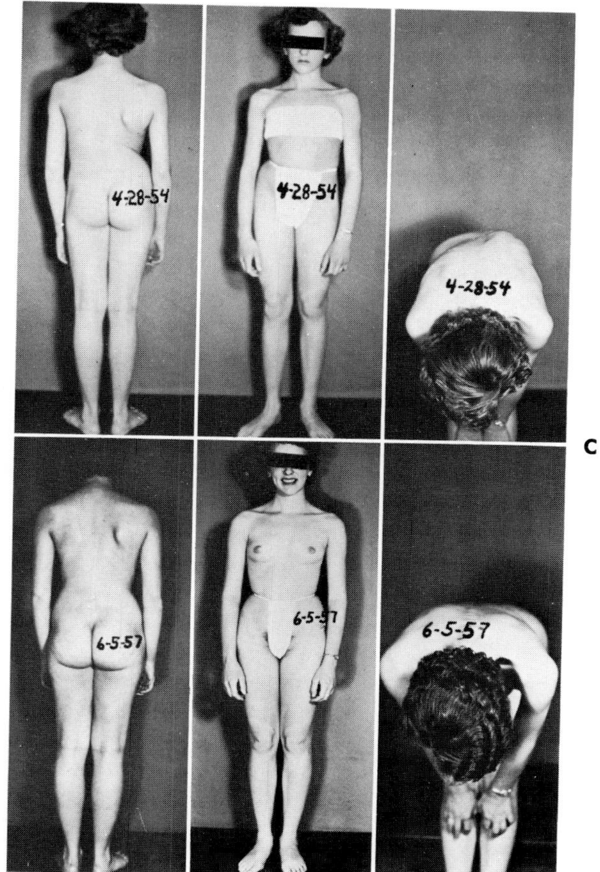

Fig. 13-8, cont'd. C, Photographs of patient, made at times of the x-ray films shown in **A** and **B.** The cosmetic improvement is striking. These curves are sometimes described as having little cosmetic deformity. They seldom surpass 70 degrees, but with this amount of curve, the asymmetry of the waist is deforming.

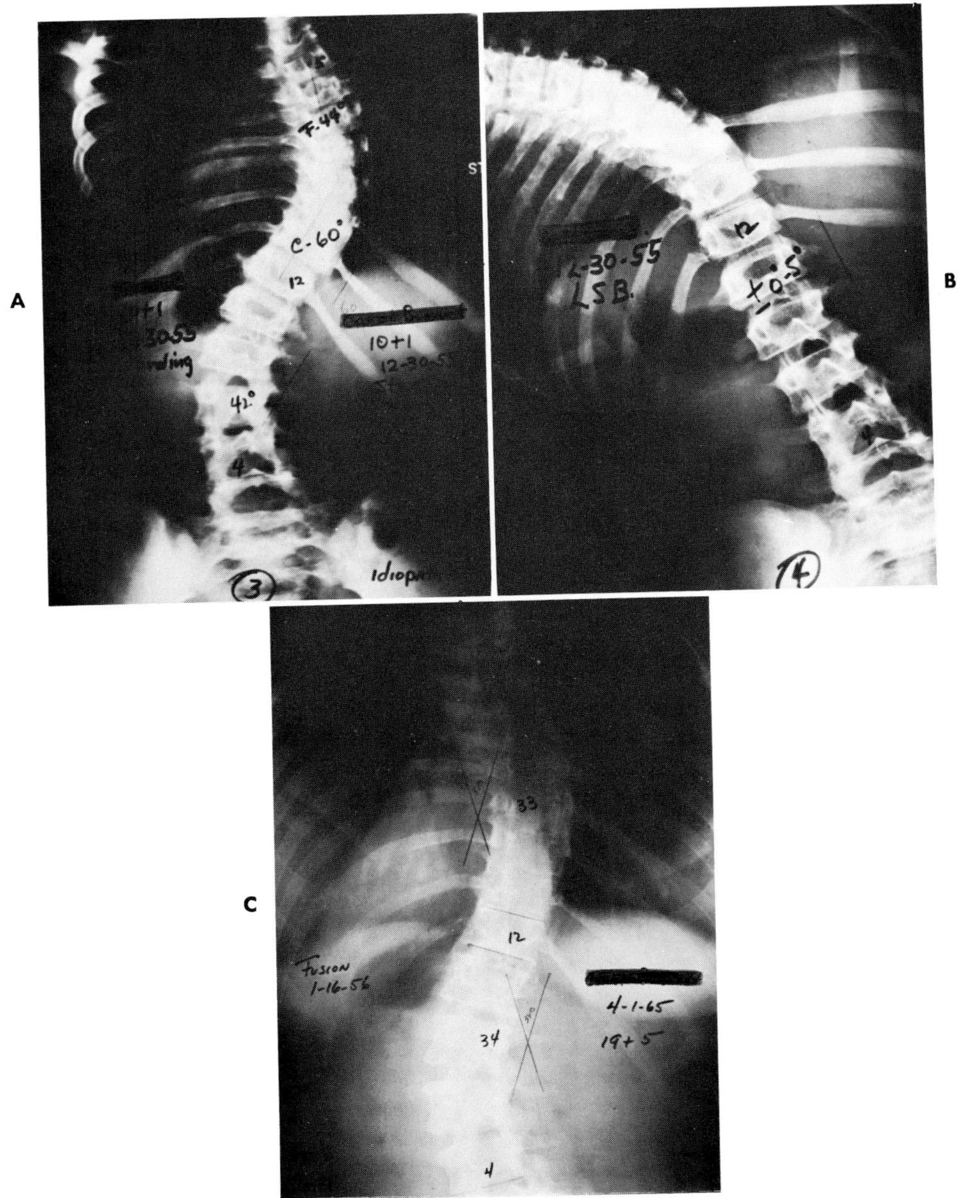

Fig. 13-9. This patient was first seen at age 9 + 5 and was "watched." The curve at that time was 45 degrees. **A,** At age 10 + 1 the right thoracic curve was 60 degrees and the left lumbar, 42 degrees. Side bending x-ray films are necessary to determine the flexible and structural components of the lower curve in planning correction and fusion. Note that T12 is a neutrally rotated end vertebra. **B,** Left side bending x-ray film shows that the left lumbar area is only minimally structural. It will not be included in the fusion. The fusion area will be T5 to T12. **C,** Nine years after the fusion, both curves are well balanced, at the same degree. The maximal correction following localizer cast correction was 25 degrees in each curve. The cosmetic appearance is good.

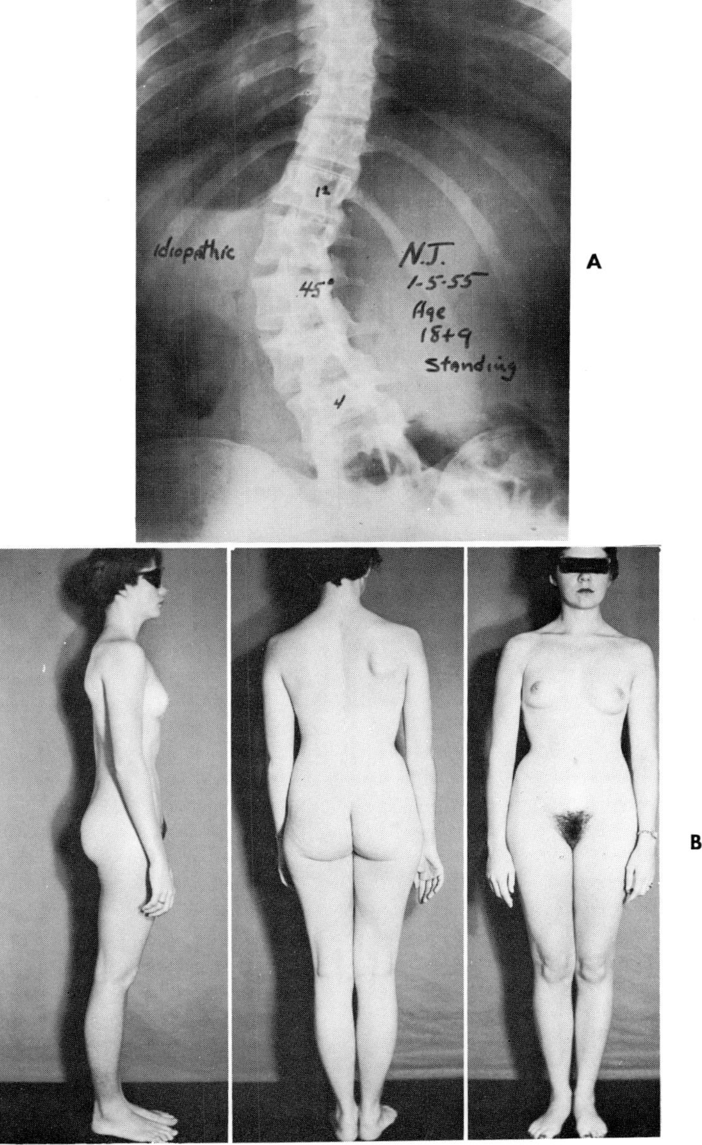

Fig. 13-10. A, Lumbar curve of 45 degrees in a skeletally mature girl. **B,** This patient, age 20, has a left curve, T12 to L4, measuring 45 degrees. Such lumbar curves are frequently not deforming, and they seldom reach severe degrees of angulation. This curve obviously need not be corrected and fused for cosmetic reasons.

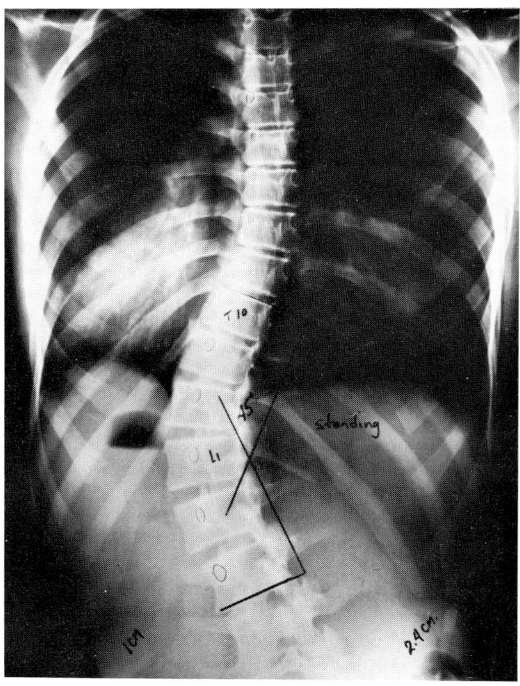

Fig. 13-11. Left thoracolumbar curve without a thoracic curve of significance. These curves are often accompanied by a low pelvis on the convex side, a feature that contributes to the deformity and to the progression. Leveling the pelvis should be included in the treatment program during growth.

such as the lumbosacral area this detail can be provided best by small "spot" films. Tomograms or special localized studies may be required, but for evaluating the curves as a whole, large 14- by 17-inch films are a necessity, even in infants. The total spine, including the entire pelvis, must be visualized. The standing view is taken whenever possible. In patients who are unable to stand, the film is made in the sitting position. The supine view supplies good bone detail but does not demonstrate the actual amount of curvature.

Technologists who are intelligent and who have acquired some knowledge of the scoliosis problem are invaluable in scoliosis treatment. Far too often inattentive and disinterested technologists will take x-ray films of only a part of a curve or will take other, unwarranted views that are of no value and only lead to unnecessary irradiation of the patient. The care of the scoliotic child takes many years and requires many x-ray examinations. Other than the crime of watching a curve progress without instituting intelligent treatment, there is nothing more harmful to the patient than the massive accumulation of unwanted and unnecessary x-ray films.

There is a real need for a better understanding of the scoliosis problem by roentgenologists. In an institution where scoliosis patients are seldom seen, interest on the part of the x-ray department must be stimulated. Even in some established scoliosis services, the x-ray departments lack interest and do not produce satisfactory films. The orthopaedic surgeon in charge of such a program must demand the facilities, technologists, and equipment to provide them consistently. There must be a special filing and storing system for scoliosis x-ray films. They must be readily available to the orthopaedic surgeon at all times during the care of the patient, both in the hospital and in the outpatient department.

Although the small child's spine is adequately viewed in its entirety on a 14- by 17-inch film, the adolescent requires a longer film, which can be supplied only by a 36-inch cassette. It is necessary to have an upright wall Bucky diaphragm. The tube to film distance should be 6 feet or longer. If good bone detail cannot be obtained at this distance, the film should be repeated at a closer distance. It is essential to obtain detail in both the anteroposterior and lateral views. If equipment is not available, two exposures with 14- by 17-inch films will include the entire spine but less satisfactorily. These films can be cut to form a composite.

Immediately after the long film is dry it must be cut transversely into two 14 by 17 film sizes. These are immediately and accurately joined by using a "packaging" tape on each side of the cut film, close by the lateral edge. Packaging tape is strong and will not break when used as a hinge. It may also be removed. "Scotch tape" or other forms of tape cannot be peeled off the film and will easily tear.

Side bending x-ray films are of value for the evaluation of the flexible and structural components of the curves. These show the patient's ability to correct the curve voluntarily in the supine position. Forcible side bending confuses the evaluation. The patient is positioned and supervised so that he will exert his own best effort. Each curve must be clearly shown. The 14- by 17-inch film is best for this purpose.

Distraction films are of value. These require the aid of two assistants pulling simultaneously. One will exert a strong pull on the head with a halter and the other will pull on the legs or pelvis. These x-ray studies determine the correctability of large major curves under forceful distraction. The test should be performed by experienced personnel, with maximal tolerated distraction. In small curves distraction films are unnecessary.

The standing anteroposterior x-ray views are taken with the body weight equally distributed and with normal posture without shoes. If there is a short leg, the weight must still be evenly distributed.

Lateral views of the spine should be taken at a 6-foot distance. The tube may be moved closer to obtain better bone detail in additional films. In growing children the thoracic spine is normally surprisingly flexible.

In a lateral x-ray study of 100 children, there was great variation in the measurement of the thoracic rounding in three positions: with arms (1) at the sides, (2) raised forward to the horizontal, and (3) held directly overhead. Uniform lateral standing x-ray views are obtained by raising the arms forward with the hands on a bar at shoulder height and maintaining normal posture. Lateral x-ray films in either the standing or the supine position must be made without twisting of the trunk. Both the shoulders must be aligned so that they are at right angles to the cassette. The pelvis must be likewise aligned. The rib prominence must not be allowed to rotate the torso and produce an oblique view of the spine. This is especially true with the patient lying down. Patients with large curves and prominent rib deformities are positioned by padding the concavity of the thorax so that each shoulder is the same height from the x-ray table. In extreme deformities the pelvis must also be aligned.

The request form for x-ray films must provide specific directions to the technologist. A request for scoliosis films should include the following:

1. There should be a standing anteroposterior view, at 6-foot distance, of the entire spine, including the pelvis and base of the skull. The size of the film will depend on the size of the patient. For good bone detail additional films may be necessary.

2. A supine anteroposterior view at 36-inch distance, including the major curve or curves, is needed. The specific area desired is to be designated on the request form. Two 14- by 17-inch films may be required in large patients.

3. Right and left supine bending films should include all curves. A right thoracic curve will be shown on a single 14- by 17-inch film. Two may be required for the upper thoracic and the left lumbar curves in larger patients.

4. A sitting film may substitute for the standing in certain paralytic patients. Specific directions should be given. Sometimes both standing and sitting views are necessary.

5. Posteroanterior films of the left wrist and hand are required for skeletal age in children. These should be requested individually and not routinely to avoid taking them on adults.

6. A "spot" lateral film of the lumbosacral spine is imperative. This should be supplemented by oblique and anteroposterior views if there is any question of abnormalities.

7. Tomograms and other special studies should be specifically ordered.

8. Evaluation of postoperative fusion areas should be by anteroposterior and both oblique views, confined to the fusion area at 36-inch distance. All such studies should be taken supine. Lateral views of a fusion are not usually informative. The area of the spine to be studied should be marked on the back with a skin pencil.

9. The technologist should review all films before dismissing the patient. All poor x-ray examinations should be repeated at once. If in doubt the technologist should ask for help in evaluating the x-ray films. Dark films that can be read only with intense light and light films that do not give bone detail must be *discarded and replaced* with good ones.

The evaluation of a scoliotic spine is the responsibility of the orthopaedic surgeon. A "reading" by the roentgenologist is necessary as a routine in all x-ray departments, but this should be delayed until the attending orthopaedist has studied and has recorded the curve measurement.

It is of utmost importance that all marking of x-ray films be done with a soft leaded pencil or a special removable marking fluid. Ink cannot be erased from x-ray film. Many measurement markings must be changed and it is imperative that they be easily removable.

Measurement of curves in scoliosis

Since a scoliotic curve is not a true arc and structural curvatures have some degree of vertebral rotation, there is no exact method of x-ray determination of the magnitude of the curve. A fractional curve has one horizontal vertebra, which is always at one end. Ferguson calls it a return to the erect. In a full curve only the apical vertebra is horizontal.

The methods of Ferguson and of Cobb are used to measure the curve on x-ray.

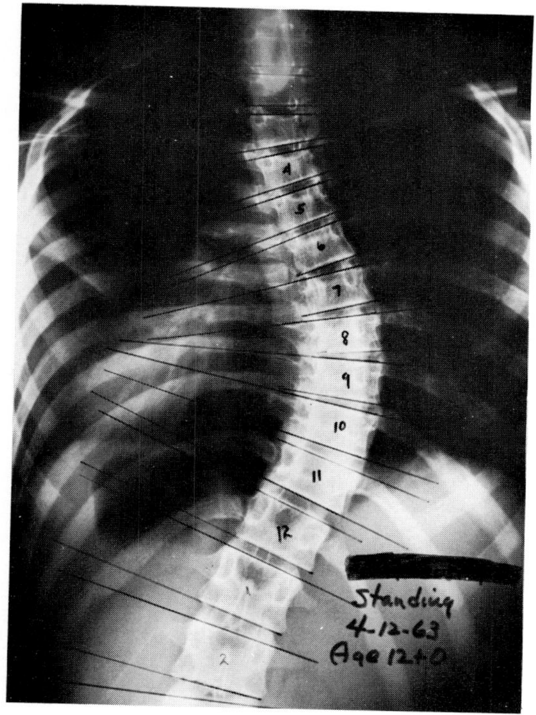

Fig. 13-12. Determination of end vertebrae of a curve. All lines on vertebral margins converge on concavity (left) between T6 and T12. The interspaces at T11-T12 and at T5-T6 are parallel. Either T5 or T6 and T11 or T12 can be designated as end vertebrae. The lines at T4-T5 and those at T12-L1 begin to diverge on the left side. These vertebrae are in the compensatory curves above and below the right major thoracic curve, T5 (or 6) to T11 (or 12).

Each has its advocates, but there is an increasing trend to adopt the method of Cobb as a standard. This is fortunate, for the two methods give widely divergent values—which can confuse the evaluation of the end results of treatment.

The end vertebrae of each curve must be selected in either method. An end vertebra is identified as the *maximally tilted vertebra*. There are several criteria for its selection.

1. If lines were drawn along the top or bottom of each vertebral body on the anteroposterior x-ray film, the last vertebra on either end that demonstrated convergence of these lines toward the concavity of the curve and divergence toward the convexity would be the end vertebra (Fig. 13-12).
2. The vertebral interspaces within a curve are wider on the convexity and narrower on the concavity. When the interspace below or above a vertebra is of uniform width, or when there is a reversal of the interspace wedging, the last vertebra on either end to participate in the interspace wedging characteristic of this curve will be the end vertebra.
3. The change in interspace wedging may not take place abruptly. At the end of a curve, particularly at the lower end, there may be a vertebra having parallel interspaces both above and below. This vertebra may be included in the curve without changing the measured angle, unless the end vertebra is wedged.

The Cobb method of measuring a curve consists of drawing lines along the lower margin of the caudad end vertebra and the upper margin of the cephalad one. It may be necessary to use other landmarks to draw lines that are perpendicular to the long axis of these vertebrae. Such lines usually meet at a point outside the x-ray field, so perpendiculars are erected from these lines and the corresponding angle is measured.

The curves above or below are measured by using the same line on the end vertebra and drawing similar lines on the other end vertebrae of the other curves. The transitional end vertebra is sometimes slightly wedged, requiring lines to be drawn on both its top and bottom. The line is selected that gives the greatest magnitude of the curve. Much confusion has arisen because some orthopaedic surgeons have identified the end vertebra as the one that is neutrally rotated, even though it may lie within an opposite curve. This can lead only to further error in evaluating results. (See Fig. 13-13.)

The margins of the interspace separating two vertebrae between two curves may appear parallel. Unless there is wedging, either of these vertebrae may be selected as an end vertebra without changing the measurement.

If a fusion is contemplated and there are two parallel end vertebrae above or below, the one farthest from the apex must be included in the fusion and should be used to measure the curve.

In evaluating the progress of nonoperative treatment, it is better to choose the one nearest the center of the major curve. The farther one will join the adjacent curve after treatment with the Milwaukee brace has been started.

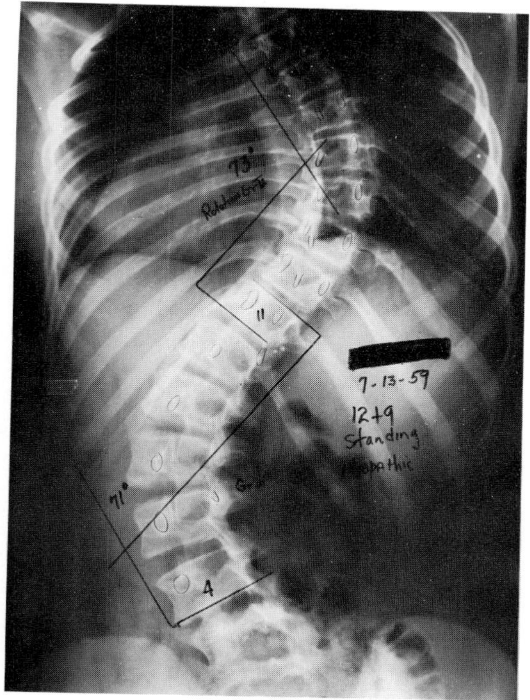

Fig. 13-13. The maximally tilted vertebra is T11. The lower margin of the body is used for erecting a perpendicular to measure the right thoracic curve and its upper margin measures the lower curve. Note that T11 is rotated to the convex side of the lower curve and is, therefore, not a neutral vertebra. Note also that L4 is the maximally tilted vertebra at the lower end of the lumbar curve, but it also is not neutral on rotation.

One of the criticisms of the Cobb method of measurement is that during correction only the ends of the curve may improve while the more rigid central portion changes very little (Fig. 13-14).

As an example, a T4 to L1 curve is measured by the Cobb method at 75 degrees. When corrected, the curve is again measured, using the same vertebrae. This curve now measures 25 degrees. On the correction film the positions of T4 and T5 are found to be reversed. They now lie within the compensation curve above. The interspace between T4 and T5, formerly wider on the right (the convexity of the right thoracic curve), is now wider on the left (the convexity of the left compensatory curve above). T6 is now the maximally tilted end vertebra of the right thoracic curve. The same findings are present at its lower end. The direction of T12 and L1 has been reversed, and T11 is now the lower end vertebra. The original curve, T4 to L1, has been shortened to a curve from T6 to T11. Most of the correction has been obtained by "bending the ends" of the original curve. The new curve, T6 to T11, measures 60 degrees. In evaluating the result of correction, should the original curve be measured again or should the shortened curve

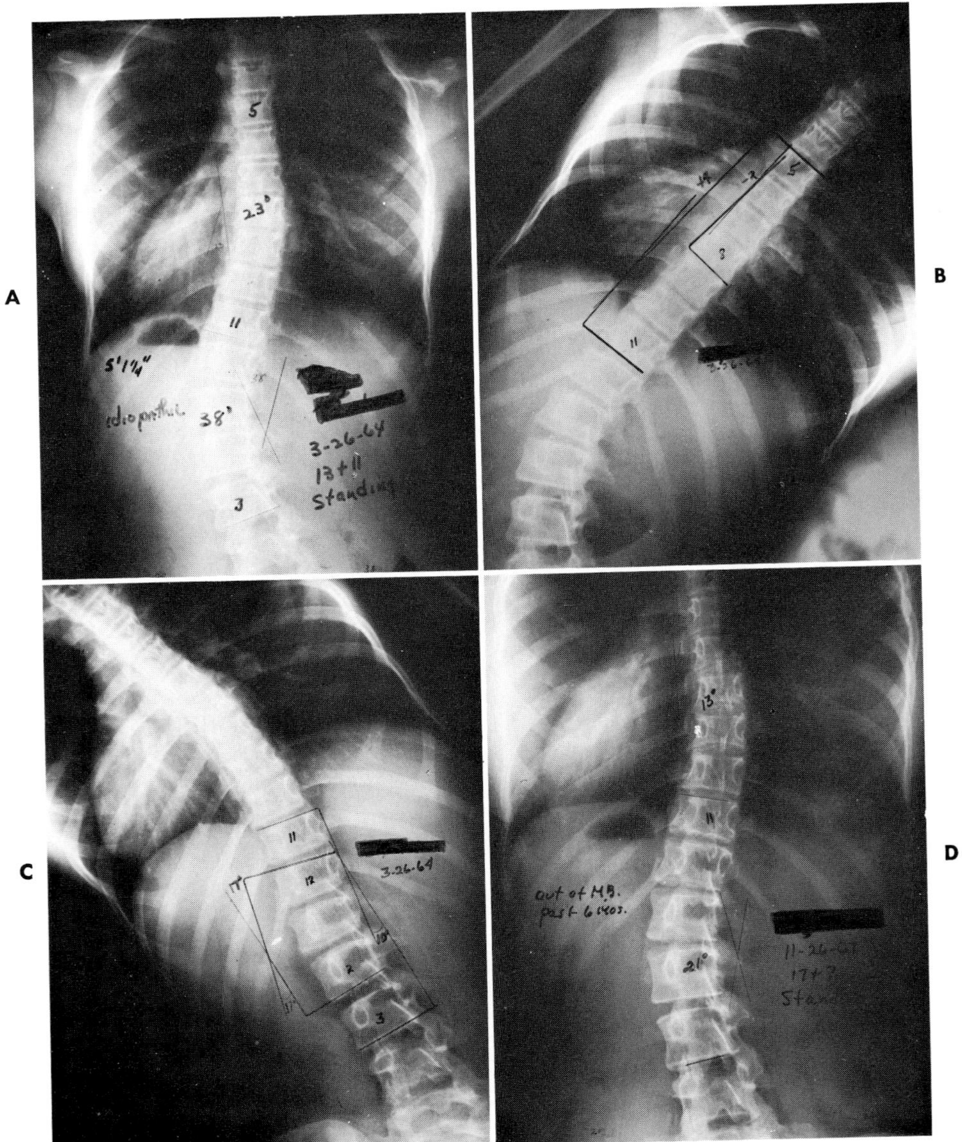

Fig. 13-14. R. F. **A,** Chronological age 13 + 11; bone age 13 + 6. Double major pattern: right, T5 to T11, 23 degrees; left, T11 to L3, 38 degrees. Pelvis is low on left by 1.3 cm. Iliac apophyses have barely appeared. Treatment recommended: Milwaukee brace. **B,** On right side bending, the right thoracic curve straightens and overcorrects on original curve, T5 to T11. The shortened structural curve is now T5 to T8 and this still measures 2 degrees. **C,** On left side bending, the thoracolumbar curve T11 to L3 has a residual curve of 10 degrees. The shortened curve T12 to L2 measures 17 degrees. **D,** Patient wore the Milwaukee brace full time for two years and was gradually weaned. This x-ray film was taken six months after the brace was discontinued. Upper curve, T5 to T11, reduced from 23 to 13 degrees (43%). Lower curve, T11 to L3, reduced from 38 to 21 degrees (44%). **E** and **F,** Lateral views, standing, show there has been no increase in thoracic lordosis by the brace treatment. The two x-ray films were taken at different distances.

be used? Obviously, there will be a discrepancy. It is possible to bend the ends of a curve so that the same end vertebrae will measure zero degrees or less. A shortened curve will still be present within the original end vertebrae.

A practical viewpoint must be adopted in evaluating the result of correction. It is axiomatic that a short curve is less disfiguring than a long one, because it is compensated better and shows its rotation and deformity less.

A double major curve pattern, right T5 to T11 and left T11 to L4, will have upper thoracic and low lumbar compensatory curves. With four short curves, compensation and balance are nearly always excellent. The cosmetic deformity is mainly through trunk shortening. There is little deformity and, even with curves of 50 or 60 degrees, no treatment may be warranted, if the patient is skeletally mature.

Long curves cause more deformity because rotation is more pronounced. There is a body list and the thorax collapses to cause a disfiguring "overhang." The greater the curve angle, the worse the cosmetic deformity. Elimination of the "overhang," reduction of length and magnitude of the curve, and lessening of the rib prominence contribute to the improved appearance. It is necessary to include all of these factors in evaluating the end result. (See Fig. 13-15.)

The same is true of some shorter right thoracic curves that measure 100 degrees or more. They sometimes collapse with "overhang." Most of these need to be stabilized by extending the fusion into the compensatory curve below. It is the rebalancing, as well as the curve correction, that gives the good cosmetic result. In some of these, stabilizing without any curve correction has been known to give cosmetic improvement.

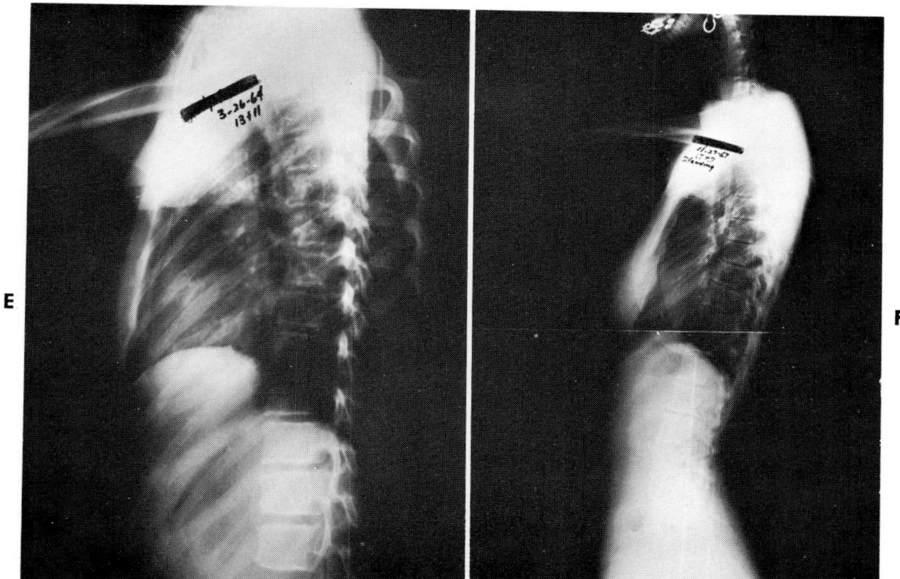

Fig. 13-14, cont'd. For legend see opposite page.

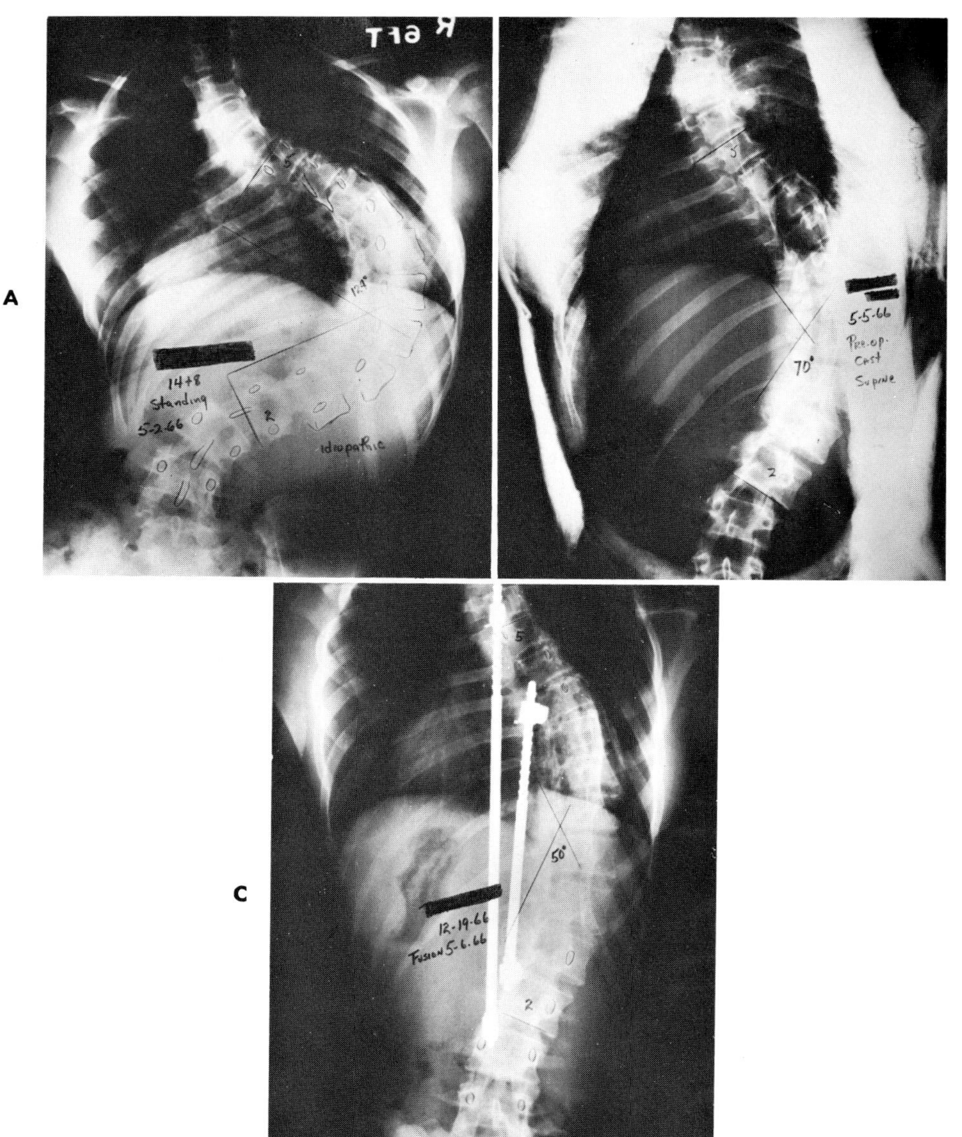

Fig. 13-15. R. B. **A,** Chronological age 14 years 8 months. Iliac apophyses capped. Bone age 15 years. Thoracic curve pattern. Rotation grade III, right convexity, maximally tilted end vertebrae T5 and L2. Cobb measurement 124 degrees, standing. Treatment indicated: *surgical.* The collapsing right thoracic pattern creates the greatest cosmetic deformity and the most angulation. **B,** Preoperative cast correction was to 70 degrees. **C,** With Harrington distraction rods, this correction was changed from 70 degrees in the cast to 40 degrees. She lost 10 degrees in the postoperative period, giving a final correction of 50 degrees.

It is therefore of practical importance to measure the amount of correction in comparison with the original curve. If desired, the shortened curve can also be measured and recorded.

Ferguson's method selects the end vertebrae of a curve in the same manner. He locates the central point of the body of each end vertebra and the vertebra at the apex of the curve. Two lines are drawn connecting these points, and the angle of intersection is measured. This is consistently a lesser angle than that obtained by the Cobb method and often it becomes unrealistic. If the end vertebra is greatly rotated, its center is not distinguishable. Curves of 140 degrees by the Cobb method will sometimes measure 70 degrees by the Ferguson. In this paper, the Cobb method will be used exclusively.

An end vertebra may or may not be neutrally rotated. On an anteroposterior x-ray film, the degree of rotation of a vertebra will be judged by the position of its spinous process and by the relative position of its oval pedicles in relation to the vertebral bodies.

If the tip of the spinous process is projected beyond the midpoint of the body toward the concavity of a curve, that vertebra is rotated toward the convexity of

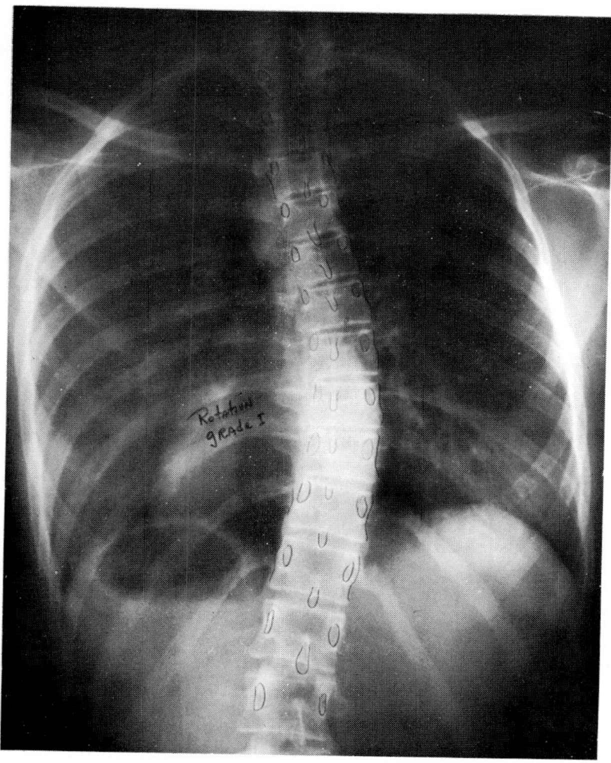

Fig. 13-16. The end vertebrae of this right thoracic idiopathic curve are T5 and T12 (maximally tilted). Rotation is grade I (minimal).

the curve. When the spinous process is in the middle of the vertebral body to which it belongs, that vertebra is not rotated and is neutral. If the outline of the spinous process were always distinct, this would be a satisfactory method of determining rotation. When the spines are poorly visualized, anomalous, or even absent as in spina bifida, this method is not applicable.

It is a more realistic and accurate method to observe also the relationship of the oval pedicle shadows to the vertebral body outline. With neutral rotation the pedicles are symmetrical within the body outline. With rotation of the body the pedicles are displaced toward the concavity of the curve. We have modified Cobb's method of grading rotation in the following manner:

Grade I. Both oval pedicle shadows lie within the vertebral body outline but both are minimally displaced toward the concavity of the curve (Fig. 13-16).

Grade II. One pedicle has narrowed in its configuration and lies on the vertebral body margin on the concavity. The other lies somewhat displaced

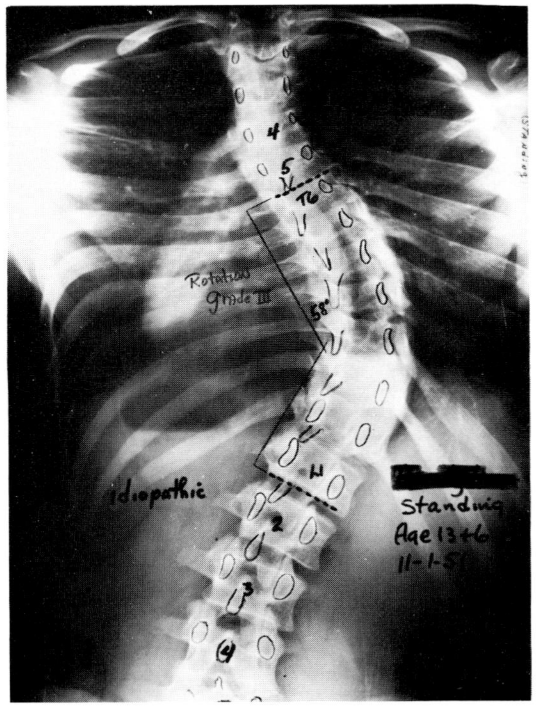

Fig. 13-17. Grade III rotation. The pedicles are displaced toward the center of the body outline. The pedicle on the concavity has disappeared, especially at the center of the curve. On the convexity the pedicle approaches the middle of the vertebral body outline. Note that rotation toward the convexity of the right thoracic curve is continued beyond the end vertebra L1. L2 and L3 are similarly rotated. L4 is neutral.

toward the concavity in relation to the vertebral body border. (See Fig. 13-18, *B*.)

Grade III. One pedicle has disappeared into the concavity. The other lies close to or at the center of the vertebral body outline and has developed a narrow configuration.

Grade IV. The remaining pedicle shadow is very narrow and lies beyond the midpoint of the vertebral body toward the concavity. The vertebral body is seen almost in lateral projection because it is rotated 30 to 45 degrees. (See Fig. 13-15, *A*.)

The maximally tilted end vertebra may not be neutral but may be rotated in the same direction as the vertebrae within the curve. (See Fig. 13-17.) This extension of rotation may reach farther to include additional vertebrae that are similarly rotated toward the convex side of the major curve, which is toward the concave side of the compensatory curve in which they lie. The level of neutral rotation is most important in determining the proper fusion area.

The value of side bending x-ray films has been questioned by many orthopaedic surgeons who have had experience in scoliosis. James does not use them, since he feels that the clinical evaluation of rotation by having the patient bend forward gives all the desired information. I believe that x-ray evaluation of flexibility of all the curves gives knowledge that is imperative in all patients who are to be given operative treatment. It is of value also in small curves in young children. The x-ray films should be taken supine while the patient bends actively as far as he can.

The measurement of side bending x-ray views requires a change in the level of the end vertebra, for the curve will usually shorten. Side bending x-ray films are taken because of the desire to evaluate the structural qualities of the curve. The shortened curve reveals this knowledge.

Selection of the fusion area

The fusion area is dependent on several factors: etiology, age of patient, type of curve pattern, and extent of vertebral rotation. The level must be accurately determined, anatomically and by x-ray verification.

The etiology of the curve will help determine the extent of the fusion. Curves of paralytic etiology, particularly those of the collapsing type, will require an extensive fusion almost routinely.

The age of the patient must be considered. The young child will usually require a longer fusion if total dependence is to be placed upon it to maintain correction. Fusions done in accordance with standards applicable to the older adolescent may result in bending of the graft and lengthening of the curve in the young child. A curve with a shorter fusion can be successfully kept in correction in the young child if prolonged external correction with the Milwaukee brace is maintained during growth.

The curve pattern must be analyzed. A double major curve pattern requires fusion of both curves. The single major curve with flexible compensatory curves requires only one curve to be fused.

Side bending x-ray films are of particular importance in the right thoracic–left lumbar pattern. The right thoracic curve will nearly always be found to have a large structural component. The left lumbar, although of similar angulation, is often found to have a large flexible component; if so, this lumbar curve will not require fusion, since its flexibility will allow it to balance and compensate the corrected and fused thoracic curve. (See Fig. 13-18.)

The extent of vertebral rotation is a determining factor. If the maximally tilted end vertebrae demonstrate neutral rotation, the fusion can be confined within

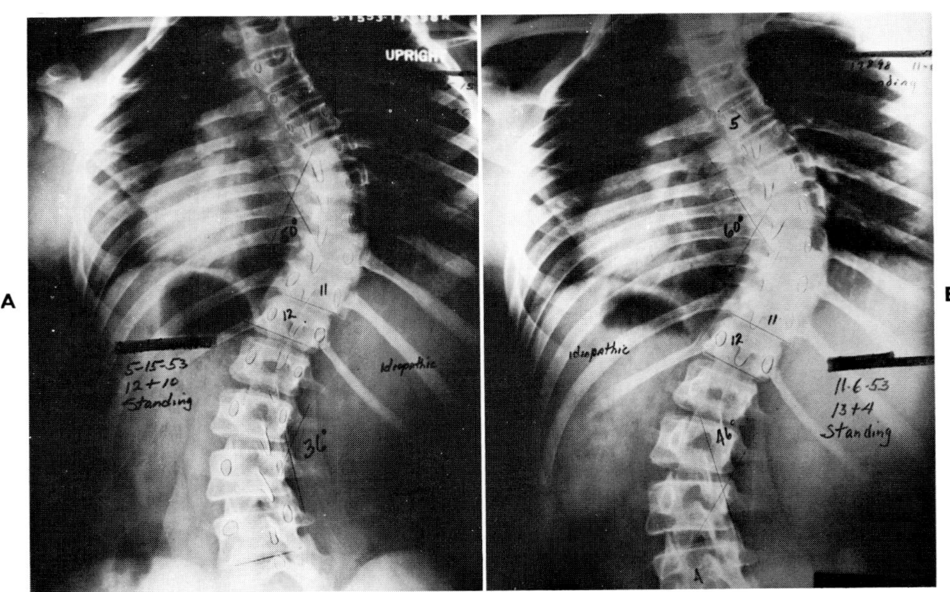

Fig. 13-18. A and **B** demonstrate clearly the fallacy of watchful expectant treatment of an idiopathic structural curve in a growing child. In a six-month waiting period, from age 12 + 10 to age 13 + 4, the right thoracic curve increased 10 degrees and the compensatory curve below likewise increased. Note that T12 (the end vertebra) is neutral (it is slightly rotated toward the left lumbar curve). T11 is neutral in rotation and is parallel to T12. The fusion area should be T5 to T12. The iliac apophyses have not appeared. **C,** This right thoracic curve is 25 degrees structural on right side bending. It is more structural than the lumbar curve and presumably it appeared first and lost its flexibility first. (Primary curve?) **D,** Flexibility is shown on side bending in the lumbar curve, which even in the shortened curve is only 10 degrees. Only the right thoracic curve will need to be fused. The minimal upper thoracic compensatory curve may be disregarded. These x-ray films were taken when the patient was first seen. It would have been wise to repeat them six months later for reevaluation of flexibility. **E** and **F,** X-ray films of a patient at one year and at eight years after localizer cast correction and fusion. Both curves are in good balance and compensation. Fusion was T4 to L1—one extra vertebra above and one below the right thoracic curve. Only the T5 to T12 area needed to be fused but the additional vertebrae in the fusion did no harm.

their boundaries. The common right thoracic pattern may be used as an example. If rotation toward the convexity is continued into one, two, or three lumbar vertebrae before a neutrally rotated segment is reached, the fusion must usually be extended to include all of these vertebrae. The rule is to fuse from neutral to neutral vertebrae.

There are some exceptions. Extended rotation beyond the curve may disappear

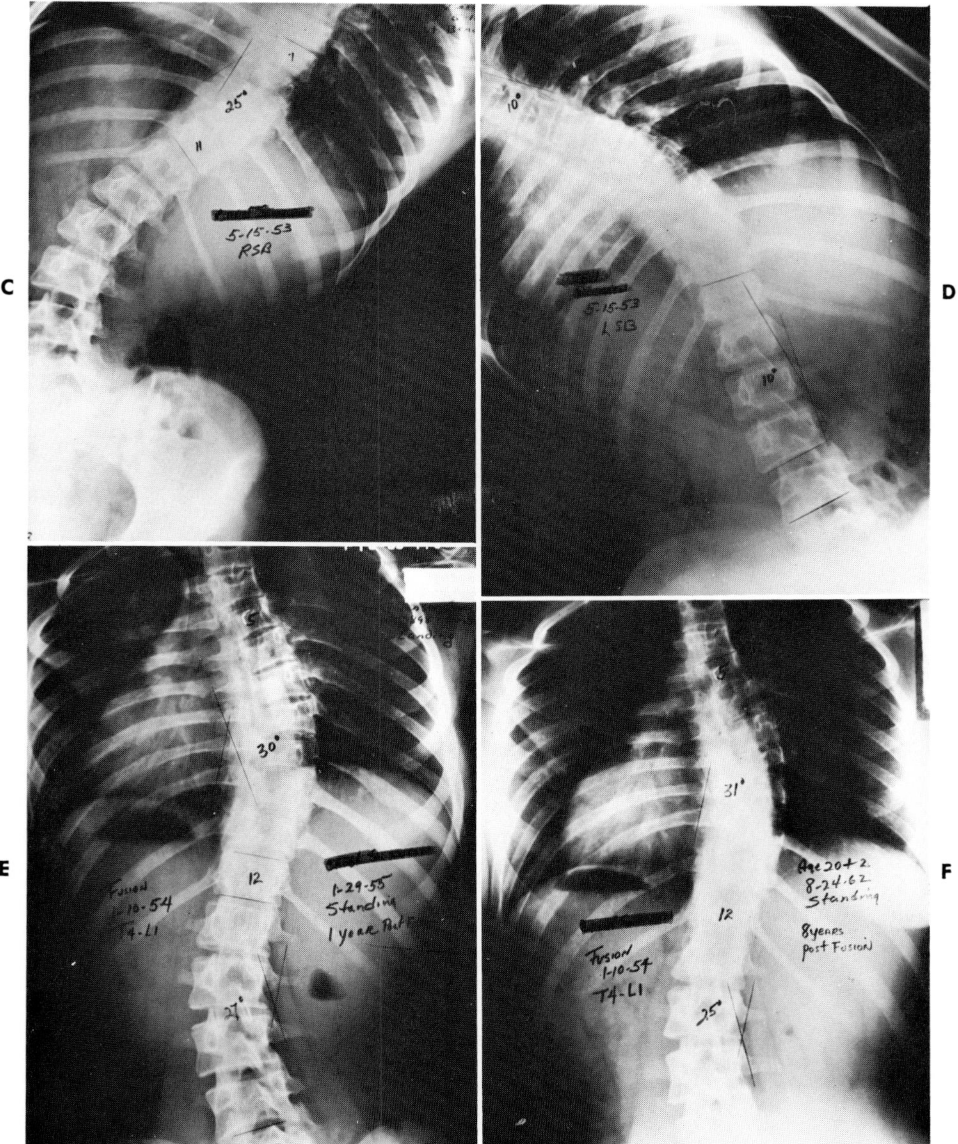

Fig. 13-18, cont'd. For legend see opposite page.

with cast correction and, on the correction films, the lower end vertebra may be neutrally rotated. (See Fig. 13-19.) When this derotation occurs, the fusion area can be safely shortened—but never by more than two segments and most often by only one.

Extended rotation below a thoracic curve must be watched for and the correct

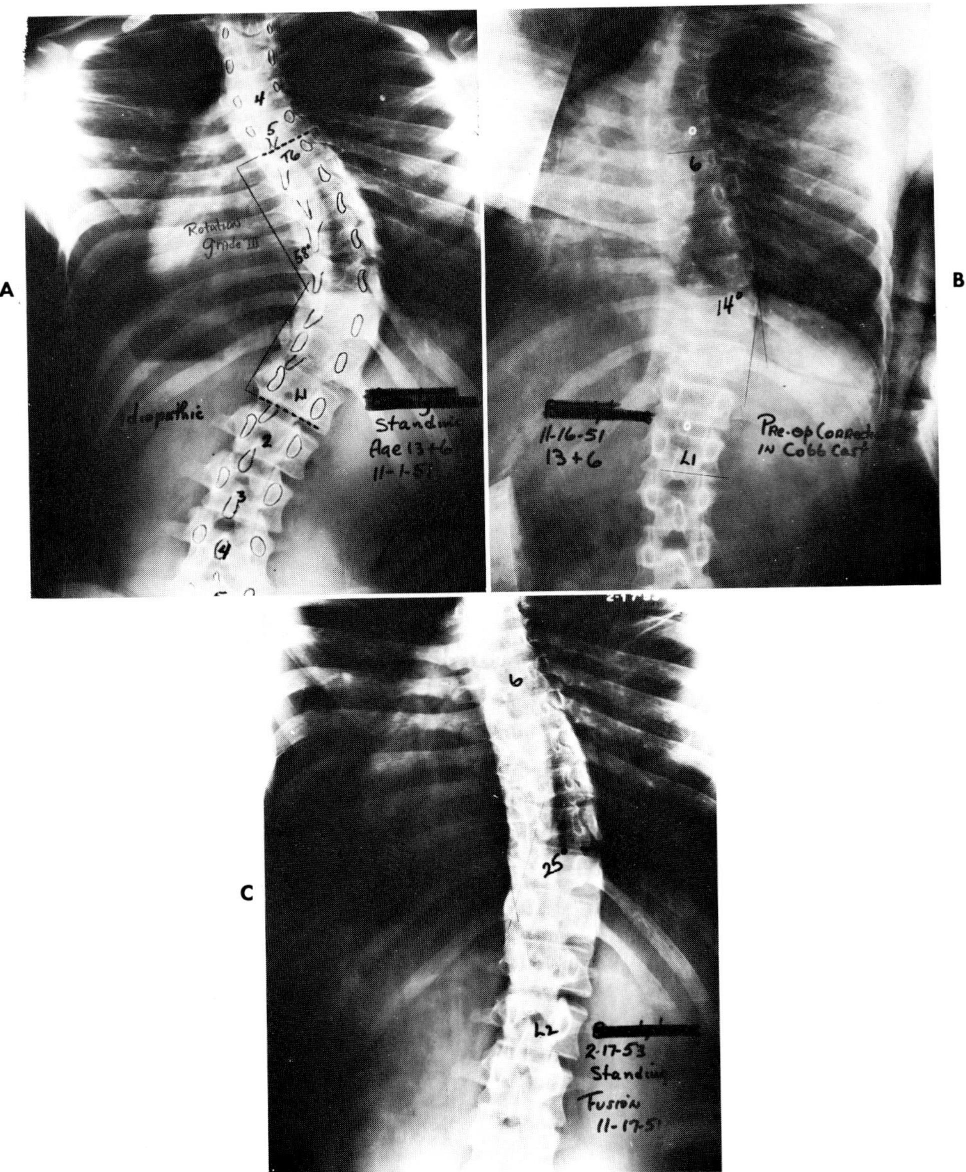

Fig. 13-19. For legend see opposite page.

fusion area selected. The penalty for not including those rotated vertebrae is the lengthening of the curve. This will nearly always lead to a severe loss of correction and to an unacceptable cosmetic result. (See Fig. 13-20.)

Extended rotation in a low lumbar or thoracolumbar curve is less likely to create such a problem. When the end vertebra is L3 and rotation includes L4 and L5, it is not necessary to fuse to the sacrum, even though this might in fact be the neutral vertebra. It is sufficient to include only one segment below the end vertebra.

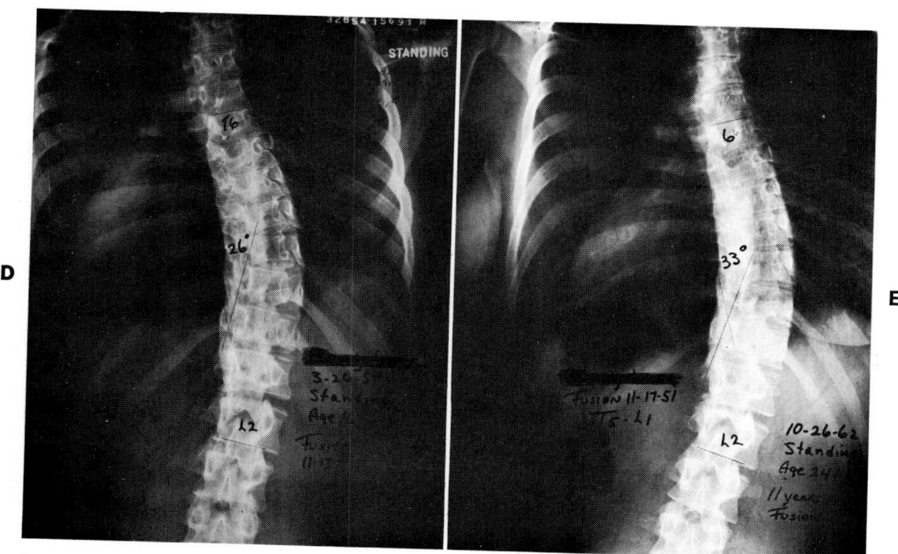

Fig. 13-19. A, A thoracolumbar curve pattern with rotation extending beyond the curve. T6 and L1 are the maximally tilted end vertebrae, but they are not neutrally rotated. Rotation continues below as far as L4 which is neutral. T6 is rotated, T5 is slightly rotated, and T4 is neutral. In planning the fusion area, it is best to fuse from neutral to neutral vertebra—in this case, from T4 to L4. Before deciding, it is best to study the rotation present in the correction film. Note that the rotation of the apical vertebrae is grade III. Spines extend beyond the body margin, and the pedicle outline has disappeared on the concavity. **B,** The preoperative Cobb type of turnbuckle cast gave noticeable derotation. L1 is now completely neutral as is also T6. This derotation permits shortening the fusion area by one or possibly two segments below. Unfamiliarity with the problem led to a decision in 1951 to shorten the fusion to include T5 to L1, which proved to be too short. **C,** Three months after the fusion the cast was changed. Already the interspace between L1 and L2 had opened toward the convexity of the curve and rotation of L2 and L3 was again present. It is now evident that the minimum fusion area should have been T5 to L2. The inclusion of L3 would have been safer. **D,** At two years after the fusion the same condition existed. There had been no further loss, but the rotation in the lumbar spine continued to extend down to L4. The patient had then been out of external support for over twelve months. **E,** Eleven years after the fusion, the further opening of the interspace wedging between L1 and L2, plus the continued torque produced by the extended wedging, has increased the total curve to 33 degrees. However, there has been no further extension of the curve and the end result is still satisfactory. In this case, fortune smiled. In most instances such an error in selecting the fusion area will lead to complete loss of correction.

The closer the curve approaches the sacrum, the less important is the extended rotation.

Fusion to the sacrum is not often indicated in idiopathic scoliosis. It is usually required when a lumbar curve is associated with a spondylolysis or a spondylolisthesis at the lumbosacral region. Other evidence of instability, such as pain in this

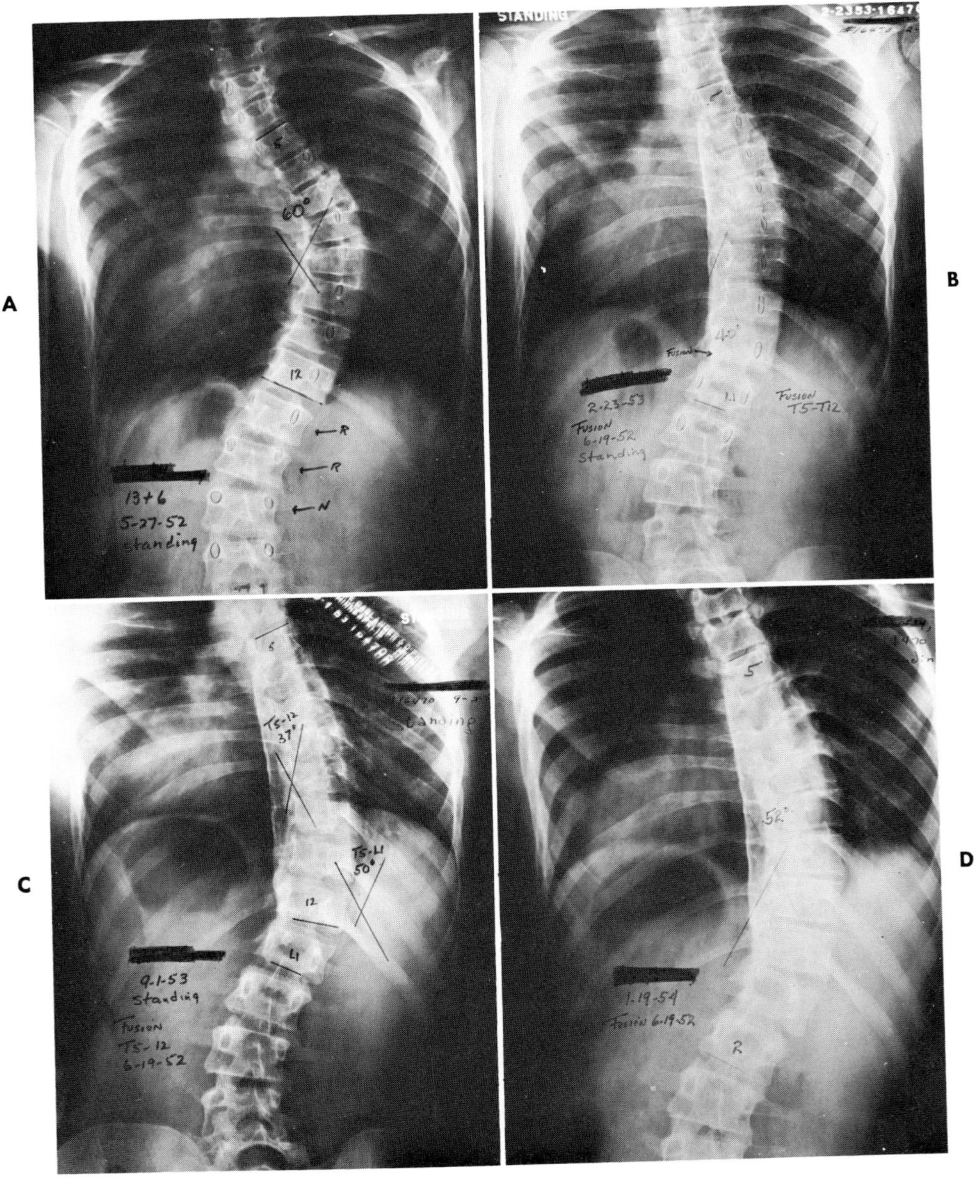

Fig. 13-20. For legend see opposite page.

area, is also an indication. All patients with scolioses should have a lumbosacral x-ray study routinely taken.

We have fused many double major curves from upper thoracic to L4 or L5, and only in rare instances has this resulted in low back disability. Fusions extended across the lumbosacral joint lead to a high percentage of pseudarthroses. To lessen this problem, it is necessary to include one or both thighs in the postoperative localizer cast and to keep the patient in bed postoperatively for six months. Unless there is a clear-cut need for lumbosacral fusion, it is probably best not to do so. Fusion of this area can be done at a later time if the indications arise, although the incidence of pseudarthroses will then be higher.

There is a special indication for lumbosacral fusion in lumbar curves treated

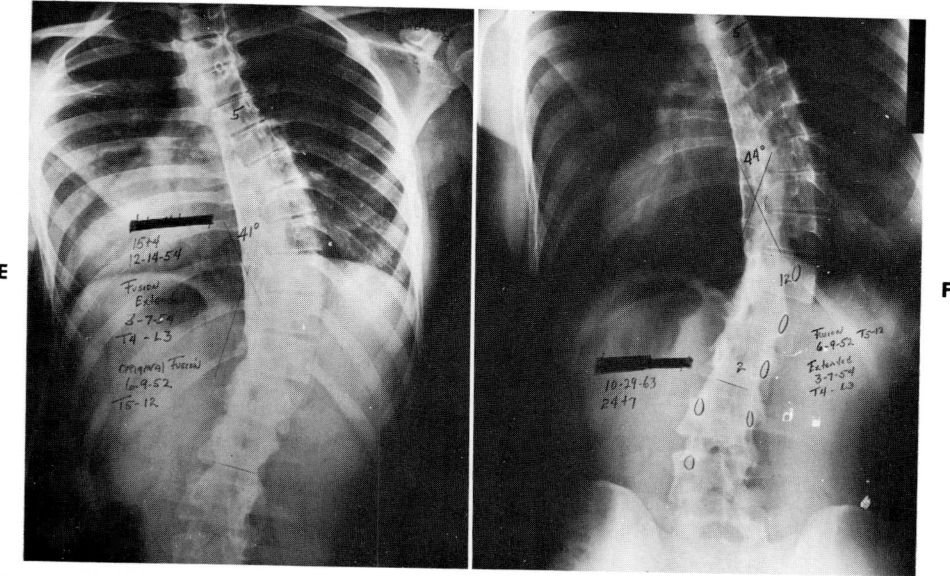

Fig. 13-20. H. McI. **A,** Age 13 years 6 months, idiopathic right thoracic curve. T5 (or T6) and T12 are the maximally tilted vertebrae of the 60-degree curve. Rotation is grade III in apical area. Note that rotation continues in the same direction to include L1 and L2, although these lie in the compensatory lumbar curve. L3 is neutral in rotation as is also L4. T5 is neutral. The fusion area should have been T5 to L3. **B,** Fusion was confined to the measured curve, T5 to T12. On removal of the cast, eight months after operation, the fusion was solid but L1 had now been added to the curve, increasing its total angulation. **C,** Fifteen months after fusion the angle of the lengthened curve had increased further. The original curve that was fused had not materially increased. **D,** Eighteen months after fusion L2 had been added to the total curve, increasing its angulation. Plans were made to attempt to recorrect the curve and extend the fusion. **E,** Curve was partially corrected in a wedging cast and the fusion was extended from T4 to L3. About 10 degrees of correction was obtained. If doing this today, we would add an osteotomy of the fusion area to obtain further correction. **F,** Considerable cosmetic improvement was obtained although the change on x-ray measurement was small. This x-ray film was taken eleven years after the original fusion and nine years after attempted recorrection and extension of the fusion.

in the Milwaukee brace. The lumbar curve occasionally includes a fourth and fifth lumbar segment that is tilted from the sacrum. This longer curve may be difficult to control with the brace. Shortening this curve by fixing L4 and L5 in relatively normal alignment to the sacrum makes correction and control of the lumbar curve easier. This can be better achieved with a cast than with a brace. Additional correction is done during surgical exposure by inserting a short threaded Harrington rod and hook assembly from the ala to a slot in the posterior pedicle where it joins the articular and transverse processes. Distraction here is effective in realigning the fourth lumbar vertebra. (See Fig. 13-21.)

Fusion is then performed, L4 to sacrum, and the localizer cast correction is maintained with the patient supine for six months. The fusion mass is then maturing and the Milwaukee brace with thoracic and lumbar pads is reapplied. Ambulation is now permitted. This method is recommended only when the thoracic curve is well controlled by the brace. It is very effective when all indications are met (Fig. 13-22).

Spondylolisthesis at L5-S1 may be associated with a scoliosis problem. There are three types:

1. An idiopathic right thoracic curve may have a flexible compensatory curve

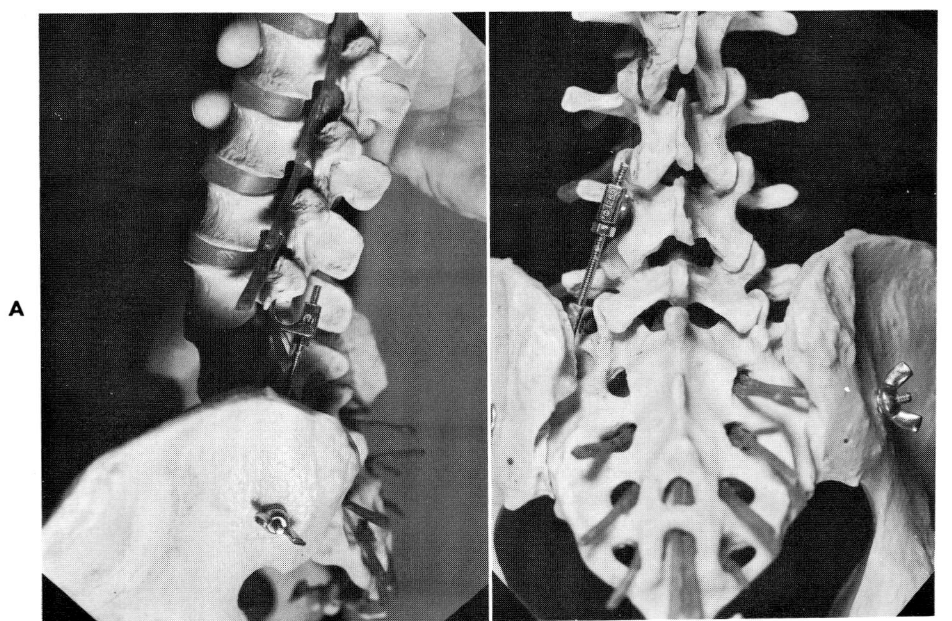

Fig. 13-21. Insertion of a short distracting threaded rod is shown on a skeleton. **A,** Insertion of the upper hook is into a slot cut into the bone at the junction of the pedicle, transverse process, and articular process, close to but not into the foramen. **B,** Lower hook seats into a slot as far laterally on the ala as possible.

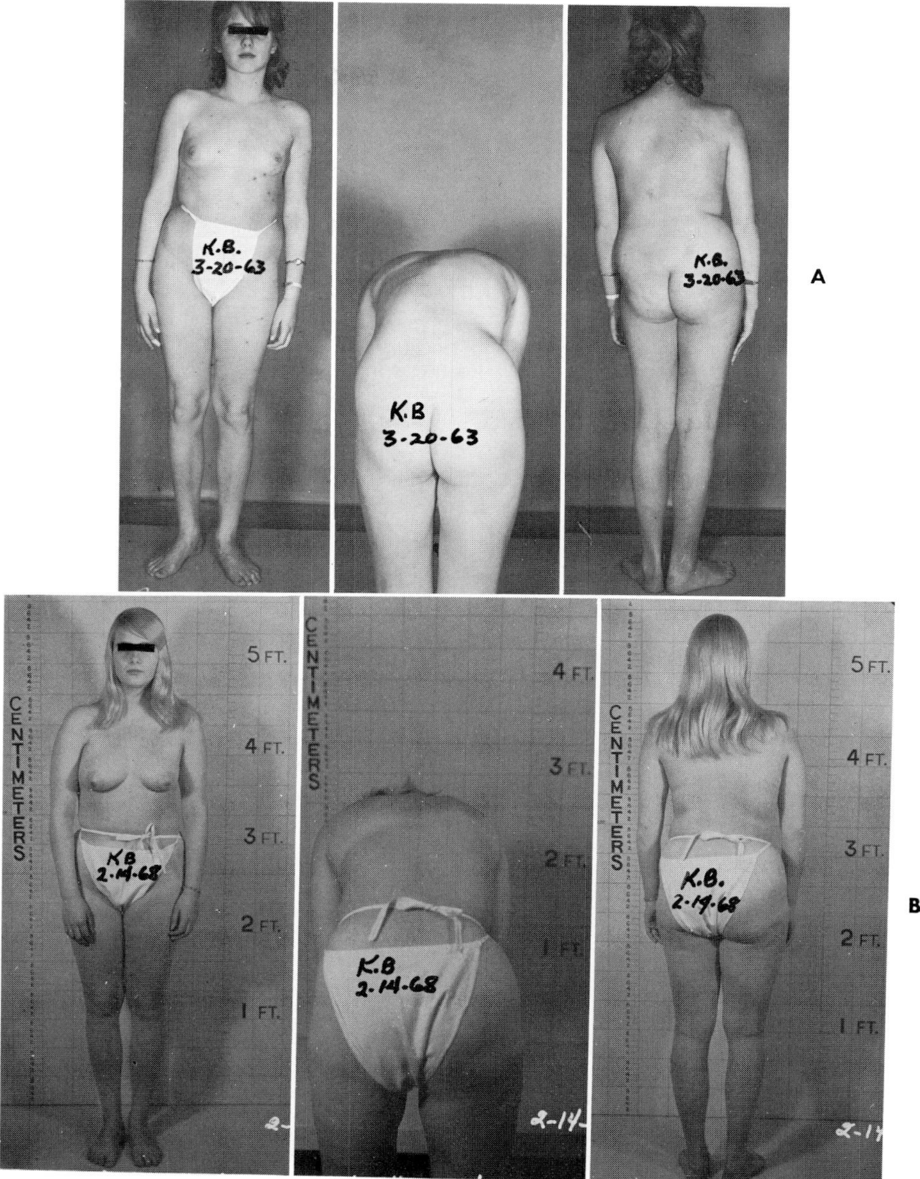

Fig. 13-22. K. B. **A,** Idiopathic curve, of double major pattern grade I, with spondylolisthesis L5-S1 contributing to L5 tilt. Left lower extremity short, contributing to increasing angulation of left lumbar curve. Treatment program included (1) cast correction (localizer) for three months while waiting for Milwaukee brace; (2) Milwaukee brace with left shoe built up 1 inch, six months; (3) cast correction, supine; (4) short Harrington rod and Milwaukee brace with left shoe buildup after L4-S1 fusion had matured; (5) shortening of right femur 1 inch. **B,** Out of brace one year. Corrections achieved: T5 to T11, from 45 to 30 degrees, and T11 to L5, from 58 to 30 degrees.

below, and there may be a spondylolysis or a spondylolisthesis in addition. In this event, the thoracic curve is treated appropriately and the lumbosacral defect is not treated unless it is symptomatic or progressive.

2. Double major curves of the right thoracic–left lumbar pattern may be present, and the spondylolisthesis or spondylolysis may be present also. If so, it may participate in and add to the rotation of the L5 vertebra. The relationship of these defects to the production of torsion and rotation of the fifth lumbar vertebra has been analyzed by several writers, most recently by Tøjner of Aalborg, Denmark, who found a torsion scoliosis associated with spondylolisthesis and spondylolysis in 30% of 237 patients.

The treatment of each patient having this combination must be individualized. If there appears to be a significant olisthetic scoliosis, it should be given cast correction and a low lumbar fusion, usually with use of a short distraction rod. The double major curve alone may require correction and fusion in addition.

3. Spondylolisthesis may cause the patient to list, and the entire spine may then deviate directly from the lumbosacral area. In an attempt to compensate, a very long thoracolumbar curve is produced. Such listing is the result of torsional forces in conjunction with muscle spasm. Hamstring contracture is present and there may be radicular pain.

Most of these deformities are diagnosed early while the list and curvature both disappear in the prone position. If the curve is still flexible, it will disappear if a corrective cast is applied; and the spine will be permanently straight if the lumbosacral spine is fused. It is sufficient to fuse from L4 to the sacrum. The spine must be held in cast correction until the fusion is mature. Early ambulation should not be permitted. Decompression of the nerve roots at the time of fusion is often indicated.

If this deformity has persisted throughout many years of growth, a structural curve will have developed and correction is no longer easily achieved. It now becomes necessary to correct and fuse the entire curve as well as the lumbosacral area. The long thoracolumbar curve is corrected best with Harrington strut bars. The lower hooks can be placed into the sacral alae or a trans-sacral bar may be used. The entire curve must be fused to the sacrum. Cast correction is necessary to align the entire fused spine over the pelvis. Lumbosacral pseudarthroses are frequent. The cast must include the thighs and the patient must be kept in bed until the fusion is solid and mature throughout.

Another special problem is the double thoracic major curve. This usually requires correction and fusion of both curves. With the upper curve less structural and rigid and the asymmetry of the neckline minimal, there are few indications for fusing the upper curve. But when this curve's structural fixation surpasses 25 degrees on side bending x-ray films, both curves should be fused. This high thoracic curve does not usually correct well by cast or Milwaukee brace. Fusion is indicated. The Harrington threaded rod of ⅛-inch thickness, its medium-sized hook (1254-1256) placed into the T1-T2 articulation and the lower hook placed around the

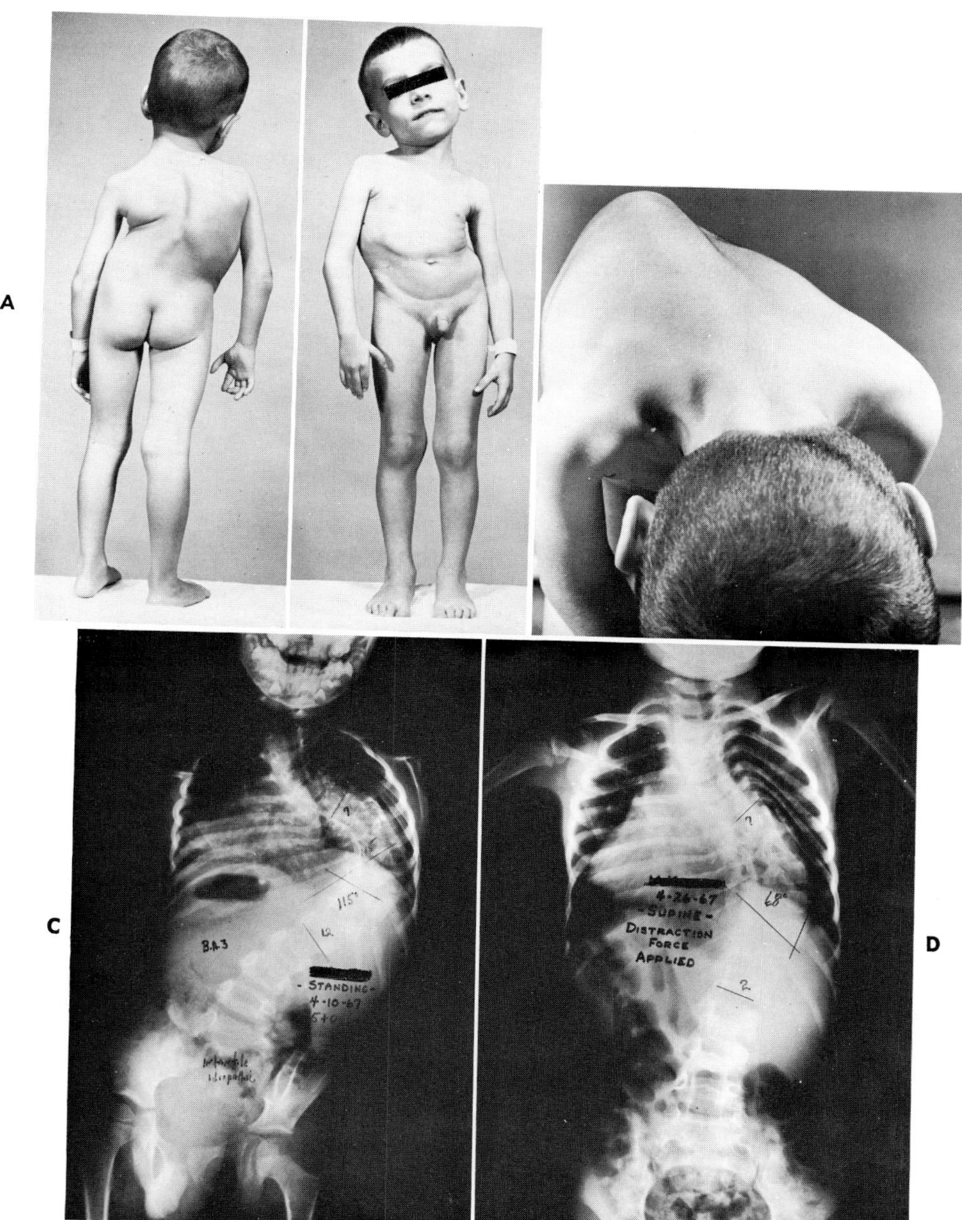

Fig. 13-23. M. K. **A,** Chronological age 5, bone age 3. Infantile idiopathic scoliosis, untreated. **B,** Rib hump of 10 cm. on forward bending. **C,** Infantile idiopathic scoliosis noted before age 1 but given only "observational treatment" progressed to 115 degrees. **D,** Distraction on x-ray table gave correction to 68 degrees.

Continued.

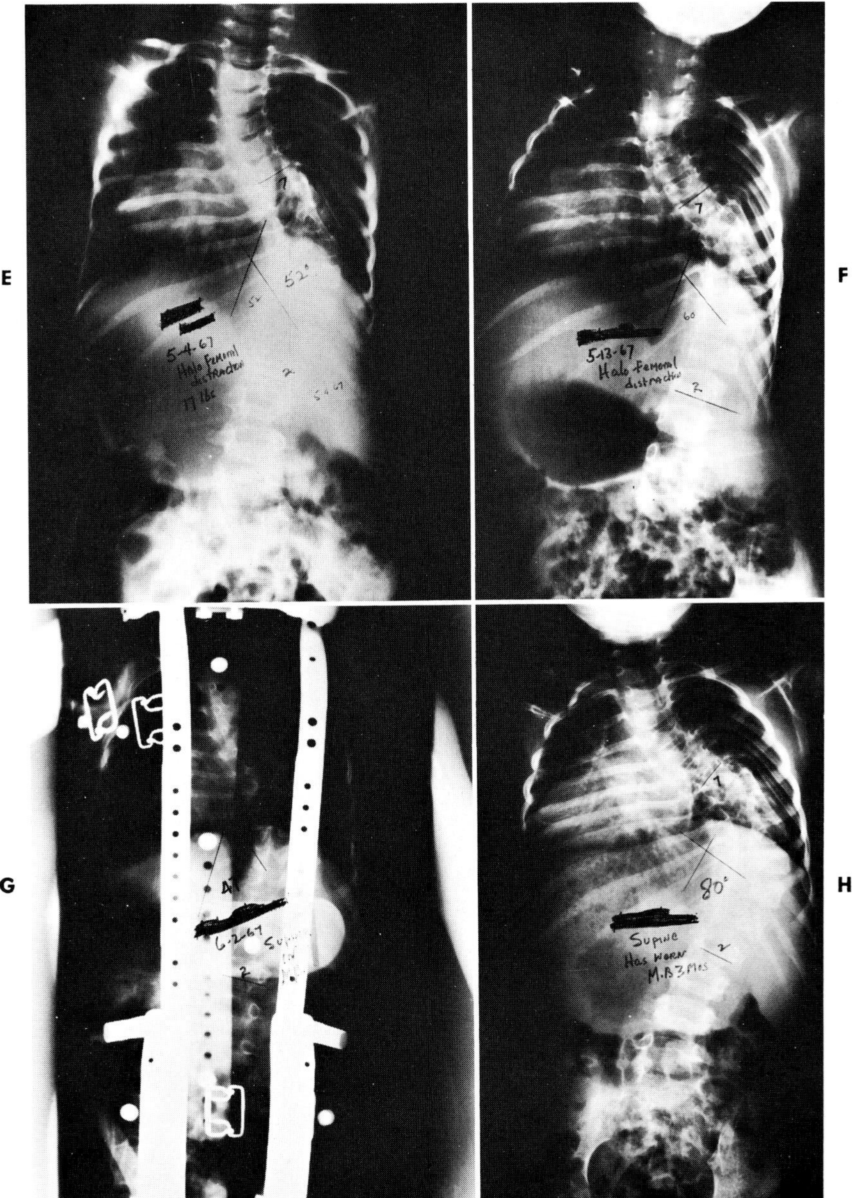

Fig. 13-23, cont'd. E, Halo-femoral (H. F.) distraction to 17 pounds was used; skull traction reduced curve to 52 degrees in two weeks. Note that the curve on initial distraction had reduced to 68 degrees. **F,** Further H. F. distraction gave no further correction. **G,** Milwaukee brace with fitted and H. F. distraction gradually discontinued. Maximum correction, patient supine in Milwaukee brace without the H. F., was to 47 degrees. Patient was allowed to go home and told to remain in bed but was unable to keep down full time in Milwaukee brace. **H,** In three months the curve, patient out of brace and supine, was 80 degrees.

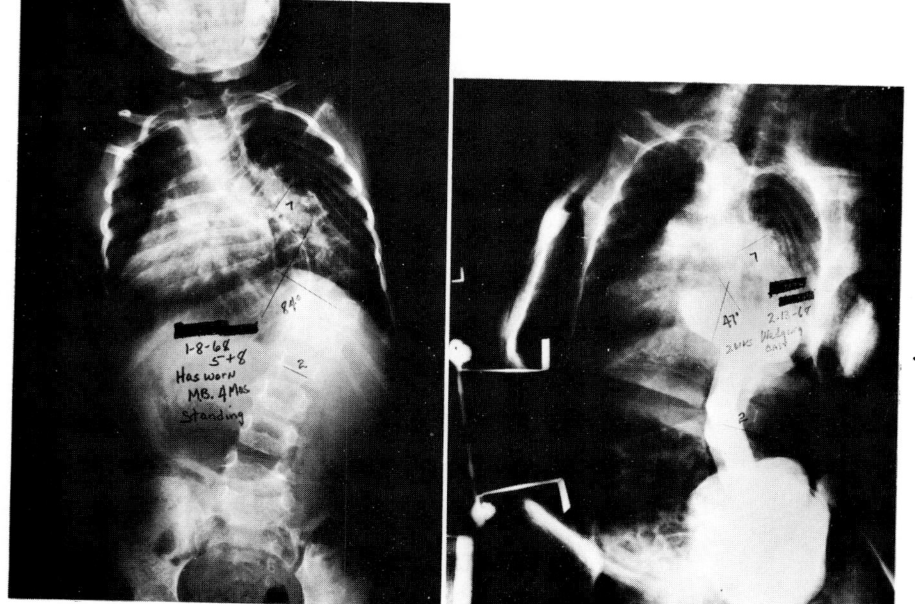

Fig. 13-23, cont'd. I, In four months the curve was still uncontrolled and measured 84 degrees. The brace was obviously not going to solve the problem. **J,** The plan of treatment was now again changed. Turnbuckles were applied on a new localizer cast and the curve corrected to 47 degrees. The patient was scheduled to come back in two months for a new preoperative localizer cast. The central five vertebrae of the major curve, T7 to L2, will be fused in maximal correction. After this fusion is mature, he will again be placed in a Milwaukee brace. The short fused segment will enhance the effectiveness of the brace and maintain good correction during the entire growth period. This case illustrates both the challenge of the problems and the ingenuity of the orthopaedic surgeon in treating severe scoliosis.

transverse process of the upper end of the lower curve, will distract and correct. It is best to place the strut bar in the lower curve first.

Summary

Idiopathic scoliosis is a problem to the orthopaedic surgeon. Knowledge of its inconsistency is essential to treatment. There is no dependable pattern of behavior, and prognosis can only be based on probabilities and particularly on experience. Experience can be obtained only when large numbers of patients with scoliosis are carefully observed, individually analyzed, and—above all—adequately treated to prevent catastrophic progression. Such experience is best obtained by the establishment of a scoliosis service in a teaching institution, under the direction of a group of orthopaedic surgeons who are intensely interested in this problem.

There will probably always be two types of problems: one is the small curve, in its early structural changes, that is discovered during growth years. In treating these the Milwaukee brace has no peer, and it is better to overtreat them than to neglect them.

The second is that of the badly deformed child whose progressive curve has been neglected (Fig. 13-23). During early years of childhood, every effort should be made to avoid surgical fusion but sometimes there is no other recourse. In older children, correction and fusion without delay is unquestionably the treatment of choice.

References

1. James, J. I. P.: Two curve patterns in idiopathic structural scoliosis, J. Bone Joint Surg. **33-B:**399, 1951.
2. James, J. I. P.: Idiopathic scoliosis: the prognosis, diagnosis and operative indications related to curve patterns and the age of onset, J. Bone Joint Surg. **36-B:**36, 1954.
3. James, J. I. P., Lloyd-Roberts, G. C., and Pilcher, M. F.: Infantile structural scoliosis, J. Bone Joint Surg. **41-B:**719, 1959.
4. Langenskiold, A., and Michelsson, J. E.: The pathogenesis of experimental progressive scoliosis, Acta Orthop. Scand. supp. 59, 1962.
5. Lloyd-Roberts, G. C., and Pilcher, M. F.: Structural idiopathic scoliosis in infancy: a study of the natural history of 100 patients, J. Bone Joint Surg. **47-B:**520, 1965.
6. Michelsson, J. E.: The development of spinal deformity in experimental scoliosis, Acta Orthop. Scand. supp. 81, 1965.
7. Ponseti, I. V., and Friedman, B.: Prognosis in idiopathic scoliosis, J. Bone Joint Surg. **32-A:**381, 1950.
8. Scott, J. C., and Morgan, T. H.: Natural history and prognosis of infantile idiopathic scoliosis, J. Bone Joint Surg. **37-B:**400, 1955.
9. Tøjner, H.: Olisthetic scoliosis, Acta Orthop. Scand. **33:**4, 1963.
10. Walker, G. F.: An evaluation of an external splint for idiopathic structural scoliosis in infancy, J. Bone Joint Surg. **47-B:**524, 1965.

14. Turnbuckle and Risser localizer casts in the correction of scoliosis: selection of patients and techniques*

Louis A. Goldstein, M.D.

The armamentarium of the orthopaedic surgeon who undertakes to treat scoliosis today should include the various methods proved to be effective in the correction of a curvature of the spine either singly or in combination. These are (1) external corrective forces: the plaster cast[4, 13] (Risser's turnbuckle wedging cast and Risser's localizer cast), the Milwaukee brace,[1, 2] and continuous traction (either halo-femoral pin traction[12] or Cotrell traction[6]); (2) instrumental correction[10] (Harrington type); and (3) wedge resection of vertebrae.[5, 14, 15]

Correction of the curvature by turnbuckle wedging cast and by localizer cast will be discussed in this paper.

Turnbuckle cast

The basic principle of the turnbuckle cast is the application of a plaster cast without corrective forces. The correction of the curvature is then obtained by turnbuckle wedging.

The allowable correction is determined from (1) the degree of fixed angulation in the compensatory countercurves as measured on roentgenograms made with the spine in bent position (Fig. 14-1, *B* and *C*) and (2) the alignment of the end vertebrae in the fusion area, as seen on the correction roentgenogram (Fig. 14-1, *D*).

Two considerations govern the allowable correction:

1. A perpendicular drawn from the middle of the inferior surface of the bottom vertebra must pass through or to the convex side of the top vertebra. If this line passes along the concave side of the top vertebra, it is indicative of overcorrection. (Fig. 14-1, *D*).

*This work was partially supported by National Institutes of Health Grant No. A-2919, United States Public Health Service.

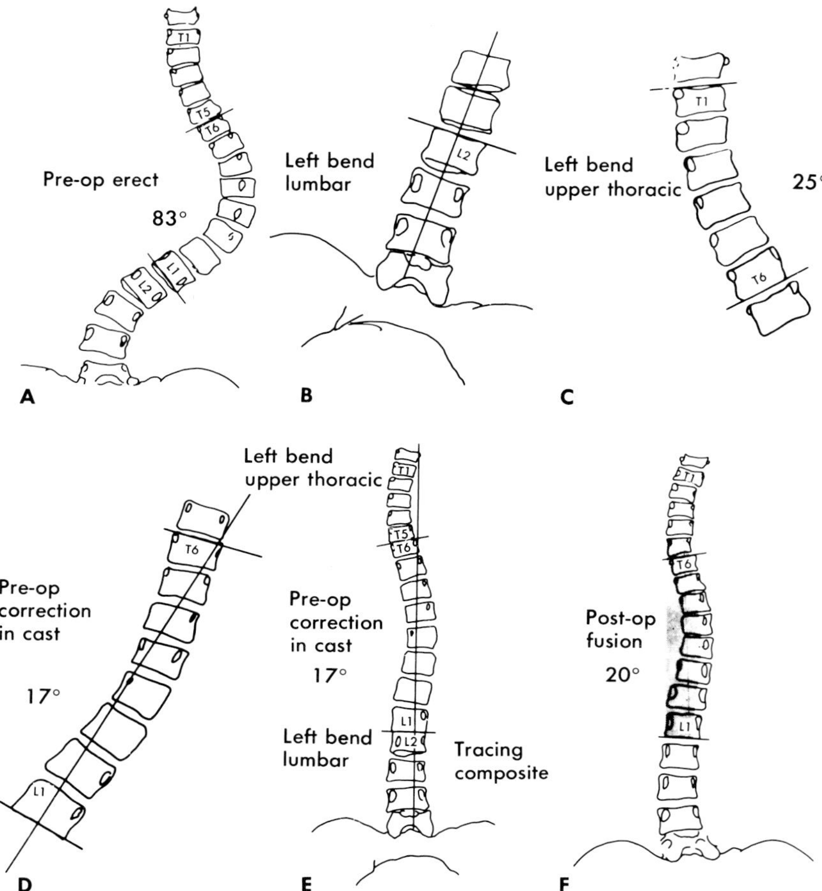

Fig. 14-1. Principles of preoperative correction of the curvature in turnbuckle plaster cast. Tracings of anteroposterior roentgenograms of the spine. **A,** Preoperative, erect. **B,** Left bending lumbar. **C,** Left bending upper thoracic. **D,** Preoperative correction of major curve in cast. **E,** Composite tracing of bending roentgenograms and of the corrected curve gives a preview of the postoperative result if the fusion is properly placed, the fusion is of proper length to maintain correction, and the fusion is solid. **F,** is based on the postoperative roentgenogram. (From Goldstein, L. A.: Clin. Orthop. **35:**100, 1964.)

2. When the correction roentgenogram with the area of fusion (T5-L1) delineated on it is superimposed on the lateral bend roentgenograms, as in Fig. 14-1, *E,* there should be good overall alignment of the fused segment and of the curves above and below. As a basic rule, the angular deformity of the major curve should not be corrected to less than the sum of the fixed angulations of the compensatory countercurves. The spine might then be unable to compensate, and an unbalanced trunk and contralateral displacement of the torso would be the result.

Technique of cast application

The plaster cast may be applied with the patient on a Goldthwait frame or on a Risser localizer table.

Early in our experience the turnbuckle cast was applied with the patient on bent Goldthwait irons as recommended by Cobb.[4, 7] The patient is placed supine on the frame which is bent toward the concavity of the major curve. This partially straightens the curves above and below the major curve to be corrected. The head is also flexed toward the same side to avoid undue tension on the neck during the correction. Over a double layer of stockinette adequate padding, Webril and soft felt, is applied. Both thighs are included in the cast and there is a headpiece, the plaster being well molded to the chin and occiput. Extra thicknesses of felt are placed in the axillary line on the convex side of the curve. This is subsequently withdrawn giving a little added room for the rib cage as the cast is wedged. Adequate padding of bony prominences, particularly iliac crests and rib rotational deformities, is important. The molding of the plaster under the chin and the occiput and on the back of the neck is done with care. If the plaster is not well molded into the hollow of the neck and over the occiput, the effect of the headpiece will be lost during the turnbuckle wedging correction because the chin can be pulled down into the neck portion of the cast. About halfway through the process of applying the plaster, aluminum hinges are placed anterior and posterior and incorporated in the plaster. These are placed in a relatively closed position with the joint of the hinge well lateral to the apex of the curve. The effect of this, combined with the carefully molded headpiece and the pelvis control by the thigh pieces, is that lateral wedging of the cast results in a distracting as well as a lateral bending force. This combination of forces is very effective in correction of the curvature.

The turnbuckle cast is now applied with the patient on the localizer table instead of the Goldthwait frame for convenience and ease of application.

Five to seven days after application, the cast is sufficiently dry for a window to be cut on the convex side and the cast to be split on the concave side as illustrated in Fig. 14-2. The turnbuckle is inserted over lugs, and correction is accomplished by turning up the turnbuckle each day as many turns as the patient will tolerate. This is gauged by two criteria: (1) complaint of discomfort on the concave side of the curve and (2) tightness of the chin against the plaster chinpiece. The more mobile curves are corrected in five to seven days. The more rigid curves may require two to three weeks for optimal correction. A complaint of pressure over any area, particularly iliac crests or the rib cage, requires immediate exposure of the area to inspect the skin and prevent pressure necrosis.

When roentgenograms show that the desired correction has been obtained, the cast is boxed in with supporting struts applied to both sides. Several days later a large window is cut in the back of the cast to allow exposure of one ilium, for removal of a large amount of iliac bone, and the area of the spine to be fused. A precordial opening and a large abdominal window are also cut in the cast preoperatively.

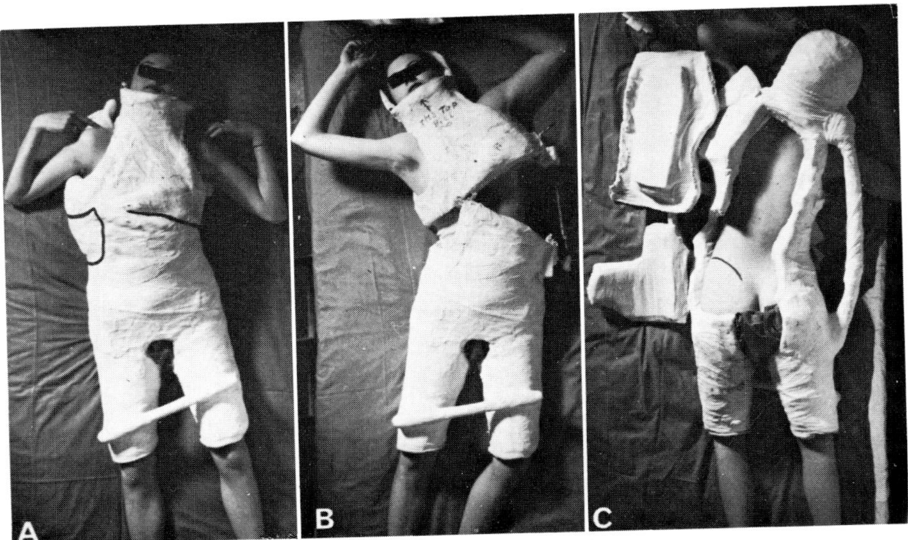

Fig. 14-2. Risser turnbuckle cast. **A,** Before correction. **B,** Turnbuckle wedging for correction of right thoracic curve. **C,** Large posterior window through which spine fusion is performed. (From Goldstein, L. A.: J. Bone Joint Surg. **48-A:**167, 1966.)

A preoperative spine marker film is made by injecting sterile methylene blue under aseptic precautions into the tip of the spinous process at or near the distal end of the fusion area. Surgery is performed through the large window in the back of the cast. Following skin suture removal, the patient is discharged home in this cast for six months in recumbency.

Selection of patients for turnbuckle cast correction

Idiopathic curves. Single major curves can be corrected in the turnbuckle cast. The turnbuckle principle, however, is not applicable for correction of combined thoracic and lumbar curves, or in the double structural thoracic curves. Also, when a long fusion is necessary because of a long, mobile curve, or when vertebrae distal to the curve are rotated into the convexity of the major curve, optimum correction cannot be obtained by turnbuckle wedging because the distal vertebrae to be included in the fusion would be in an overcorrected position. These curves require a localizer cast.

Paralytic curves. A single major curve, with or without pelvic obliquity, is corrected by turnbuckle cast. When there are two structural curves to correct and stabilize, the turnbuckle cast cannot be used.

Congenital curves. A single major curve, with or without pelvic obliquity, can be treated by turnbuckle cast. The turnbuckle cast is often very useful both as a supplementary correction force and as the major correction modality after osteotomy of congenital unsegmented bars.

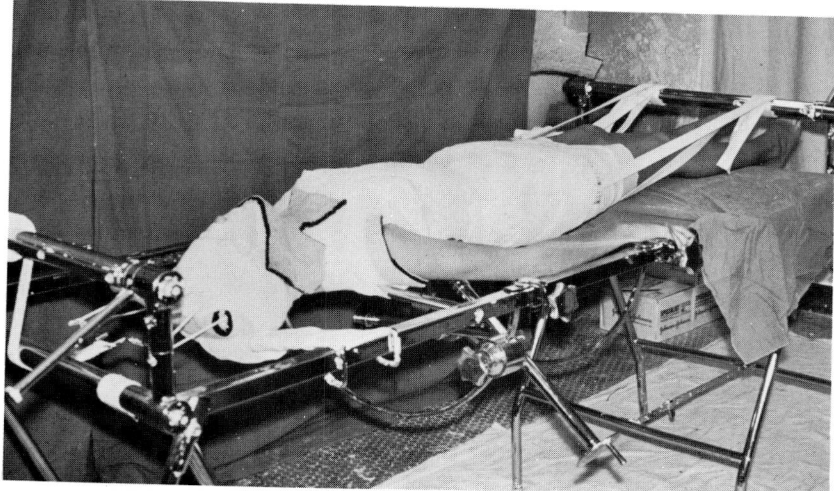

Fig. 14-3. Localizer cast application. Patient is in position on Risser localizer table for application of a localizer cast. The pelvic girdle between two layers of wax paper is applied over padding and can be easily withdrawn after the cast is completed. Increasing head halter and pelvic traction is applied, to patient tolerance. The localizer is adjusted below the apex of the rib cage deformity for correction of a right thoracic curve. The plaster is applied with the patient under the influence of the distraction and lateral pressure forces.

Localizer cast

The localizer cast has in great part replaced the turnbuckle cast for correction of scoliosis. The localizer cast is different from the turnbuckle cast in that the corrective forces are applied by head and pelvic distraction along with lateral pressure just prior to and during application of the plaster cast so that at completion of the cast the correction has been accomplished. Further correction can be obtained either by applying serial casts or by wedging the initial cast.

Technique of cast application

There are several techniques of application of the localizer cast. The method we have used is as follows: The patient is placed on a Risser localizer table. Webril applied firmly and smoothly to the torso is used as the basic padding. This is supplemented by 1-inch foam rubber under the sacrum and occiput and by soft felt molded to the iliac crests, back of the head, and shoulder girdle. A moistened felt pad is molded to the chin, mandible, and anterior neck. A disposable Zimmer head halter and a canvas pelvic girdle are applied with padding between two layers of waxed paper. Pelvic and halter traction is then gradually increased to patient tolerance. (See Fig. 14-3.) The localizer is adjusted over the apex of the thoracic curve, with an opposite localizer either over transverse processes of the lumbar curve or over the lateral aspect of the opposite hip to balance the patient. Circular plaster is then applied, starting at the pelvis. The molding is into the waist area soft tissues rather than over the iliac crests, avoiding pressure against these crests. After the pelvic portion has been well molded and while it is setting, the application of the plaster is continued up over the thorax and shoulders. The headpiece is then applied, with careful molding about the chin and mandible, the back of the neck, and the occiput. The corrective forces are maintained until the plaster has set. If the thighs are to be included in the cast, this is done before the patient is removed from the table. When the curve is to be corrected by cast alone, either turnbuckle or localizer, we have included both thighs in the plaster to get a better grasp on the pelvis. When the localizer cast is used in association with instrumentation of the spine, the cast does not include the thighs.

Surgery is performed in the cast through a large window that exposes one ilium and the area of spine to be fused, as with the turnbuckle cast (Fig. 14-4,*A*). A precordial window is also cut, and a large window is fashioned over the abdomen to reduce pressure on the abdominal contents when the patient is prone during surgery. Recently we have introduced the practice of cutting a lid from the chin and anterior neck region; this allows direct laryngoscopy and easy intubation, eliminating the need for blind endotracheal intubation for anesthesia. (See Fig. 14-4, *B*.)

Patients are discharged home in this same cast, with the removable lids plastered

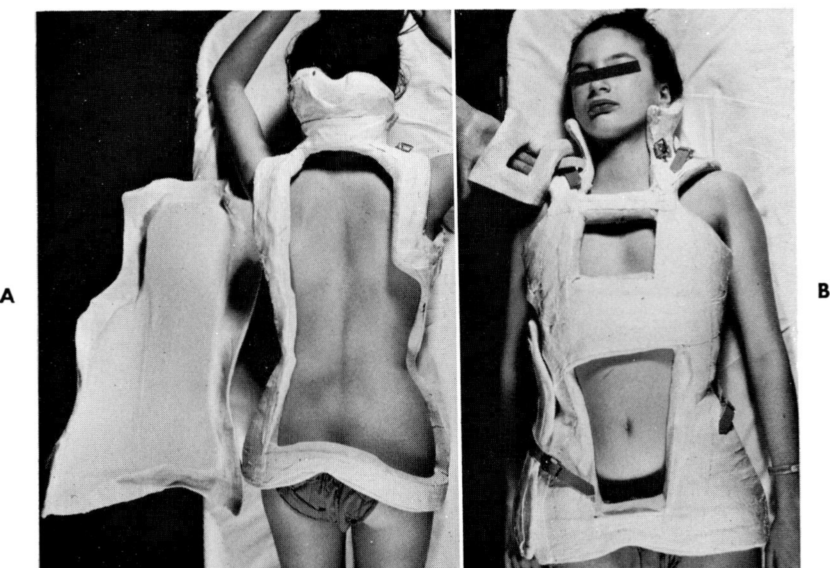

Fig. 14-4. Preoperative localizer cast. **A,** Large posterior window through which fusion is performed allows wide exposure of one ilium, for removal of a large amount of iliac bone graft, as well as the area of the spine to be fused. **B,** Front of the localizer cast, showing the large abdominal window that minimizes pressure on abdominal contents when patient is prone during surgery. The chin-neck trap door allows direct laryngoscopy for intubation for anesthesia. The precordial window is also shown.

in; or a new cast is applied under corrective forces at about two weeks postoperative, depending on the condition of the cast.

Selection of patients for localizer cast correction

A localizer cast is used for uncomplicated curves in idiopathic, paralytic, and congenital scolioses. Its limitation is chiefly the inability to get optimum correction in the severe rigid curves, of any etiology, that require supplementary corrective forces or in paralytic and congenital scolioses with pelvic obliquity.

Selection of the fusion area

The minimum fusion area has been defined[3] as the region including all vertebrae in the major curve. If one considers the minimum fusion area in a particular patient as that area of the spine requiring stabilization to maintain correction, then one must take into account the rotation of the vertebrae at and beyond the ends of the curve. Moe[11] has pointed out that all vertebrae rotated into the convexity of the major curve should be included in the fusion area and that, preferably, the fusion should extend from neutral vertebra above to neutral vertebra below. It is essential, therefore, that the minimum fusion area in any particular patient

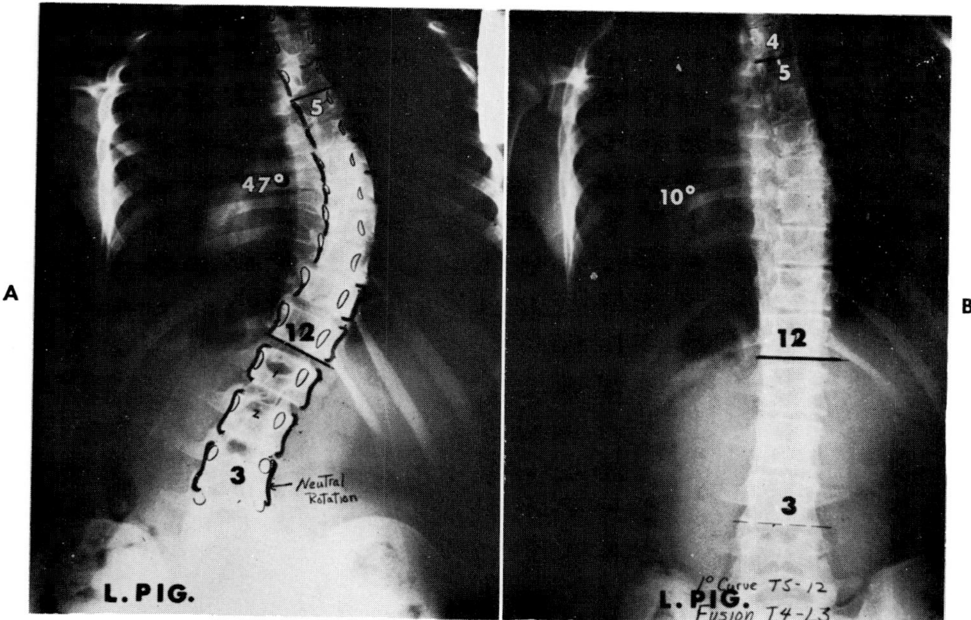

Fig. 14-5. A, Preoperative film. Major curve, fifth to twelfth thoracic vertebra. First and second lumbar vertebrae are rotated toward the convexity of the major curve. **B,** Postoperative view. Spine fusion extends from the fourth thoracic to the third lumbar vertebra, from neutrally rotated vertebra above to vertebra in neutral position below. (From Goldstein, L. A.: J. Bone Joint Surg. **48-A:**167, 1966.)

include not only those vertebrae within the major curve, but also all those beyond this curve which are rotated toward its convexity.

In the patient whose roentgenograms are shown in Fig. 14-5, the major curve extends from the fifth to the twelfth thoracic vertebra as determined by their tilt toward the concavity of the curve. (See Fig. 14-5, *A*.) Proximally the fifth thoracic

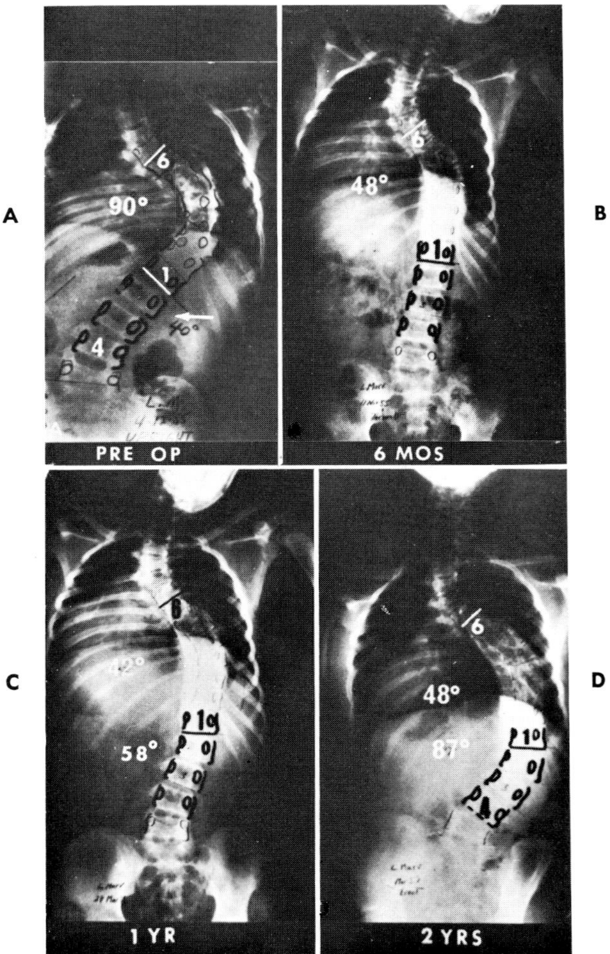

Fig. 14-6. Lengthening of curve. **A,** Preoperative erect roentgenogram. Major curve, sixth thoracic to first lumbar vertebra. Second, third, and fourth lumbar vertebrae are rotated toward the convexity of the major curve. **B,** Six months postoperative. The fusion extends from the sixth thoracic to the first lumbar vertebra (major curve alone). **C,** One year postoperative. Extension of the major curve to include the second and third lumbar vertebrae. **D,** Two years postoperative. Increase of the deformity, owing to further distal extension of the curve to the fourth lumbar vertebra. Correction within the fused major curve is maintained. The fusion was too short. (From Goldstein, L. A.: J. Bone Joint Surg. **48-A:**167, 1966.)

vertebra is rotated toward the convexity of the curve, and the fourth thoracic vertebra is in neutral rotation. Distally, the first and second lumbar vertebrae are rotated toward the major curve's convexity and the third lumbar vertebra is in neutral rotation. In this patient the fusion must extend from the fourth thoracic through the third lumbar vertebra (Fig. 14-5, *B*). Its failure to do so will result in lengthening of the curve distally after mobilization of the patient, even though the fusion is solid and correction is maintained within the confines of the major curve.

In another patient, the preoperative roentgenogram (Fig. 14-6, *A*) shows the second, third, and fourth lumbar vertebrae to be rotated toward the major curve's convexity. Following turnbuckle cast correction, the fusion extended from the sixth thoracic through the first lumbar vertebra (major curve alone). Follow-up roentgenograms (Fig. 14-6, *B* to *D*) showed recurrence of deformity, caused not by loss of correction within the confines of the fused major curve but by too short a fusion that allowed the curve to lengthen to include the fourth lumbar vertebra.

The roentgenogram of a third patient (Fig. 14-7, *A*) shows the end vertebrae, T4 and T11, in neutral rotation. Fusion of the major curve alone in this patient will effectively maintain correction (Fig. 14-7, *B*).

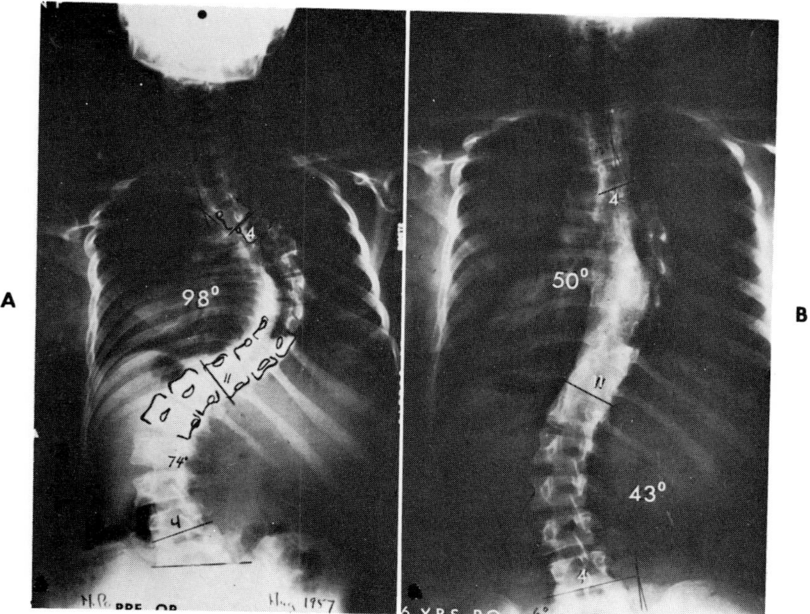

Fig. 14-7. A, Preoperative x-ray film. Major curve, fourth to eleventh thoracic vertebra. The eleventh thoracic vertebra is in neutral rotation. The twelfth thoracic vertebra is rotated into the convexity of the lumbar curve. Fusion of the major curve alone, fourth to eleventh thoracic vertebra, is permissible. **B,** Six years postoperative. Fusion extends from the fourth to the eleventh thoracic vertebra. Correction is maintained. (From Goldstein, L. A.: J. Bone Joint Surg. **48-A:**167, 1966.)

Table 14-1. Final results: correction and loss averages in 110 patients with solid fusion*

Type and no. of patients	*Original curve (Degrees)*	*Correction of pre-operative curve (Degrees)*	*Correction (Percent)*	*Final correction (Degrees)*	*Loss of correction (Degrees)*	*(Percent)*
Idiopathic						
Main thoracic (55)	75	42	56	38	4	9
Main lumbar (3)	56	38	70	37	1	4
Thoracolumbar (17)	65	44	67	41	3	8
Combined thoracic and lumbar (5)	76	35	44	32	3	10
Cervicothoracic (1)	55	23	42	20	3	13
Paralytic (16)	81	48	57	44	3.5	8
Congenital (13)	73	37	54	33	4	9

*From Goldstein, L. A., and Evarts, C. M.: Further experiences with the treatment of scoliosis by cast correction and spine fusion with fresh autogenous iliac bone grafts, J. Bone Joint Surg. **48-A:**962, 1966.

Present treatment program

Instrumentation[9, 10] has been used in our program since December, 1961, at first in selected patients only; then its indications gradually broadened as we gained experience. For three years we have used preoperative cast correction followed by instrumentation in the cast, for whatever further correction can be obtained, along with fusion for stabilization of the spine in the corrected position. These patients have a new localizer cast applied under moderate halter and pelvic traction two weeks after operation, and in this they are discharged home.

Results of treatment in turnbuckle and localizer plaster casts

In 1966 Goldstein and Evarts[9] reported results of the treatment of scoliosis by cast correction and spine fusion in 120 consecutive patients under 20 years of age. Sixty-five of these patients underwent correction in the turnbuckle cast and fifty-five were corrected in a localizer cast. Patients were followed from two to thirteen years. Ten pseudarthroses occurred in 120 patients in whom 125 fusion operations were performed, an incidence of 8%. Eight pseudarthroses occurred in patients with idiopathic scoliosis and two in patients with congenital curvatures. These results are summarized in Table 14-1.

Statistics represent only one facet in the analysis of the end results of treatment. The quality of correction of the clinical deformity is important. This depends in significant measure on the type and degree of deformity, as well as on the effectiveness of the treatment. (See Figs. 14-8 to 14-10.)

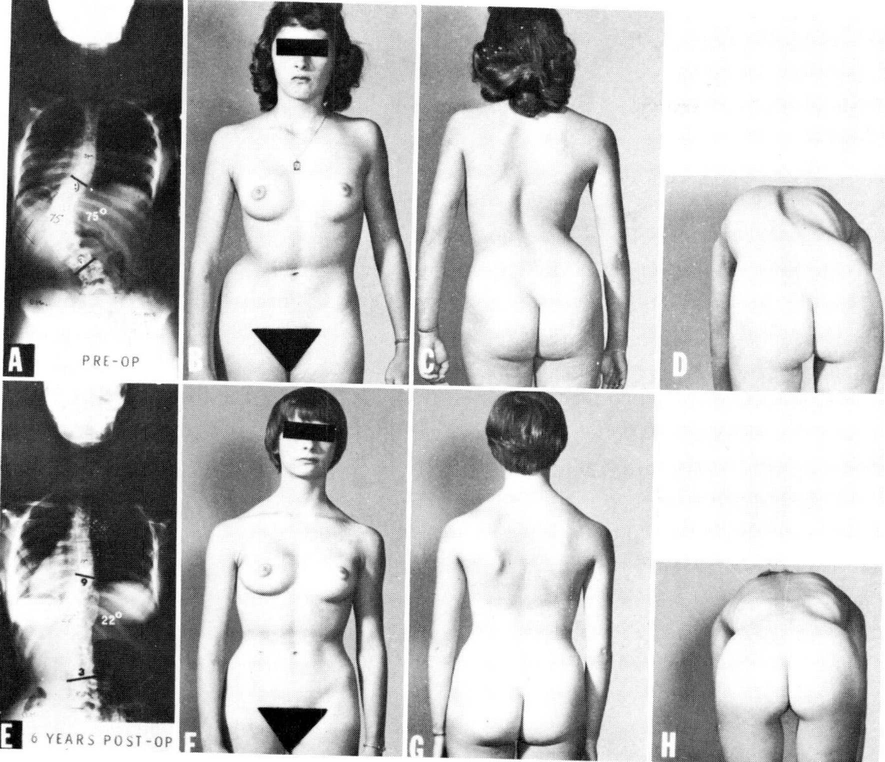

Fig. 14-8. Mobile idiopathic thoracolumbar scoliosis without structural rib deformity. Upper row of figures is preoperative; lower row, postoperative. (From Goldstein, L. A.: J. Bone Joint Surg. **48-A:**167, 1966.)

Summary

The plaster cast is useful both as a major and as a supplementary correction force for the reduction of scoliotic curves. The turnbuckle cast is particularly useful in the correction of single major curves, for rigid curves, and for curvatures associated with pelvic obliquity. The localizer cast can be used for correction of single or double curves, but it is not an adequate correction appliance for the reduction of rigid curves or of curvatures associated with pelvic obliquity. The localizer cast is also useful for preliminary correction either prior to instrumentation or preliminary to further correction to be obtained by the wedging principle.

Our present treatment of choice for idiopathic scoliosis is a single preoperative localizer cast followed by instrumentation and fusion in the cast.

For optimum correction of the curvature in a particular patient the method of choice will depend upon the type and degree of deformity. The surgeon must be knowledgeable in the use of the various methods of correction that have been proved effective.

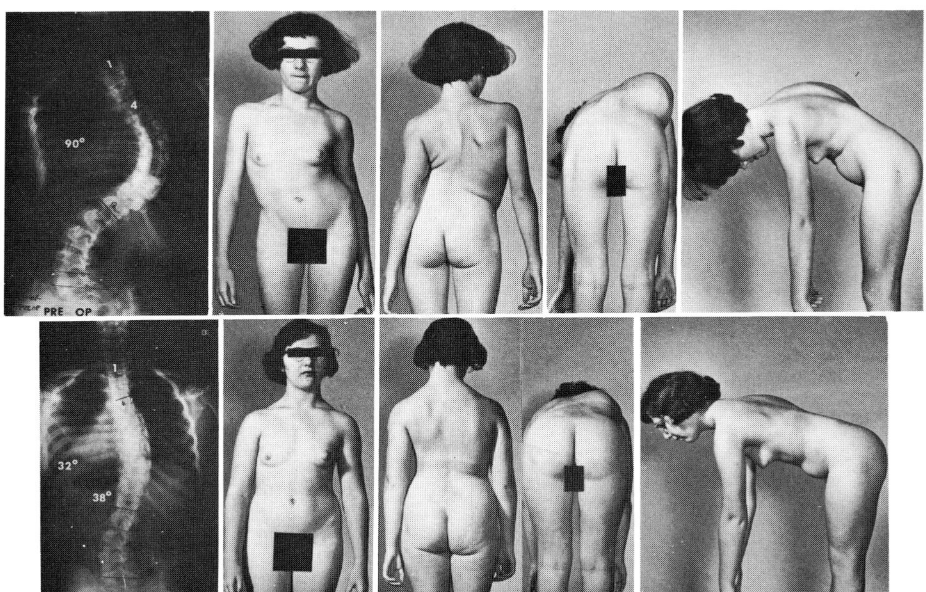

Fig. 14-9. Severe idiopathic thoracic scoliosis. The absence of angular rib deformity allows a remarkable reduction in the rotational rib prominence. Upper row of figures is preoperative; lower row, postoperative. (From Goldstein, L. A.: J. Bone Joint Surg. **48-A:**167, 1966.)

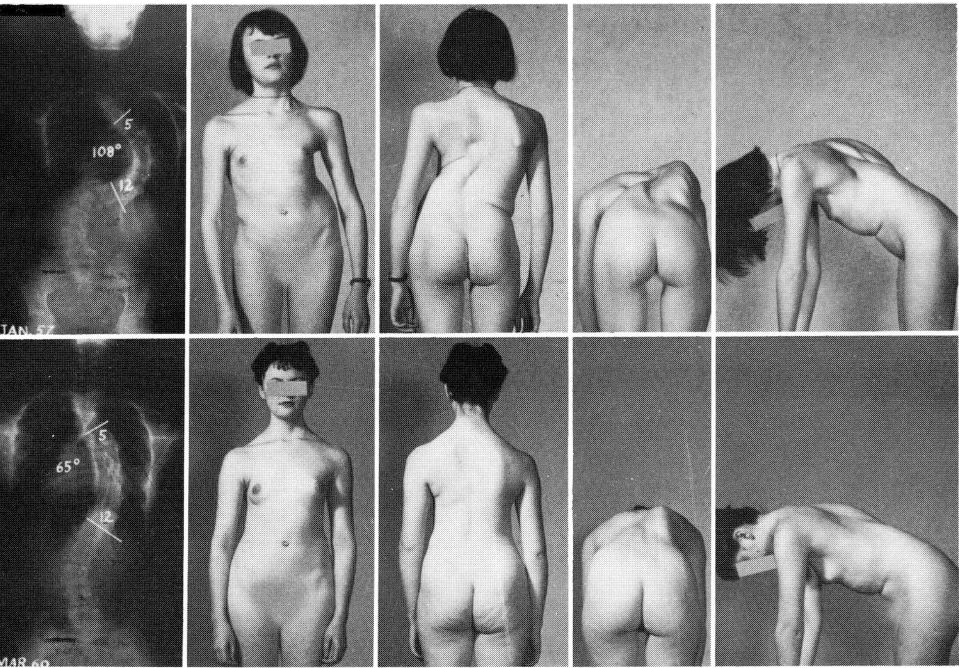

Fig. 14-10. Severe idiopathic thoracic scoliosis with structural rib angulation. Upper row of figures is preoperative; lower row, postoperative. (From Goldstein, L. A.: J. Bone Joint Surg. **48-A:**167, 1966.)

References

1. Blount, W. P.: Scoliosis and the Milwaukee brace, Bull. Hosp. Joint Dis. **19:**152, 1958.
2. Blount, W. P., and Moe, J. H.: Non-operative treatment of scoliosis with the Milwaukee brace. In American Academy of Orthopaedic Surgeons, Instructional Course Lectures, unpublished.
3. Butte, F. L.: Scoliosis treated by the wedging jacket; selection of the area to be fused, J. Bone Joint Surg. **20:**1, 1938.
4. Cobb, J. R.: Technique, after-treatment, and results of spine fusion for scoliosis. In American Academy of Orthopaedic Surgeons, Instructional Course Lectures, Ann Arbor, 1952, J. W. Edwards Co., vol. 9, pp. 65-70.
5. Compere, E. L.: Excision of hemivertebrae for correction of congenital scoliosis; report of two cases, J. Bone Joint Surg. **14:**555, 1932.
6. Cotrell, Y.: Personal communication, 1952.
7. Goldstein, L. A.: The surgical treatment of scoliosis, Springfield, Ill., 1959, Charles C Thomas, Publisher, p. 19.
8. Goldstein, L. A.: Surgical management of scoliosis. In American Academy of Orthopaedic Surgeons, Instructional Course Lectures, J. Bone Joint Surg. **48-A:**167, 1966.
9. Goldstein, L. A., and Evarts, C. M.: Further experiences with the treatment of scoliosis by cast correction and spine fusion with fresh autogenous iliac bone grafts, J. Bone Joint Surg. **48-A:**962, 1966.
10. Harrington, P. R.: Treatment of scoliosis; correction and internal fixation by spine instrumentation, J. Bone Joint Surg. **44-A:**591, 1962.
11. Moe, J. H.: A critical analysis of methods of fusion for scoliosis; an evaluation in two hundred and sixty-six patients, J. Bone Joint Surg. **40-A:**529, 1958.
12. Perry, J., and Nickel, V. C.: Total cervical spine fusion for neck paralysis, J. Bone Joint Surg. **41-A:**37, 1959.
13. Risser, J. C., Lauder, C. H., Norquist, D. M., and Craig, W. A.: Three types of body casts. In American Academy of Orthopaedic Surgeons, Instructional Course Lectures, Ann Arbor, 1953, J. W. Edwards Co., vol. 10, pp. 131-142.
14. Von Lackum, H. L., and Smith, A. DeF.: Removal of vertebral bodies in the treatment of scoliosis, Surg. Gynec. Obstet. **57:**250, 1933.
15. Wiles, P.: Resection of dorsal vertebrae in congenital scoliosis, J. Bone Joint Surg. **33-A:**151, 1951.

15. Concave rib resection and ligament release for correction of idiopathic thoracic scoliosis*

Louis A. Goldstein, M.D.

The evaluation of the end result of the surgical treatment of scoliosis depends upon the type and degree of deformity present preoperatively as well as the effectiveness of treatment. The result of treatment should be judged not only by the degree and percent of correction of the curvature that is maintained but also by the quality of the correction of the rib cage deformity.

The severity of rib cage deformity is not necessarily directly related to the degree of lateral angulation of the spine (Fig. 15-1).

Curvatures of identical degrees may vary in the degree of structural change, and the structural change influences the potential correctability regardless of the method of correction used (Fig. 15-2). All curve measurements were made by the Cobb method.[1]

From October 1963 to August 1967, 72 patients with idiopathic thoracic scoliosis have had special treatment in the concavity of the curve in addition to other correction measures in an effort to improve the quality of correction of the rib cage deformity.

Seventeen patients had concave segmental rib resection,[2] 13 with rib osteotomy[1] or costotransversectomy[3] supplementing Harrington instrumentation[3] for correction of the curvature. Fifty patients had a single preoperative localizer cast,[3, 4, 6] concave ligament release, and instrumentation. Five patients had concave ligament release with instrumentation but without preoperative localizer cast.

Technique

The segmental rib resection, rib osteotomy, and costrotransversectomy were done through the midline incision used for the spine fusion. The reflection of the

*This work was partially supported by National Institutes of Health Grant No. A-2919, United States Public Health Service.

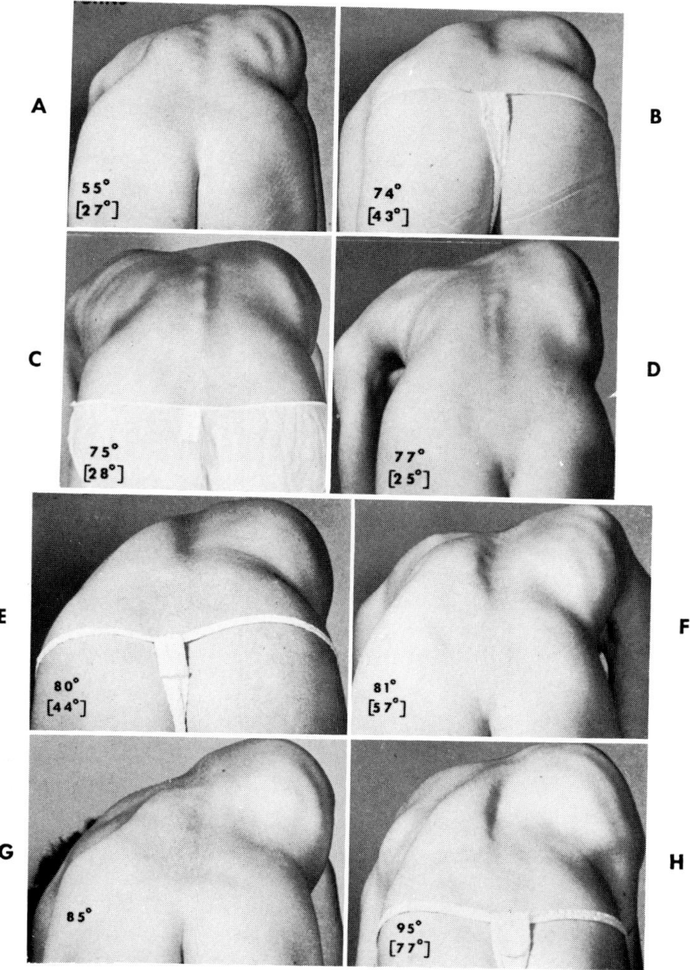

Fig. 15-1. Profile views of rib cage deformity, demonstrating the variability in severity of the thoracic cage deformity in relation to degree of lateral angulation of the spine. The top numeral in each frame represents the lateral angulation of the major curve in the erect position. The number in brackets is the residual angulation on bend radiograph. **A** and **B** have very favorable types of rib cage deformity for any method of correction. **D** with a 77-degree curve shows moderately severe structural rib changes on the convex and concave ribs, whereas **C,** with an almost identical angulation, shows no rib angulation. The restoration of rib cage symmetry in **D** will not approach the quality of correction obtainable in **C** regardless of the method of correction. Likewise, **E** (with absence of structural rib angulation) has a much more favorable type of deformity to correct than **F,** who shows structural changes in convex and concave ribs. Although the rib cage asymmetry in **G** is severe, the rounded convexity means a high degree of correction potential. The same is true with the 95-degree curve of **H.**

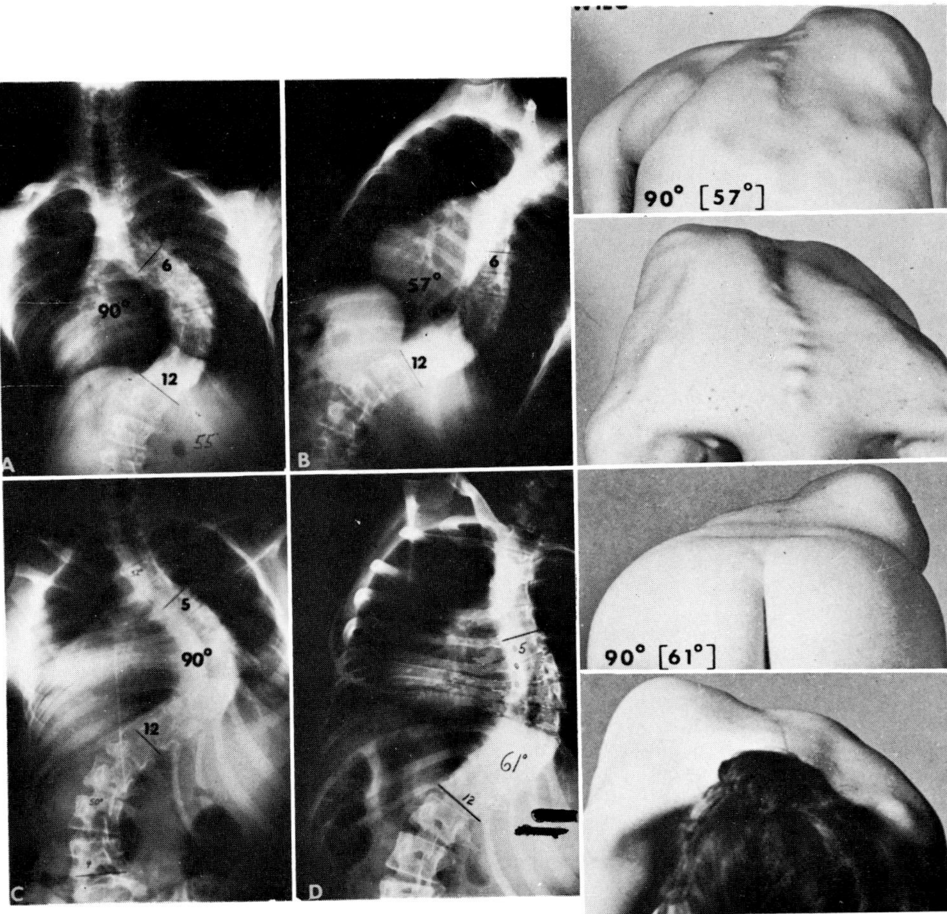

Fig. 15-2. Two patients with 90-degree idiopathic thoracic curves. **A** and **C,** Anteroposterior films made in erect position. **B** and **D,** Right bending roentgenograms showing more severe structural rib cage changes in **D;** the ribs remain closely approximated at the apex of the curve. Caudad and cephalad profile views of the rib cage deformity are shown to the right of the roentgenograms of each patient, demonstrating the difference in type of deformity and degree of angulation. (**C** and **D** from Goldstein, L. A.: J. Bone Joint Surg. **48-A:**167, 1966.)

soft tissue structures further laterally exposing the ribs in the concavity of the curve allowed the removal subperiosteally of a 1½-inch segment of rib from four or five levels. (See Fig. 15-3.) In several patients a separate incision was used lateral to the midline incision for the segmental rib resection prior to exposure of the spine through the usual midline incision.

The ligament release procedure consists of complete circumferential reflection of ligaments off the transverse processes in the concavity of the curve. The ligament reflection is carried out to the tips of the transverse processes at all levels in the concavity of the curve. (See Fig. 15-4.)

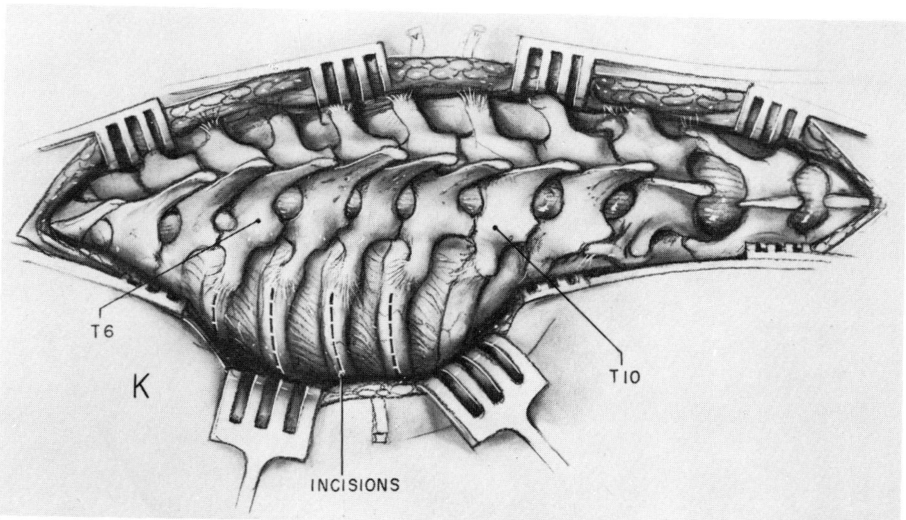

Fig. 15-3. Exposure for spine fusion with rib resection. The soft tissues on the concave side of the curve are widely retracted allowing exposure of about 2 inches of four or five ribs at the apex of the curve. The dotted lines indicate incision through periosteum for subperiosteal resection of one and one-half rib segments. (Reprinted from Atlas of Pediatric Surgery, edited by R. R. White, from Section on Orthopaedic Surgery by L. A. Goldstein and R. B. Dickerson. Copyright 1965, McGraw-Hill Book Co., New York, used by permission of publisher.)

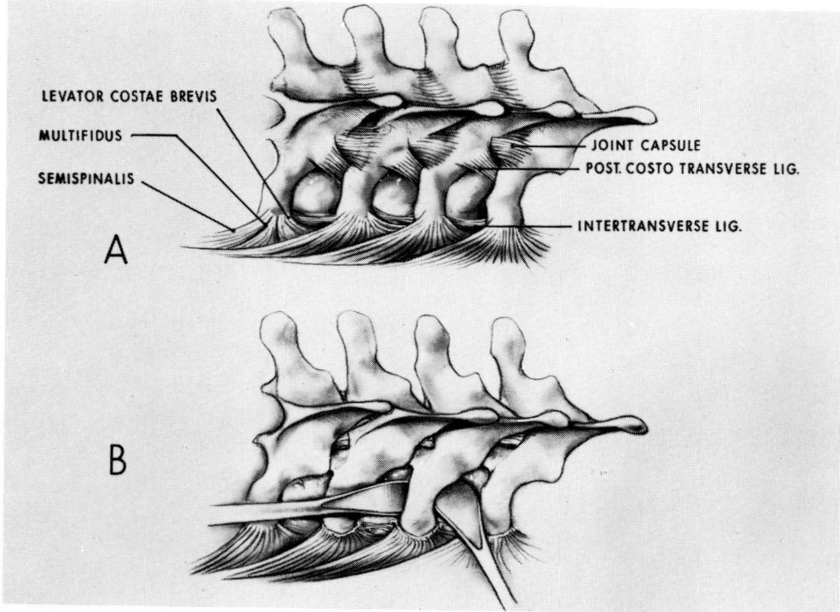

Fig. 15-4. Concave ligament release. **A,** The small muscle attachments and ligaments usually visualized in the exposure of the spine for fusion. **B,** After reflection of all soft tissue structures off laminae, articular processes, and tranverse processes.

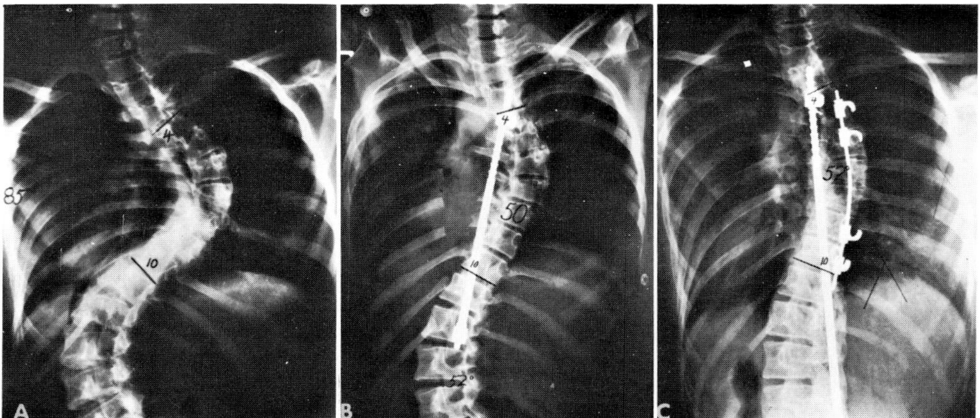

Fig. 15-5. Idiopathic scoliosis, curve correction by rib resection and instrumentation. **A,** An 85-degree right thoracic curve. **B,** Seven days after subperiosteal resection of 1½-inch segments of five concave ribs and instrumentation of the thoracic curve, film shows wide separation of rib stumps and good spread of distal rib fragments. **C,** One-year postoperative film shows bony union of approximated rib stumps and some loss of correction of the improved rib cage symmetry noted in **B.** (A second-stage procedure was performed two weeks after stage one, with insertion of a longer rod for correction of the lumbar curve as well as the thoracic curve. The spine was fused from T4 to L4.)

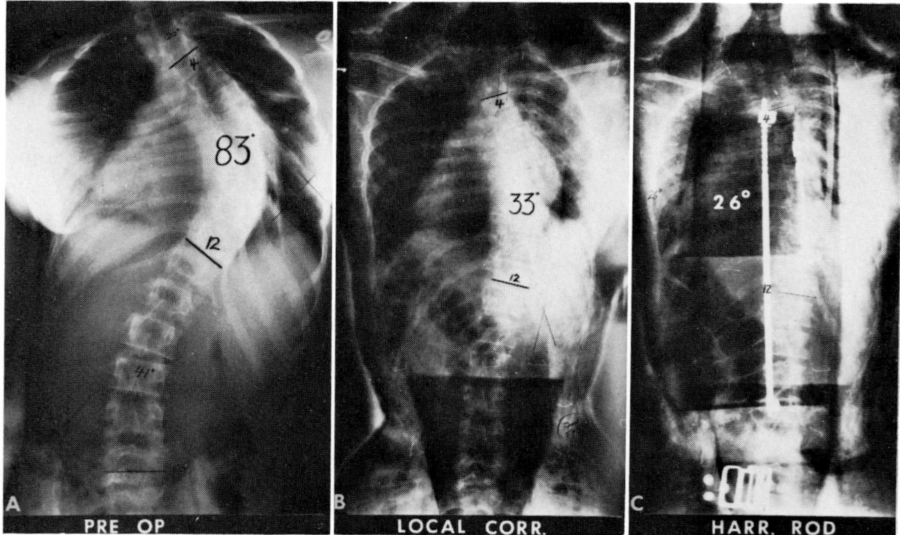

Fig. 15-6. Correction of curvature by localizer cast, concave ligament release, and instrumentation. **A,** Precorrection roentgenogram. **B,** After localizer cast correction. **C,** After concave ligament release, further correction, and internal fixation with instrumentation and fusion.

Films made during the first postoperative week after segmental rib resection show wide separation of the rib stumps and good separation of the distal rib fragments, creating improved rib cage symmetry as illustrated in Fig. 15-5, *B*. Rib stumps, however, gradually approximate so that at the end of three to four weeks they are in contact and usually go on to bony union. This results in some loss of the improvement in rib cage symmetry that occurred immediately after operation. (See Fig. 15-5, *C*.) It was because of this and increased morbidity that we abandoned the rib resection technique and now perform the concave ligament release.

The 17 patients who had rib resection or costotransversectomy were operated on between October 1963 and October 1964. The 55 patients reported in this

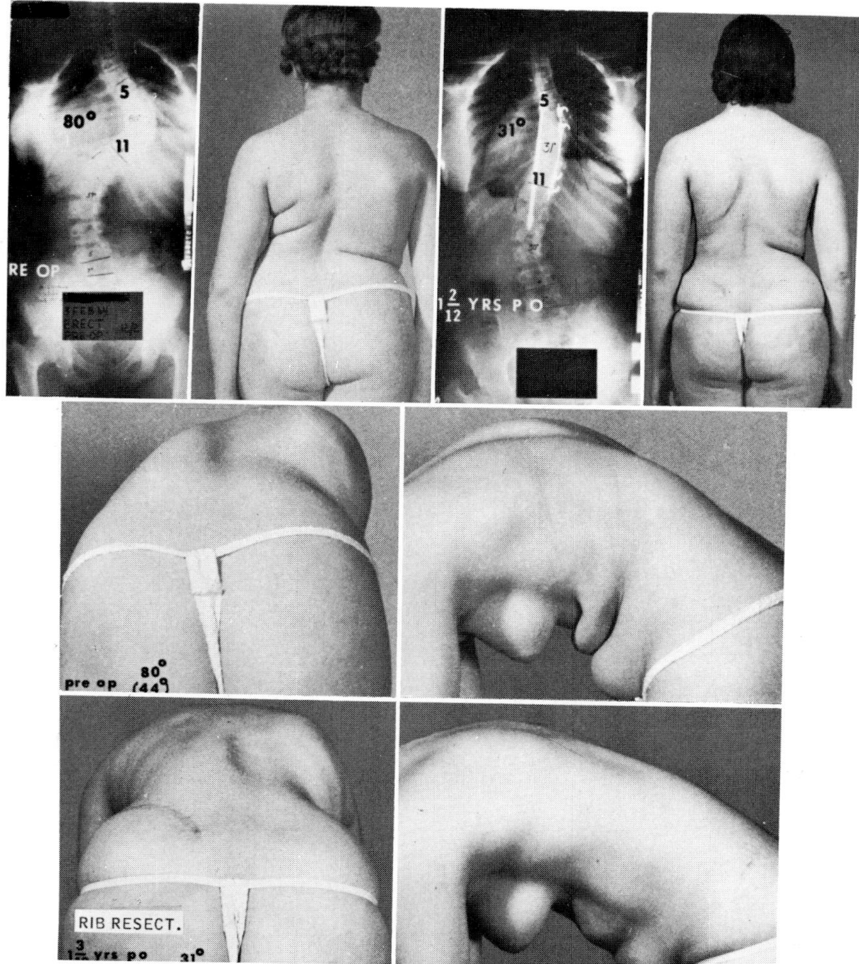

Fig. 15-7. Idiopathic thoracic scoliosis. Correction by rib resection and instrumentation. The absence of angular rib deformity allows restoration of excellent rib cage symmetry. Upper row of figures is preoperative; lower row, postoperative.

paper who had ligament release were operated on between November 1964 and August 1967.

Selection of patients

Concave rib resection was done in those patients who showed severe structural rib cage changes in addition to persistence of approximation of the ribs at the apex of the concavity of the curve on bend roentgenogram (Fig. 15-2, *C* and *D*).

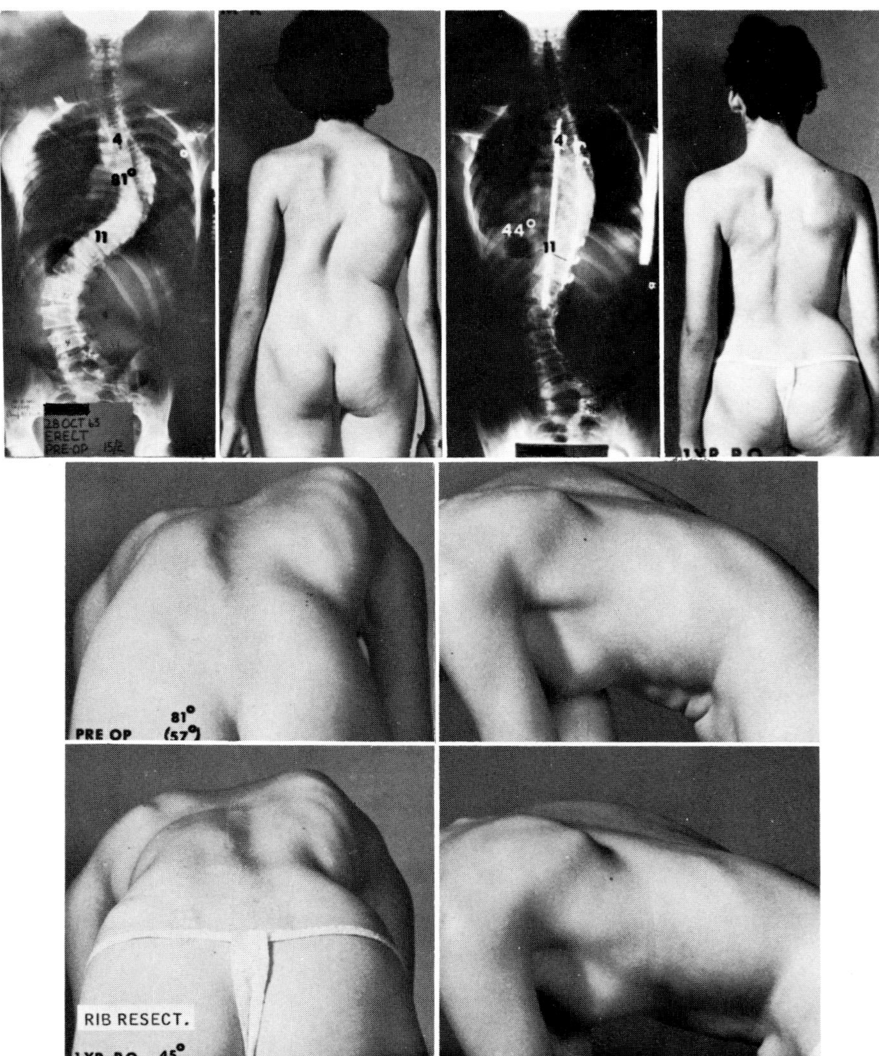

Fig. 15-8. Idiopathic thoracic scoliosis, with structural rib angulation on the convex side and structural rib depression at apex on concave side (thoracic valley). Correction by rib resection and instrumentation. Upper row of figures is preoperative; lower row, postoperative.

Concave ligament release is now done on all patients with thoracic curves that are corrected surgically. This treatment of the concave structures is supplemented by instrumentation in all cases. (See Figs. 15-4 and 15-6.)

Rib resection and instrumentation

There were 17 patients in this group. The average initial curve measured 73 degrees. An average of 41 degrees or 56% correction was obtained. The lesser percentage of correction obtained in these seventeen curves is indicative of the greater degree of structural change present preoperatively as compared with the patients in the other groups. The average loss of correction was 2.5 degrees or 6%. (See Figs. 15-7 and 15-8.)

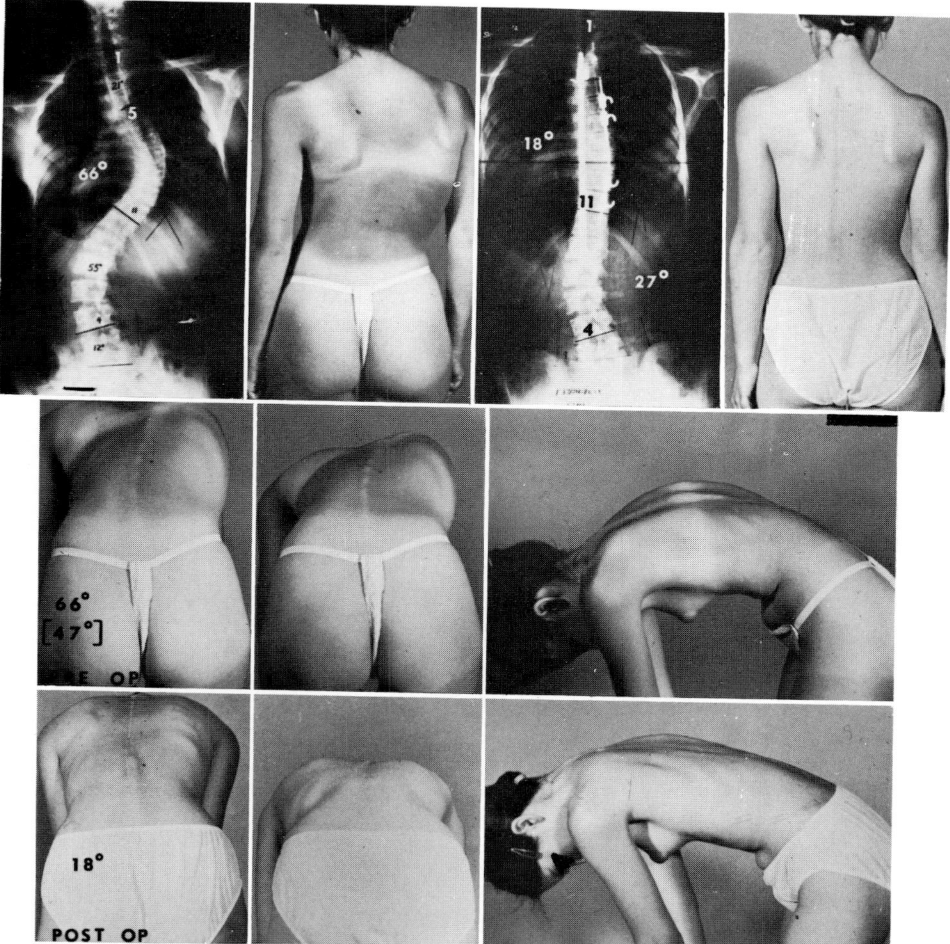

Fig. 15-9. Moderately severe idiopathic thoracic scoliosis. Correction by preoperative localizer cast, concave ligament release, and instrumentation. Upper row of figures is preoperative; lower row, postoperative.

Concave ligament release and instrumentation

Five curves had an average initial curve of 69 degrees. Average correction obtained was 42 degrees or 61%. The average loss of correction was 2.4 degrees or 6%.

Preoperative localizer cast, ligament release, and instrumentation

Fifty curves were in this group (Fig. 15-6). The average initial curve was 64 degrees, and average correction obtained by the single preoperative localizer cast was 30 degrees or 47%. Final correction obtained after concave ligament release and instrumentation in the cast was 41 degrees or 64%. Nineteen of these curves have been followed for eighteen months or longer and show an average loss of correction of 2.9 degrees or 6%. (See Figs. 15-9 and 15-10.)

It is interesting to compare the above results with correction obtained by instrumentation alone and by cast alone. Thirty-one curves were corrected by instrumentation alone. An average initial curve of 66 degrees was corrected an average of 37 degrees or 56%. In the cast correction series[5] fifty-five idiopathic thoracic curves with an average initial curve of 75 degrees were corrected an average of 42 degrees or 56%.

The average age of patients in the instrumentation group was 14.2 years and in the cast group, 13.4 years.

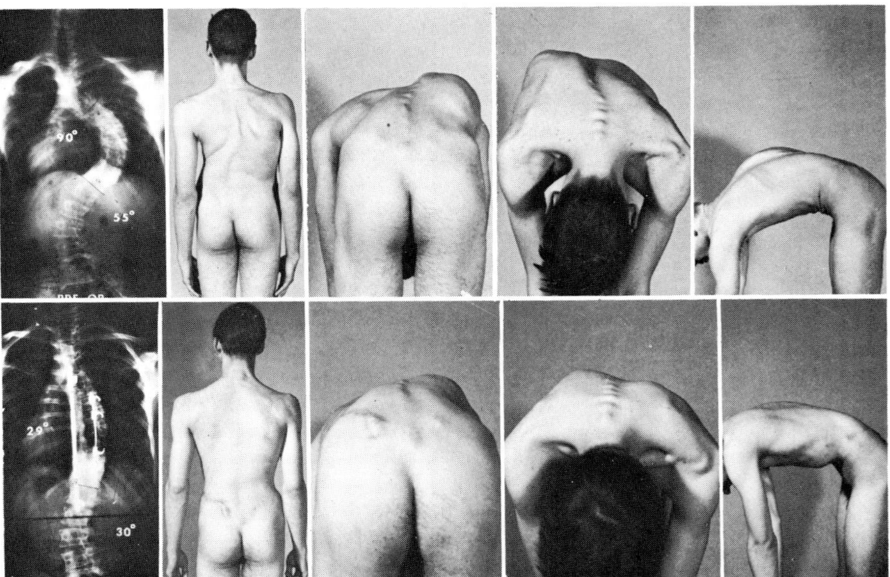

Fig. 15-10. Severe idiopathic thoracic scoliosis. Correction by preoperative localizer cast, concave ligament release, and instrumentation. Views in upper row are preoperative; lower row, postoperative.

Postoperative localizer cast (Fig. 15-11)

A large window is cut on the side of the concavity of the curve. The lid is removed for segmental breathing exercises to encourage maximum expansion of the depressed concave ribs during the period of cast immobilization. The axillary sling prevents the shoulder from dropping toward the concavity of the curve when the lid is removed for the exercises.

Complications

Morbidity related to rib resection and ligament release was studied.

The postoperative chest radiographs of the 17 patients who had rib resection or costotransversectomy showed pleural fluid in 8 patients. In 5, the pleural effusion was slight and required no special treatment. Three patients had open tube

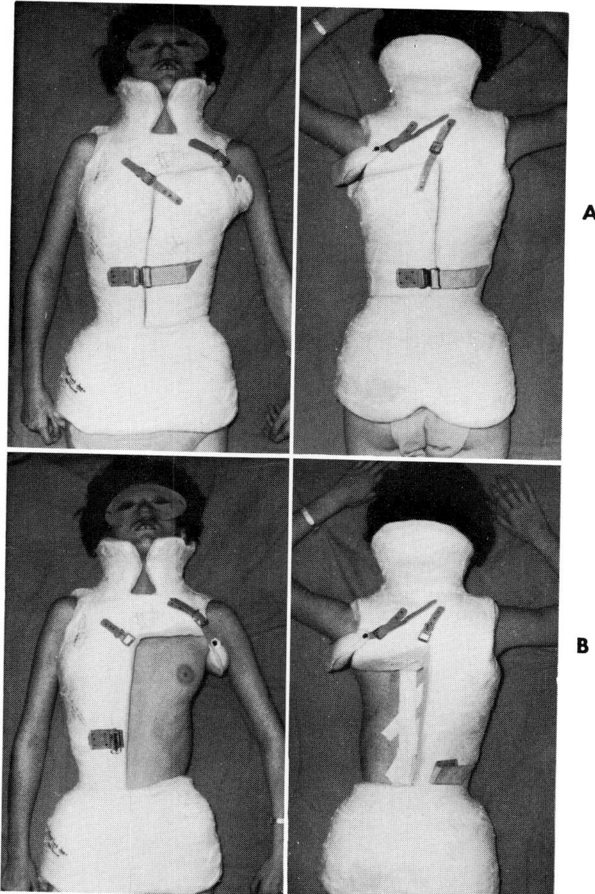

Fig. 15-11. Postoperative localizer cast. **A,** Breathing window lid buckled in place. **B,** Lid out for segmental breathing exercises. (From Goldstein, L. A.: J. Bone Joint Surg. **48-A:** 167, 1966.)

drainage of the pleural cavity. All patients recovered although one had a stormy postoperative course. Four patients had evidence of lower lobe atelectasis; all resolved.

In one patient who had concave ligament release the periosteal elevator accidentally perforated the pleura at one level. The pleural rent was sealed off. Postoperatively the patient had no evidence of pneumothorax and there were no postoperative complications.

Summary

Since October 1964 the treatment of choice for correction of idiopathic thoracic scoliosis at the University of Rochester Medical Center[3, 4] has been a single preoperative localizer cast followed by surgery performed through a large window in the cast, concave ligament release, and instrumentation for whatever further correction can be obtained. The spine is stabilized in the corrected position by fusion at the same time. Rib resection has been abandoned because concave ligament release has a lower morbidity and is more effective than rib resection in supplementing correction forces to restore rib cage symmetry.

Experience to date indicates that the combination of preoperative localizer cast, concave ligament release, and instrumentation results in the best correction of the angular deformity of the spine as well as clinical improvement of the rib cage deformity.

References

1. Cobb, J. R.: Outline for the study of scoliosis. In American Academy of Orthopaedic Surgeons, Instructional Course Lectures, Ann Arbor, 1948, J. W. Edwards Co., vol. 5, pp. 261-275.
2. Flinchum, D.: Personal communication.
3. Goldstein, L. A.: Surgical management of scoliosis. In American Academy of Orthopaedic Surgeons, Instructional Course Lectures, J. Bone Joint Surg. **48-A:**167, 1966.
4. Goldstein, L. A.: Results of treatment of idiopathic scoliosis by Harrington instrumentation and spine fusion with large amounts of fresh autogenous bone grafts; submitted for publication. Paper read at the American Orthopaedic Association Meeting, June, 1967.
5. Goldstein, L. A., and Evarts, C. M.: Further experiences with the treatment of scoliosis by cast correction and spine fusion with fresh autogenous iliac bone grafts, J. Bone Joint Surg. **48-A:**962, 1966.
6. Harrington, P. R.: Treatment of scoliosis; correction and internal fixation by spine instrumentation, J. Bone Joint Surg. **44-A:**591, 1962.
7. Risser, J. C., Lauder, C. H., Norquist, D. M., and Craig, W. A.: Three types of body casts. In American Academy of Orthopaedic Surgeons, Instructional Course Lectures, Ann Arbor, 1953, J. W. Edwards Co., vol. 10, pp. 131-142.

16. Osteotomy of the fused scoliotic spine and use of halo traction apparatus

Albert C. Schmidt, M.D.

There have been many different surgical procedures used during the past thirty years in the correction of scoliosis. Compere[3] corrected congenital scoliosis by excising a hemivertebra in two cases in 1932. Surgery consisting of wedge resection, osteotomy on the concave side of a vertebra, or removal of hemivertebra has since been described by various authors.[1, 13, 14]

Marino-Zucco[8] advised resection of the rib prominence, correction of the spinal curvature, fixation with special stainless steel plates, and arthrodesis on the concavity or the convexity depending on the age of the patient. Novak[11] favored fixation of the spine with a wire passed around the spinous processes, the thoracic transverse processes or the cervical neural arches. Smith and associates[12] reported 3 cases in which stapling was performed on the convex side of the curve in congenital scoliosis. Conclusions were that this procedure was applicable only in infants or very young children.

Gruca[5] has employed a spring screw device on the concave side or a pulling spring on the convex side. In the rigid curves he has inserted both, in addition to using spine fusion. Harrington,[6] on the other hand, uses a distraction rod on the concave side with a compression rod on the convex side, and he also fuses the corrected curve. An attempted unilateral vertebral epiphyseal arrest, by utilizing an inlay type of bone graft on the convex side of the major thoracic curve combined with the destruction of a portion of the vertebral epiphyseal cartilage adjacent to the graft, was unsuccessful in four consecutive cases, according to McCarroll and Costen.[9]

Meiss[10] of the Hague reported one case of a previously fused paralytic scoliosis with marked decompensation which was improved after an osteotomy was performed at one level.

Osteotomy of the fused scoliotic spine enables one to rehabilitate a deformed, decompensated spine in cases where the disability would otherwise remain permanent. This was first brought to my attention when a previously fused scoliotic patient fell, fracturing his graft. Spontaneous healing of the graft occurred, but not until considerable correction had been lost. It was thought that correction of the deformity might be accomplished by osteotomizing the solid column. The operation was successful, establishing that the procedure is, indeed, warranted in such cases.

The most obvious disability of scoliosis is decompensation and foreshortening of the torso. The foreshortening is usually due to a marked angular deformity of a long curve. With the "coiling" of the spinal column within an already foreshortened torso, various bodily functions may be greatly impaired, frequently shortening the life-span of the individual by many years. It may be expected that these long-term deleterious effects would be reversed by an osteotomy.

If the patient is paralytic and is fused before much rotation has occurred, the osteotomy can be quite simple. If, however, there is an acute angular deformity at the apex of a curve, the spine may be rotated to such an extent that the fused column may rotate into the sagittal plane instead of remaining in a coronal plane. When the latter condition exists, osteotomy at that level may be most difficult.

It has been my policy to osteotomize the graft at either two or three levels. If the angular deformity is great and the fused column is long, use of three levels is indicated. The number of osteotomy levels is, therefore, dependent upon (1) the degree of the fused curve, (2) the length of the fused column, and (3) the rigidity of the osteotomized column. A paralytic fused curve without much rotation, when osteotomized, usually can be corrected readily, but a congenital scoliosis as a rule is resistant to correction.

The amount of correction obtained at each osteotomy level contributes to the total correction. A previously fused congenital scoliosis in which there was inadequate length of fusion, inadequate correction, or recurrence of the deformity may present quite a problem. Not infrequently a segment of the fused column will include several malformed vertebral bodies that are firmly united, representing a solid bony column. Occasionally a solid bony bar can be demonstrated at the apex of the curve on the concave side. In this particular situation the ideal level of osteotomy is usually at the first free joint, both proximal and distal to the congenital fused vertebral column. In selected cases it is possible to divide the bar. The surgeon should be able to demonstrate motion at the osteotomized level after the fused column has been divided. If no motion is apparent, choose another level. In addition to the conventional anteroposterior roentgenograms for evaluation of a scoliotic spine, lateral view of the fused column should also be included. Oblique roentgenograms are occasionally indicated. Careful review of the roentgenograms of a congenital scoliosis is mandatory.

Operative procedure

Exposure of the entire fused column is preferable. Selection of the levels and number of osteotomy sites has already been discussed. If possible, it is preferable to have the osteotomized segments of equal length. However, in an unbalanced curve, the osteotomies should be concentrated where the angulation is the greatest. There will be three segments if osteotomized at two levels, four if divided at three levels. A specific osteotomy level is determined by locating the two intervertebral

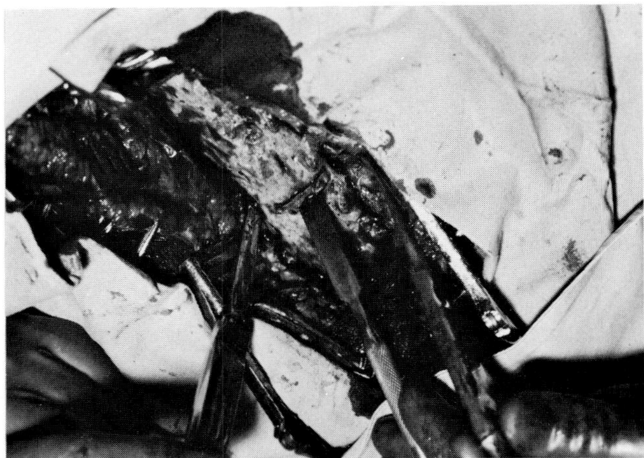

Fig. 16-1. Note Hedblom elevators inserted in the intervertebral foramina, designating the location of the osteotomy.

foramina common to that particular level. The location of the foramina is accomplished by inserting blunt curved instruments such as spatula, Hedblom elevator, or dural retractors as shown in Fig. 16-1.

A fused spinal column usually consists of a dense outer table and an inner one of lesser density. The outer table can be divided with an osteotome or rongeur. The osteotome, when used, should be angulated at about 45 degrees to the fused column, as a safety measure.

The next important step is to break through the inner table. The point of entry into the spinal canal is preferably located some distance from the lateral margins. This is best accomplished by using a long curet that can be controlled by using both hands. When the inner table is punctured, the dura is carefully retracted and the remainder of the osteotomy is then undertaken. Additional protection of the dura is also obtained by maintaining the retractors in the intervertebral foramina. An alternate method of removing the inner table is to begin at the lateral margin or the roof of the intervertebral foramina with a rongeur. It is preferable to employ a distractor to break the last few bony connections. By this method, free motion of the fragments should be demonstrated. The osteotomized level should consist of a trough about 5 mm. in width. (See Fig. 16-2.)

The bone chips, which were removed, are then loosely placed in the trough, avoiding excessive pressure on the dura. Additional bone can be placed over the defect by removing slivers from the solid columns. Since the segmentation of the graft is the result of an osteotomy, solid bony union can be expected.

Postoperative correction

Correction of the deformity should be gradual, especially in patients with congenital scoliosis, where the margin of safety is already limited. Very often, these

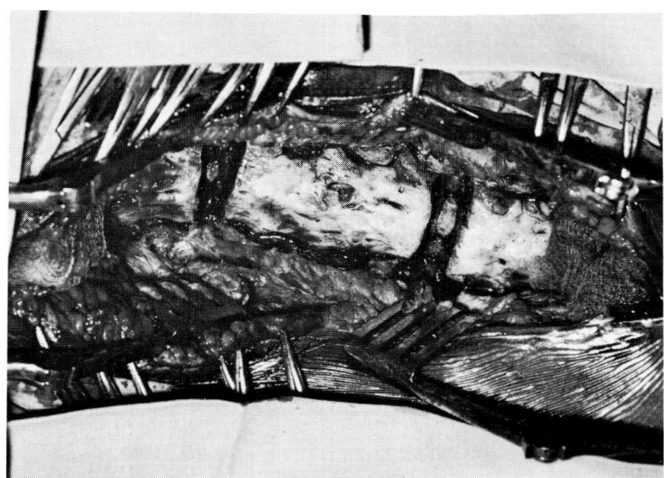

Fig. 16-2. This photograph shows the two osteotomy areas. The light area at the base is the dura.

have preexisting neurological deficits, which may increase with too rapid or too forceful reduction of the deformity. Catastrophic complications have been reported in instances where correction was too rapid.

The patient should be mentally alert before correction is undertaken. A careful check of motor and sensory deficits is mandatory at that time. Therefore, it is suggested that forcible correction be delayed for a period of a few days following osteotomy.

The apparatus used for correcting the osteotomized column should be one that is familiar to the operator. The conventional Milwaukee brace has been employed in a few of our patients. In the rigid cases skeletal distraction in combination with the Milwaukee brace was utilized. Considerable force, as much as 40 pounds of distraction, may be necessary in some instances.

Case reports

Case 1

In January of 1945, when P. P. was 6 years old, he was first seen because of a marked C type scoliosis. The spinal curvature followed an episode of poliomyelitis six months previously. In July of 1946, the curvature was corrected by means of the Milwaukee brace followed with a two-stage spinal fusion from T1 to L2, inclusive.

In May of 1947, he gave a history of falling on two different occasions, two weeks apart. The angular deformity at that time is illustrated by the roentgenogram in Fig. 16-3. A lateral view of the spine on this date revealed a fracture at the junction of T9 and T10 (Fig. 16-4). At this point he had lost no correction. The angular deformity at the fracture site gradually increased and six months later, be-

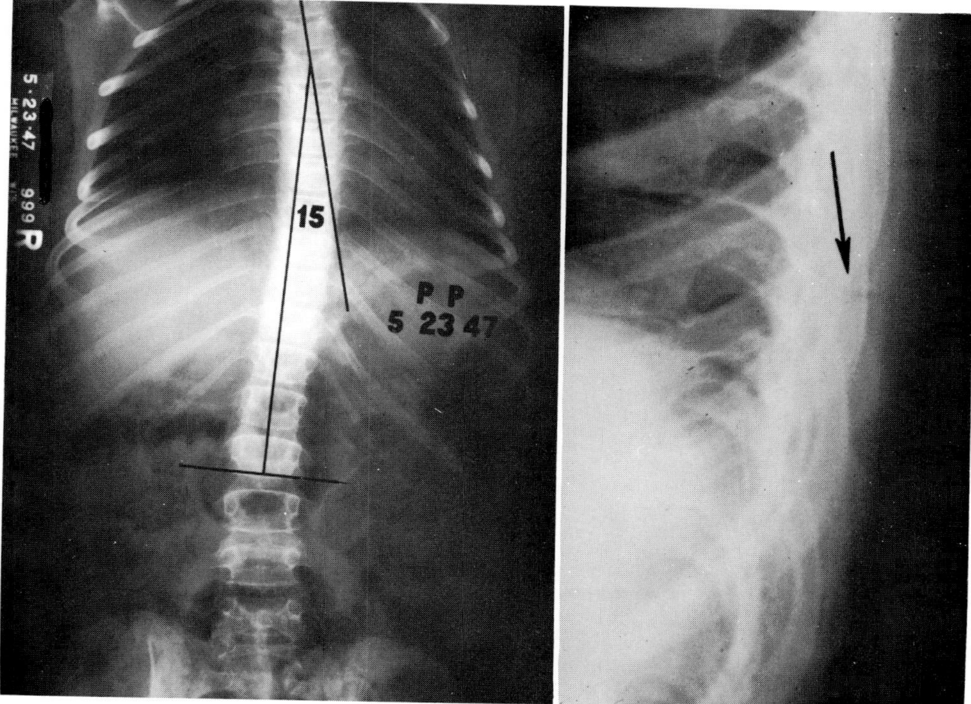

Fig. 16-3

Fig. 16-4

Fig. 16-3. Roentgenogram taken immediately after last fall.
Fig. 16-4. Roentgenogram, lateral view, showing fracture of fusion area.

cause of suspected pseudarthrosis, the spine was explored with the intention of regrafting the area. However, exploration revealed an exuberant bony bridge with solid fusion of the involved segment. At six months after the fall and for the following four years the angulation remained unchanged. It was my assumption that if a loss of correction resulted following a fracture of a fused scoliotic column, then the reverse should hold true—namely, that correction of an angular deformity is possible following a spinal osteotomy.

On July 3, 1951, osteotomies were performed at two levels, producing three separate segments. Since the patient was paralytic and had originally been fused before much rotation had occurred, the osteotomy was relatively simple.

The fused column that originally was 15 degrees and had increased to 34 degrees (Fig. 16-5) was reduced to 18 degrees with an osteotomy, as shown on the roentgenogram in Fig. 16-6.

Case 2

Fig. 16-7 shows a 13-year-old female, M. L., who suffered from poliomyelitis at the age of 7 and two years later underwent a spinal fusion from T8 to L4. Four

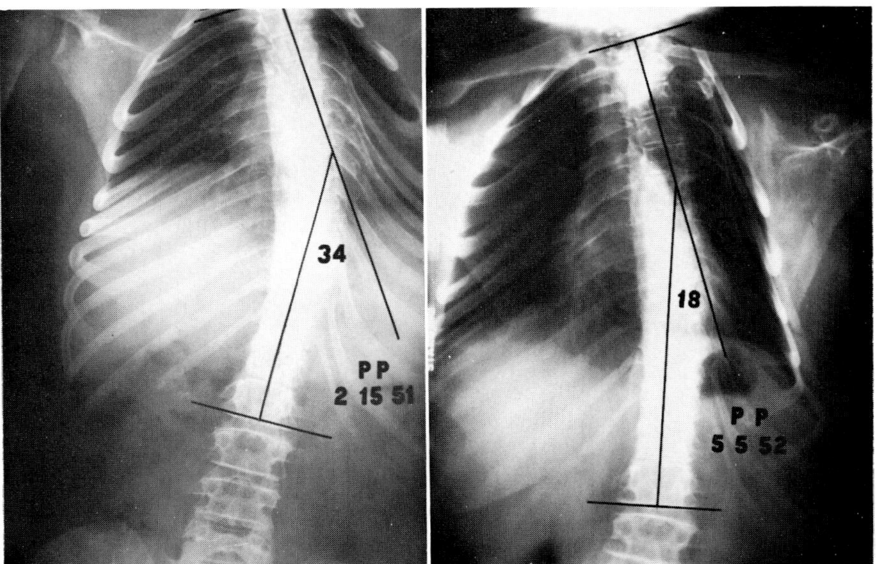

Fig. 16-5 Fig. 16-6

Fig. 16-5. Roentgenogram showing increased angular deformity and decompensation prior to the osteotomy.
Fig. 16-6. Roentgenogram ten months following the osteotomy.

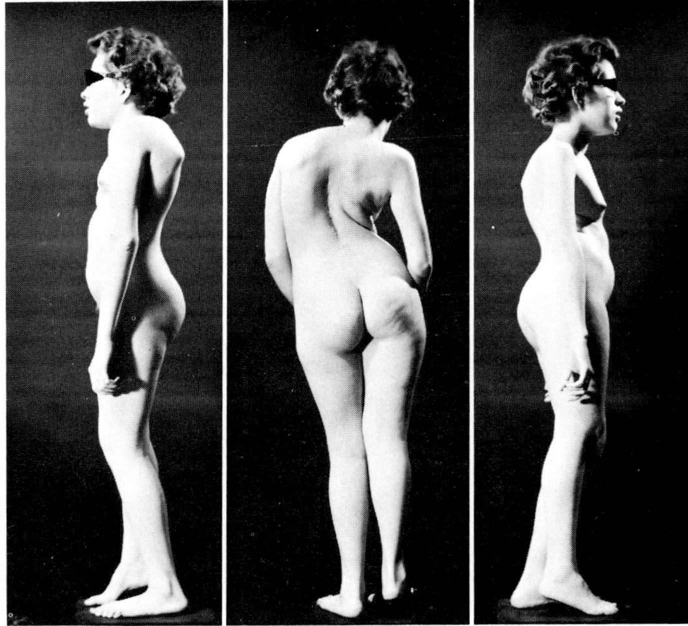

Fig. 16-7. Photographs showing marked pelvic obliquity, foreshortening of torso, and elevation of left heel.

years later she was referred to me because of marked decompensation. Note the pelvic obliquity, foreshortening of the torso, and elevation of the left heel. The body of T7 and the interspace betwen T7 and T8 which is at the junction of the fused and the unfused area reveal considerable wedging (Fig. 16-8). The unfused portion was so rigid that it was impossible to change it much, if any.

Fig. 16-9 represents the first case in which skeletal distraction was incorporated

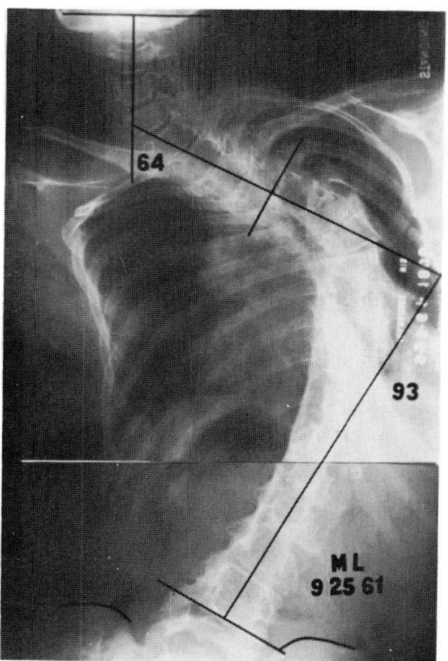

Fig. 16-8. Roentgenogram prior to osteotomies and extension of fusion. Observe the marked wedging of T7 and the interspace between T7 and T8.

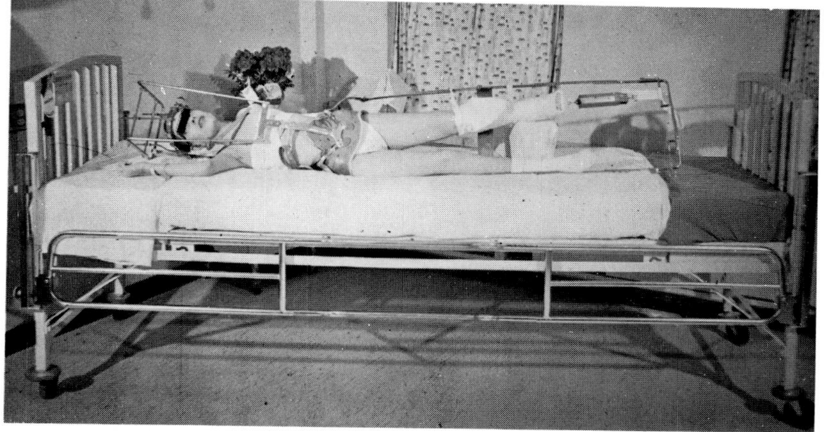

Fig. 16-9. Photograph of Milwaukee brace incorporating the halo apparatus and Kirschner wire through tibia, utilizing skeletal distraction. Traction was applied only to the high side.

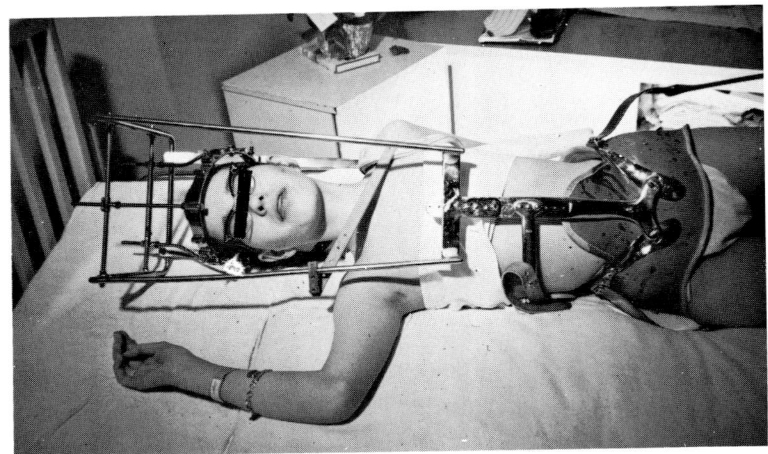

Fig. 16-10. Photograph showing halo and outrigger attached to Milwaukee brace.

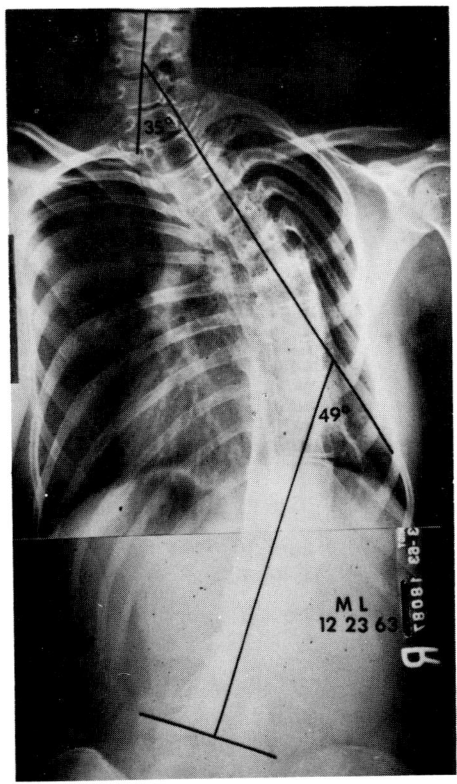

Fig. 16-11. Roentgenogram two years following osteotomies and extension of fusion area.

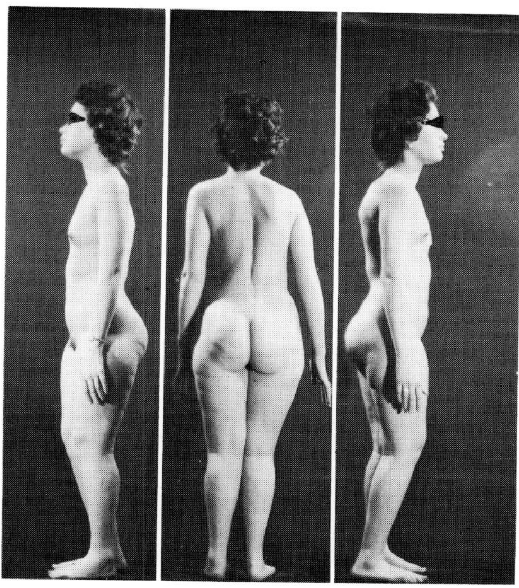

Fig. 16-12. Photographs two years following surgery.

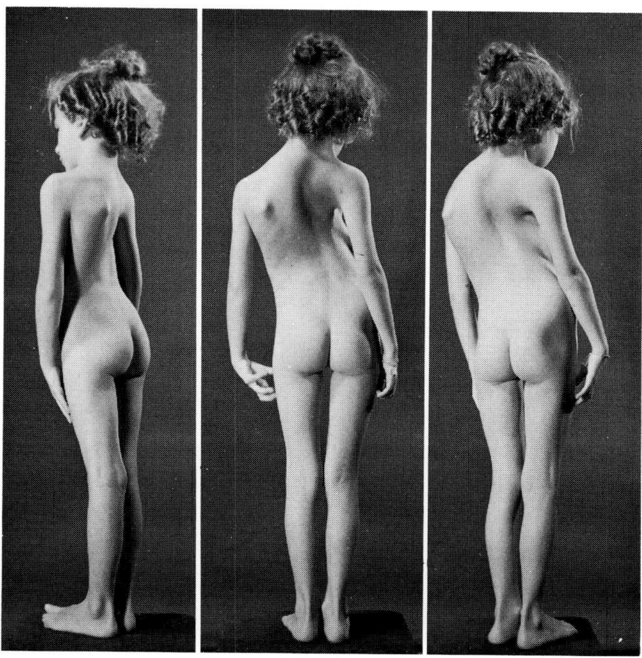

Fig. 16-13. Photographs showing flattened right chest due to absence of ribs.

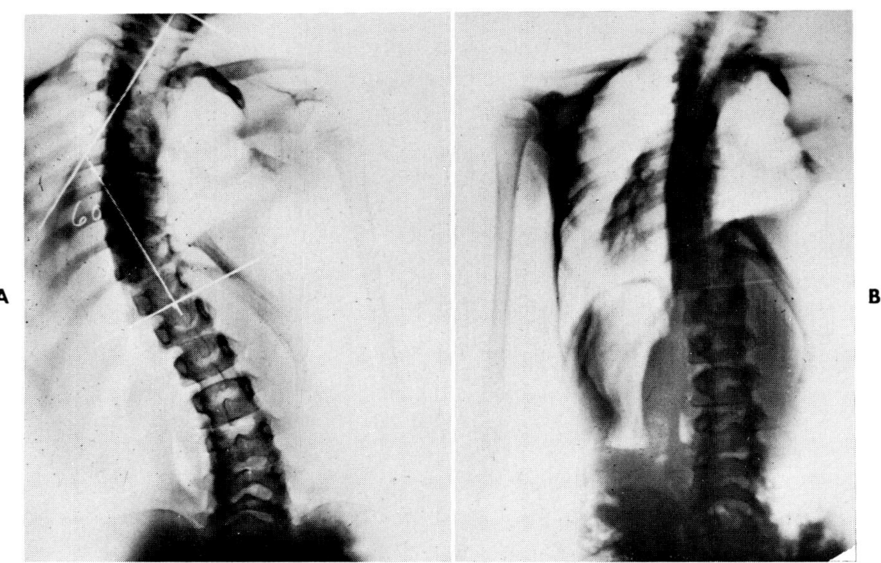

Fig. 16-14. Roentgenograms of T. H. **A,** Prior to surgery. **B,** Seven months following correction and fusion.

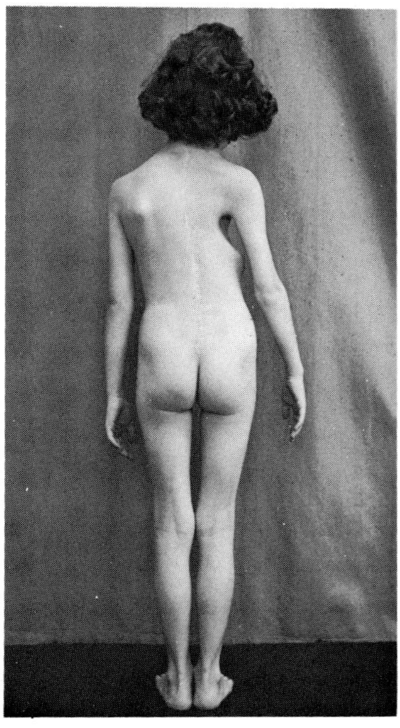

Fig. 16-15. Seven months following fusion, showing reasonably good correction.

into the Milwaukee brace.[2] To correct the pelvic obliquity, traction was applied on the high side. A short leg cast included a heavy Kirschner wire that was inserted through the tibia. This was attached to an outrigger containing a scale. Instead of a Kirschner wire, I now use a heavy Steinmann pin.

Fig. 16-10 shows the halo[4] connected to an outrigger attached to the Milwaukee brace. The fusion was extended from T8 to T2, the fused column being osteotomized at two levels. Thirty pounds of traction was applied for a period of six weeks.

A roentgenogram two years following surgery is shown in Fig. 16-11 and a photograph taken at the same time, in Fig. 16-12.

Case 3

T. H., a 7-year-old girl with congenital scoliosis, had multiple deformities (Fig. 16-13). There were only a few ribs on the right, all of which were deformed. Laminae and pedicles on the same side were also absent from T1 to T9, and there were no spinous processes at the same level. Some deformities also existed at C6 and C7. Fig. 16-14, *A*, is a roentgenogram before correction; *B* is a film made after correction with the conventional Milwaukee brace and fusion from C7 to L1,

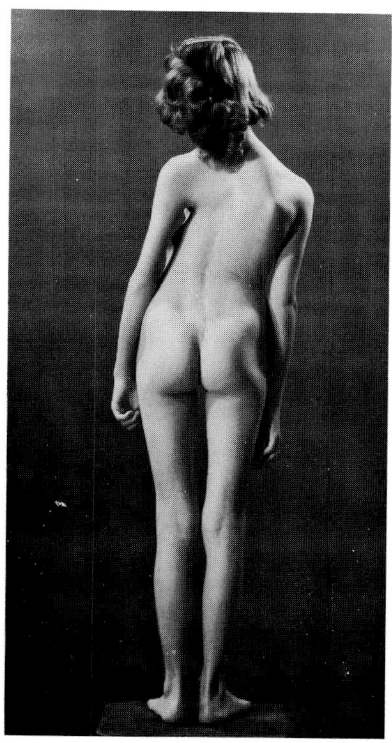

Fig. 16-16. Photograph three years following fusion reveals marked decompensation.

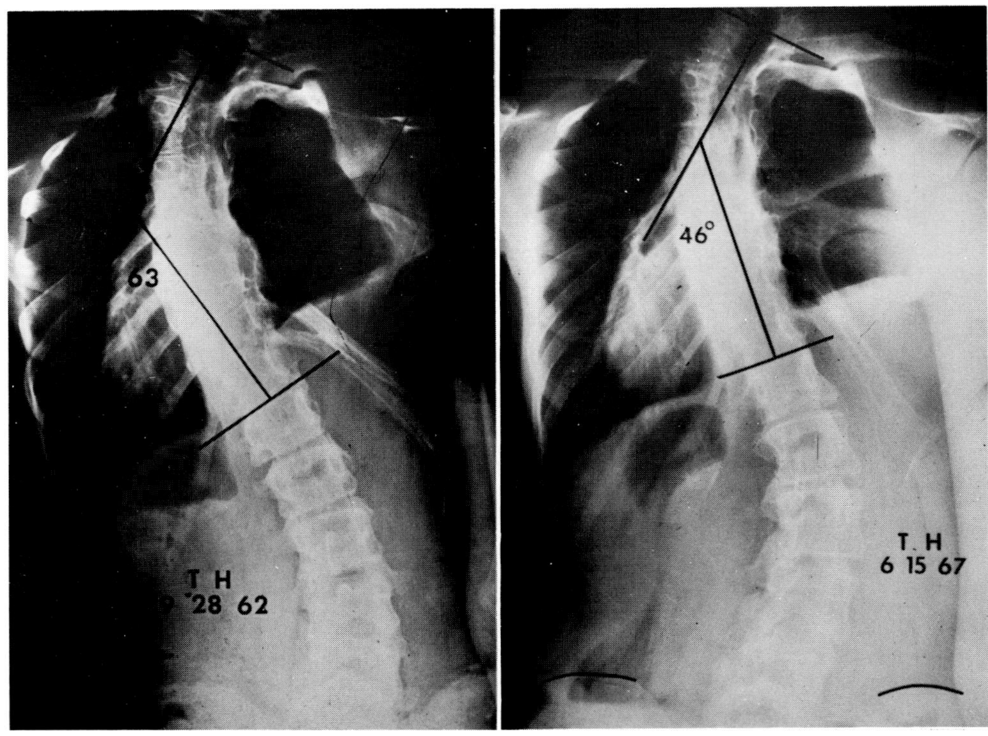

Fig. 16-17 Fig. 16-18

Fig. 16-17. Roentgenogram three years following fusion.
Fig. 16-18. Roentgenogram five years following osteotomies at three levels.

seven months postoperative, at which time the brace was removed. A photograph, also made seven months after operation, shows reasonably good correction (Fig. 16-15). Fig. 16-16 is a photograph three years later, demonstrating decompensation increased. The roentgenogram in Fig. 16-17 demonstrates a recurrence of the deformity, which undoubtedly was due to the absence of many bony structures on the right. The only available structures for fusion from T1 to T9 were the facets.

Fig. 16-18 is a roentgenogram showing the correction obtained, five years following a second series of osteotomies at three different levels, utilizing skeletal distraction as previously described. Forty pounds of skeletal traction for a period of six weeks produced an abducens paralysis on the left which cleared up in about two months. Fig. 16-19 is a photograph of the patient 5½ years following the last osteotomies. She was advised to wear the brace until maturity.

Case 4

M. W. (Fig. 16-20) was first seen by me in 1960 at the age of 6 years because of increasing deformity of the spine. The scoliosis, infantile idiopathic in type, with

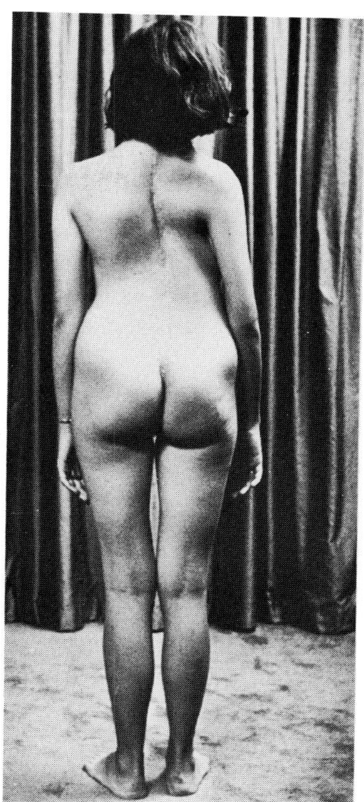

Fig. 16-19. Photograph five years following last surgery.

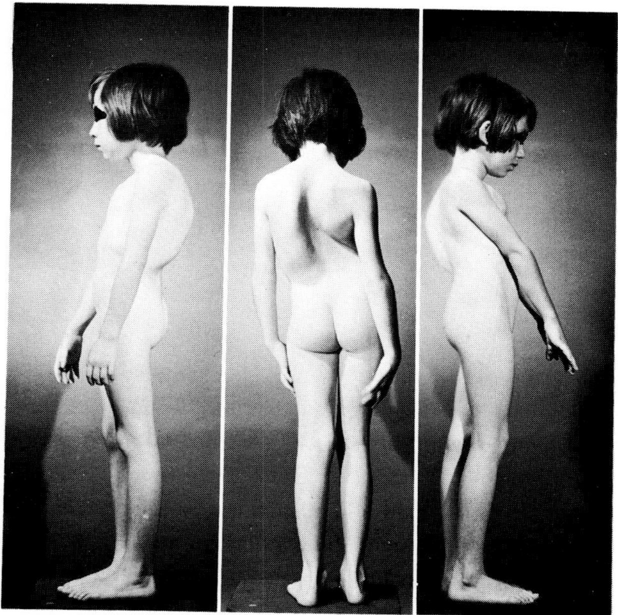

Fig. 16-20. Photographs showing left thoracic curvature common in infantile idiopathic scoliosis.

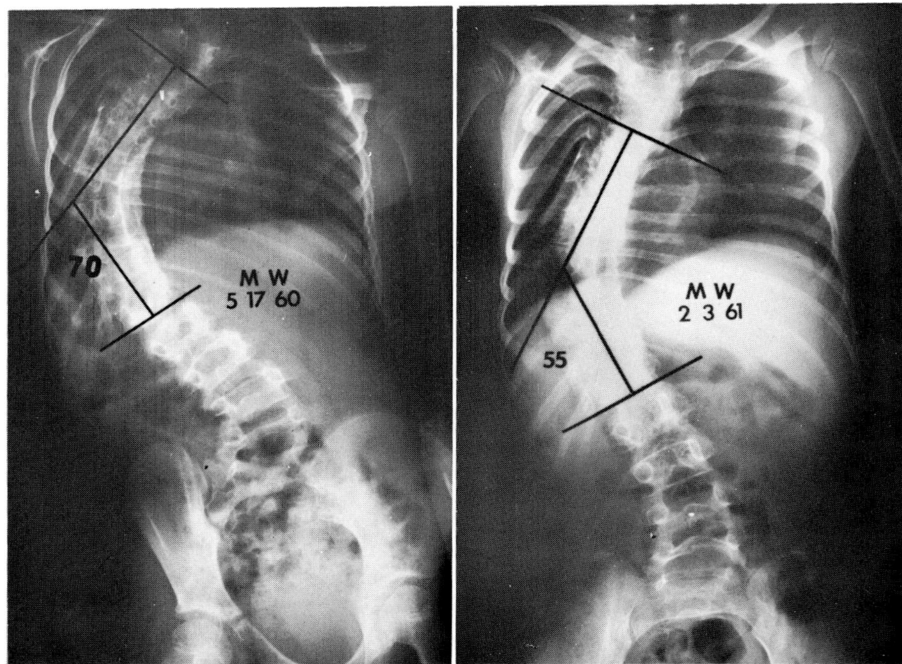

Fig. 16-21 Fig. 16-22

Fig. 16-21. Roentgenogram at age 6 years, demonstrating recurrence of deformity.
Fig. 16-22. Roentgenogram six months following original osteotomies; brace was discontinued at that time.

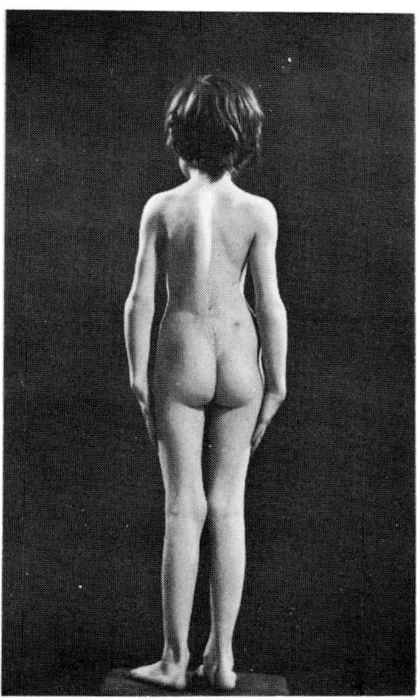

Fig. 16-23. Photograph at tıme brace was discontinued.

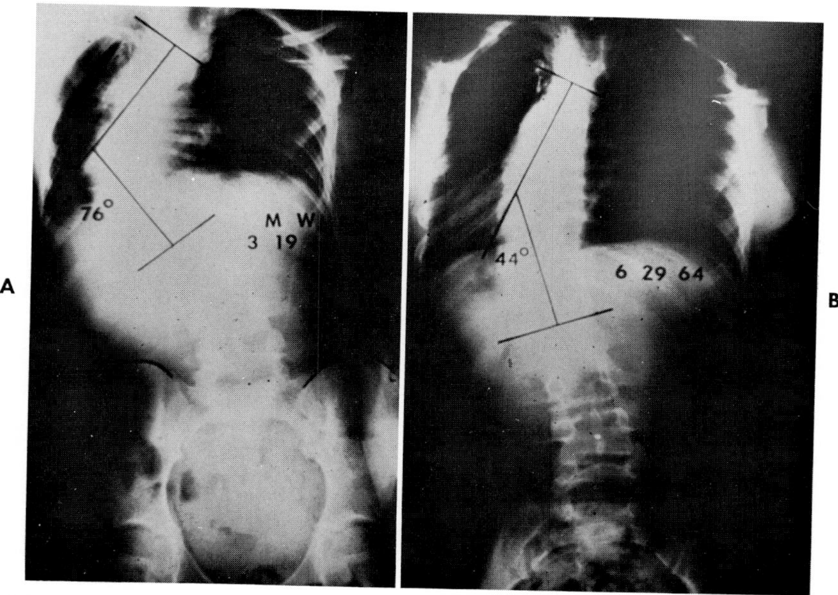

Fig. 16-24. A, Roentgenogram one year following removal of brace. Note the foreshortening of the torso, bending of the graft, and marked decompensation. **B,** Roentgenogram following second series of osteotomies. Note the elongation of the torso.

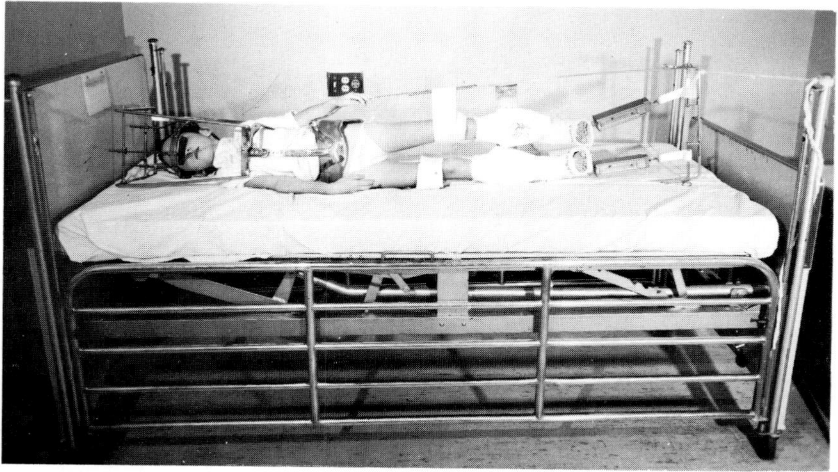

Fig. 16-25. Photograph showing skeletal distraction in combination with Milwaukee brace. Equal traction on both legs.

a left thoracic curvature, was first noted at the age of 1 year. At the age of 3 years the curve had increased to 90 degrees so fusion from T4 to L1 was undertaken with correction of the curve down to 40 degrees (Fig. 16-21). A roentgenogram three years following the original surgery demonstrated a rapidly increasing curve. Osteotomies were performed at two levels in the summer of 1960. The curve was then reduced from 70 to 55 degrees (Fig. 16-22) with the conventional Milwaukee brace. The brace was removed six months after these osteotomies, revealing satisfactory correction and compensation. Fig. 16-23 is a photograph immediately after

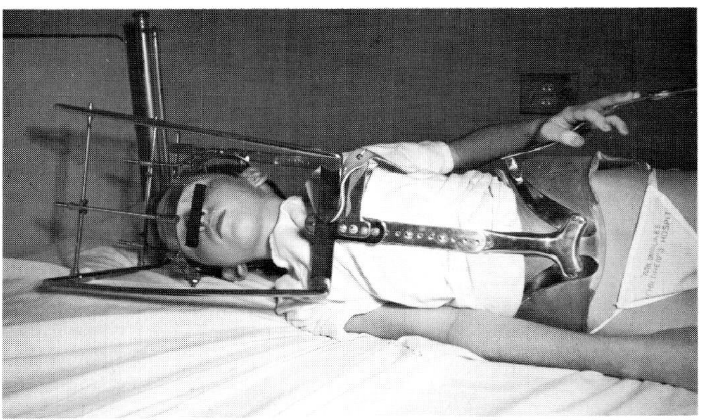

Fig. 16-26. Close-up view of halo and outrigger.

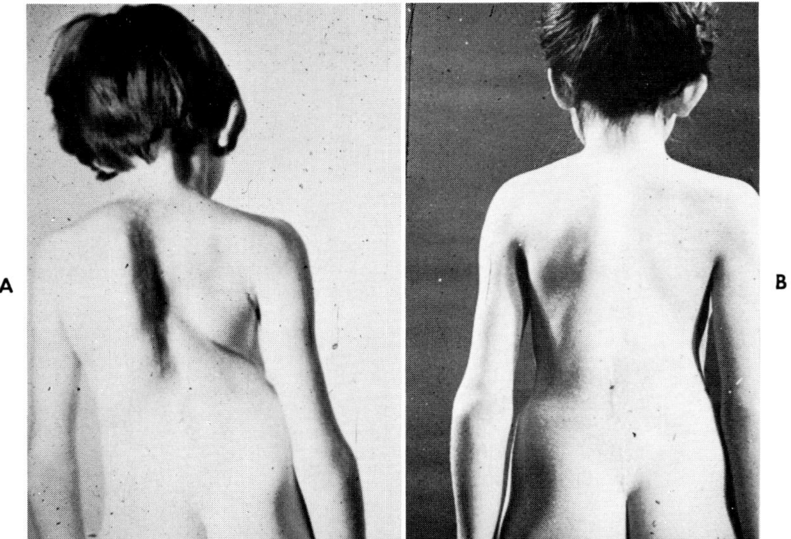

Fig. 16-27. A, Photograph just prior to last series of osteotomies. **B,** Photograph one year following surgery.

removal of brace. Fig. 16-24, *A*, is a roentgenogram taken 1½ years after operation, and one year after removal of brace, indicating that the fused column had again lost correction due to bending. In addition to the increase in lateral curvature, kyphosis and lordosis had increased proportionately, producing an extreme foreshortening of the torso. At the age of 8, a second series of osteotomies were performed at three levels, reducing the curvature from 76 to 44 degrees with skeletal distraction. In Fig. 16-24, *B*, note the elongation of the torso. The patient was placed in skeletal distraction apparatus that applied equal traction to both legs (Fig. 16-25). Fig. 16-26 shows a close-up of the halo. Fig. 16-27, *A*, is a photograph just prior to the last series of osteotomies and Fig. 16-27, *B*, one year following surgery.

Fig. 16-28 shows a roentgenogram taken at the age of 14, six years following the last surgery. Fig. 16-29, a photograph taken at the age of 13, reveals good compensation. Because of loss of correction without a corrective apparatus in the past, this patient will undoubtedly have to remain in the Milwaukee brace until the end of her growth period. It is an established fact that an infantile idiopathic scoliotic patient with a solid fusion will rapidly lose correction, because of bending of the graft, unless some supportive apparatus is worn.

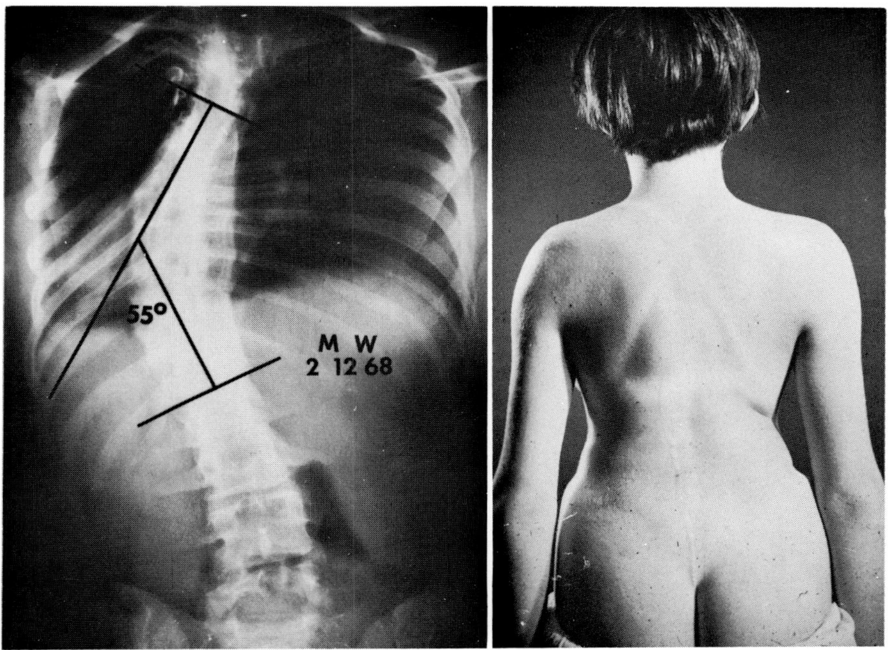

Fig. 16-28 **Fig. 16-29**

Fig. 16-28. Roentgenogram six years postoperative at the age of 14.
Fig. 16-29. Photograph at the age of 13.

References

1. Bertrand, P.: Notions nouvelles dans le traitement chirurgical des scolioses graves, Rev. Chir. Orthop. **38:**33, 1953.
2. Blount, W. P., Schmidt, A. C., Keever, E. D., and Leonard, T.: The Milwaukee brace in the operative treatment of scoliosis, J. Bone Joint Surg. **40-A:**511, 1958.
3. Compere, E. L.: Excision of hemivertebrae for correction of congenital scoliosis; report of two cases, J. Bone Joint Surg. **14:**555, 1932.
4. Garrett, A. L., Perry, J., and Nickel, V. L.: Stabilization of the collapsing spine, J. Bone Joint Surg. **43-A:**474, 1961.
5. Gruca, A.: Pathogenesis and treatment of idiopathic scoliosis, J. Bone Joint Surg. **40-A:** 570, 1958.
6. Harrington, P. R.: Treatment of scoliosis; correction and internal fixation by spine instrumentation, J. Bone Joint Surg. **44-A:**591, 1962.
7. James, J. I. P., Lloyd-Roberts, G. C., and Pilcher, M. F.: Infantile structural scoliosis, J. Bone Joint Surg. **41-B:**719, 1959.
8. Marino-Zucco, C.: Scoliosis, J. Bone Joint Surg. **36-B:**686, 1954.
9. McCarroll, H. R., and Costen, W.: Unilateral vertebral epiphyseal arrest, J. Bone Joint Surg. **42-A:**965, 1960.
10. Meiss, W. C.: Spinal osteotomy following fusion for paralytic scoliosis, J. Bone Joint Surg. **37-A:**73, 1955.
11. Novak, V.: Operative treatment of scoliosis, J. Bone Joint Surg. **36-B:**687, 1954.
12. Smith, A. DeF., von Lackum, W. H., and Wylie, R.: An operation for stapling vertebral bodies in congenital scoliosis, J. Bone Joint Surg. **36-A:**342, 1954.
13. von Lackum, H. L., and Smith, A. DeF.: Removal of vertebral bodies in the treatment of scoliosis, Surg. Gynec. Obstet. **57:**250, 1933.
14. Wiles, P.: Resection of dorsal vertebrae in congenital scoliosis, J. Bone Joint Surg. **33-A:** 151, 1951.

Author index

A

Adkins, E. W. O., 135
Albee, F. H., 132
Albright, F., 168

B

Babinski, F. F., 85
Bailey, R., 51
Barr, J. S., 87, 88, 112, 132
Bauer, G. C. H., 173
Bauman, G. I., 85, 86
Beadle, O. A., 88
Bickell, W. H., 158
Blount, W. P., 188
Brashear, R., 23, 26
Brissaud, E., 85
Brown, J. E., 67, 68
Brown, T., 79, 133
Bucy, P. C., 86
Burns, B. H., 112

C

Chandler, F. A., 86
Cobb, J. R., 243
Compere, E. L., 87, 265
Costen, W., 265
Cotugno, D., 84
Coventry, M. B., 89, 132
Cushing, 85

D

Dandy, W. E., 86
Danforth, M. S., 84, 85, 86
Delorme, T., 26
Duvall, G., 64

E

Evarts, C. M., 250

F

Farfan, H. F., 4, 59, 60, 64
Fick, R., 87
Fielding, J. W., 48
Foerster, R. E., 185
Frankel, V. H., 1
Freiberg, A. H., 86, 89
Friberg, S., 56, 112, 151
Friedman, B., 204

G

Galante, J. O., 4
Garber, J. N., 18
Garvin, P. J., 90
Geist, E. L., 87
Ghormley, R. K., 86
Goldner, J. L., 111
Goldstein, L. A., 241, 250, 254
Goldthwait, J. E., 85
Gotten, N., 12
Gruca, A., 265

H

Hadley, L., 102
Hansen, H. J., 66
Harmon, P., 112, 125
Harrington, P. R., 265
Hasbe, K., 151
Hawk, W. A., 112
Hendry, N. G. C., 89
Hessing, 188
Heyman, C. H., 87
Hibbs, R. A., 85, 132
Hippocrates, 188
Hirsch, C., 56, 88, 89, 90, 116
Hoover, N. W., 132, 135, 136
Hult, L., 56, 63
Humphries, A. W., 112

I

Inkley, S. R., 180
Inman, V. T., 88

J

James, J. I. P., 196, 227
Jefferson, G., 20
Jenkins, J. A., 112
Junghans, H., 4

K

Katz, S. F., 84
Kelly, R. P., 136
Key, J. A., 86
Keyes, D. C., 87
Kilian, H. F., 143
Klieger, B., 147
Knutsson, F., 64, 90
Kohler, R., 90

Kohn, G., 7
Kolliker, A., 87

L

Lafferty, F. W., 173
Lane, 112
Lasègue, C. H., 85
Lindblom, K., 56, 89
Lloyd-Roberts, G. C., 196, 197
Londorzey, 85
Lowe, L., 87
Luck, J. V., 87

M

Macnab, I., 10, 63, 97
Marino-Zucco, C., 265
McCarroll, H. R., 265
McCollum, D. E., 111
Meiss, W. C., 265
Mensor, M. C., 64
Mercer, W., 112
Michele, A. A., 73
Mixter, W. J., 87, 112, 132
Moe, J. H., 190, 196, 247
Moore, 112
Morgan, 196
Morris, J. M., 79, 80

N

Nachemson, A., 4, 80
Nordin, B. E. C., 171
Norton, P. L., 79, 133
Novak, V., 265

O

Ober, F. R., 87
Osler, W., 1

P

Pedersen, H. E., 26, 88
Pennell, G., 7
Pilcher, M. F., 196, 197
Ponseti, L. V., 204
Putti, V., 84

R

Raney, F., Jr., 80
Reifenstein, E., Jr., 168
Reynolds, F. C., 84
Rissanen, P. M., 90
Roche, M. B., 149, 151
Roofe, P. G., 88
Rosenberg, N., 147, 151, 162
Rowe, G. G., 149, 151

S

Saunders, J., 88
Schajowicz, F., 56
Schmidt, A. C., 265
Schmorl, G., 4, 86
Schneider, R. C., 26
Schultz, 146
Scott, J. C., 67, 196
Smith, A. DeF., 265
Smith, L., 67, 68
Smith-Petersen, M. N., 85, 86
Speed, K., 112
Spencer, G. E., Jr., 168
Splittoff, C. A., 60
Stauffer, R. N., 132
Steindler, A., 87
Stewart, T. D., 149, 151, 163
Sullivan, C. R., 158
Sullivan, J. D., 60

T

Thompson, W. A., 135
Truchly, G., 135

U

Urbaniak, J. R., 111
Urist, M., 153

V

Valleix, F. L., 84
Verbrugge, J., 90
Vesalius, A., 87
Vinke, T. H., 86
Virchow, R., 84
Von Luschka, H., 85, 87

W

Walker, G. F., 197
Watkins, M. B., 135
Whitman, A., 86
Williams, P. C., 78, 86, 87, 89
Wilson, P. D., 84, 86
Wiltse, L. L., 54, 143

Subject index

A

Abnormal female pelvis, in differential diagnosis of low back pain, 73
Acceleration-extension injuries; *see* Whiplash injuries
Aneurysm of aorta, in differential diagnosis of low back pain, 71
Annulus fibrosus, 2, 87, 97
Anterior disc excision and interbody spine fusion for chronic low back pain, 111
  anatomy and physiology, 116
  anterior and posterior fusion compared, 113
  choice of procedure, 114
    for degenerative disc disease in lumbosacral interspace, 114
    for protrusion of disc with nerve root compression, 114
    for spondylolisthesis, 115
  classification of patients, 119
  complications, 127
  diagnostic studies, 117
  essentials for success, 112
  functional results, 129
  guidelines for future treatment, 129
  history, 112
  postoperative management, 126
  study material and procedure, 112
  technique, 125
Arachnoiditis of cauda equina, in differential diagnosis of low back pain, 72
Arthritic spine, injuries to, 35
Atlas
  congenital abnormalities of traumatic origin, 37
  Jefferson's fracture, 20
    from hyperextension of neck, 21
    in posterior arch, 21, 23
Axis
  congenital anomalies of traumatic origin, 42
  spondylolisthesis, traumatic, 26

B

Biomechanics; *see also* Loading
  mechanical properties of tissues, 2
Biomechanics—cont'd
  new ideas and techniques, 1
  substructures, 4
    osseous, relative motion, 5
Brittle failure of substructures, 5
Burns test for malingering, 73

C

Centroid in kinematics, 6
Cervical and lumbar symptoms, correlation between, 67
Cervical spine
  acceleration-extension injuries; *see* Whiplash injuries
  dislocations, 18
    cock-up, 30
    without fracture, 29
  fractures; *see* Fractures of cervical spine
  treatment of injuries, 48
Charcot spine in differential diagnosis of low back pain, 70
Chemonucleolysis for intractable sciatica, 81
Chymopapain for relief of sciatic pain, 67
Cock-up dislocation of cervical spine, 30
Compression fractures
  in differential diagnosis of low back pain, 69
  in osteoporosis, 168, 170
Congenital anomalies of traumatic origin, 37
  atlas, 37
  axis, 42
Cord tumor in differential diagnosis of low back pain, 72

D

Disc degeneration; *see also* Intervertebral disc
  distinguished from herniation, 109, 110
  in low back pain, 54, 57
    correlation with heavy work, 56
    heredity as factor, 66
    personality types, 67
    primary instability heralding onset, 64
    vacuum phenomenon as evidence, 60
  pathogenesis of symptoms, 97
    damage to posterior joints, 109

Disc degeneration—cont'd
pathogenesis of symptoms—cont'd
disc narrowing, 102
extraforaminal entrapment of nerve root, 107
facet impingement, 105
mechanism of breakdown, 97
pedicular kinking, 106
root compression, 104
segmental hyperextension, 100
segmental instability, 97, 100
segmental spinal stenosis, 106
signs on x-ray study, 107
summary of symptom types, 110
Discogenic disease; *see* Disc degeneration
Discs
herniation, 109, 110
intervertebral; *see* Intervertebral disc
space infection, in differential diagnosis of low back pain, 69
Diverticulitis, in differential diagnosis of low back pain, 71

E

Elasticity of tissues, determination of, 4
Enchondroma, 86
physolipherous, 85

F

Facet syndrome, 86
Fatigue failure of substructures, 5
Fibrosis, retroperitoneal, in differential diagnosis of low back pain, 71
Flat feet and low back pain, 65
Flexed thigh test for malingering, 74
Flip test for malingering, 73
Forces and loads, 1; *see also* Loading; Loads
Fractures of cervical spine
arthritic spine, 35
atlas (Jefferson's fracture), 20
from hyperextension of neck, 21
in posterior arch, 21, 23
axis
odontoid process, 23
spondylolisthesis, 26
causes, 18
examination and evaluation of damage, 19
in head injury, 20
roentgenography, 20
fusion, 26, 30, 35, 48, 53
treatment of injuries, 48
of vertebral bodies, single and multiple, 32
Fusion
for altered disc function, 55
for cervical spine derangements, 26, 30, 35, 48, 53
for disc disease, 81
for low back pain, 111; *see also* Anterior disc excision and interbody spine fusion
for pseudoarthritis repair, 134, 135

G

Gallie fusion of cervical vertebrae, 48
Genitourinary disease, in differential diagnosis of low back pain, 72
Gout in differential diagnosis of low back pain, 69

H

Heredity and disc degeneration, 66
Hoover test for malingering, 74
Hormonal therapy for osteoporosis, 171, 179
Hyaline cartilage plate, 97
Hydrostatic pressure in disc tissue, 4
Hysteresis loop, 2, 4

I

Iatrogenic neurosis, 15
steps for avoidance, 15-17
Idiopathic scoliosis
age of onset, 196
casts for correction
localizer, 245
results of treatment, 250
turnbuckle, 241
concave rib resection and ligament release
complications, 263
concave ligament release and instrumentation, 262
postoperative localizer cast, 263
preoperative localizer cast, ligament release, and instrumentation, 262
rib resection and instrumentation, 261
selection of patients, 260
technique, 254
curves
combined thoracic and lumbar primary, 212
compensatory, 204, 205
development as flexible, 199
double primary, 204
combined thoracic and lumbar, 209
double thoracic major, 207
functional, 199
major, 205
postural, 204
primary, 204
right thoracic, 205
-left thoracolumbar, 212
secondary, 205
evaluation by x-ray, 213
fusion, 234
infantile, 196
aggressive treatment, 199
detection of curves, 199
natural history of patient, 197
treatment with Denis Browne tray, 197
juvenile and adolescent, 199
measurement of curves, 219
selection of fusion area, 227
spondylolisthesis with, 234

Iliac artery obstruction, in differential diagnosis of low back pain, 71
Instant center in kinematics, 6
  and disc disease, 7
Intervertebral disc; *see also* Disc degeneration
  aging process, 89
  loading effects, 4
  major parts and mechanism, 97
  past observations, 86 et seq.
  as unit in spinal system, 88

J

Jefferson's fracture of atlas, 20

K

Kinematics, 5
  centroid and instant center, 6
  location of rotation point, 6
Knuttson phenomenon, 99, 100
Kyphosis of thoracic spine, 64

L

Laminectomy
  for cervical fracture, 20, 23
  for intractable sciatica, 81
Leg length differences, relation to low back symptoms, 65
Ligamentum annulus, 4
List test for malingering, 74
Litigation neurosis, 10
  follow-up after court action, 11, 12
  iatrogenic, 15
Loading, 1; *see also* Loads
  assessment of failure, 5
  deformation data, 4
  effects, 2, 4
  functional, 8
  multidimensional, 4
  structural strength formula, 5
Loads
  from elastic restraints, 7
  from external effects, 7
  from joint reactions, 8
  from motion, versus motion from, 7
  from muscle activity, 8
Localizer cast for correction of scoliosis, 245
  application technique, 245
  postoperative, 263
  preoperative, 262
  selection of fusion area, 247
  selection of patients, 247
Lordosis, lumbar, and low back pain, 60
Low back pain
  age at onset, 55
  anatomy and physiology, 116
  arthritic intervertebral joints, 55
  asymmetrical orientation of facet joints, 60
  conservative treatment, 76
    braces or corsets, 79
    exercises, 77, 78
Low back pain—cont'd
  conservative treatment—cont'd
    routine care, 78
    shoe lifts, 80
    spinal fusion, 81
    traction, 81
  correlation with heavy work, 56, 57
    compensation, 57
  differential diagnosis, 68
  disc degeneration *(q.v.),* 56
  discography, 81
  electromyography, 81
  etiology, 55
  frequency, 56
  kyphosis of thoracic spine, 64
  leg lengths as factor, 65
  lumbago, 54
  lumbar insufficiency, 54
  lumbar lordosis, 60
  lumbarization, 59
  lumbosacral tilt, 61
  malingering, 73
  manifestations, 54
  neurological deficit, 65
  pars interarticularis defects, 63
  pathogenesis of symptoms; *see* under Disc degeneration
  postural foot deformities, 65
  restricted motion of spine, 64
  ruptured disc in thoracic spine, 64
  sacralization, 59
  sacrum, level between ilia, 62
  sciatic tension tests, 65
  sciatica *(q.v.),* 54, 55
  significance, 56
  spondylolisthesis *(q.v.),* 63
  spondylolysis, 63
  spontaneous subsidence, 56
  structures causing, 54, 55
  surgery
    anterior disc excision and interbody spine fusion *(q.v.),* 111
    for elderly, 82
    standard operations, 111
  tender spinous processes, 65
  thoracic spine conditions, 63
  thoracolumbar scoliosis, 63
  tropism, 60
Lumbago
  defined, 54
  diagnosis, 85
  as stage of low back pain, 55
Lumbar insufficiency in low back pain, 54
Lumbar lordosis and low back pain, 60
Lumbarization and low back pain, 59
Lumbosacral pain; *see* Low back pain, manifestations
Lumbosacral strain and instability, 54, 55; *See also* Low back pain
Lumbosacral tilt and low back pain, 61
Lumbosciatic syndrome, correlation with cervical pain, 67

M

Malingering by low back pain patients, 73
  tests for, 73 et seq.
Marie-Strümpell arthritis in differential diagnosis of low back pain, 69
Metastatic malignancy in differential diagnosis of low back pain, 71
Milwaukee brace for scoliosis, 188, 189, 193, 194
Motion and loading, 7, 8
Motor unit as substructure, 4
Multiple back operations
  decision to reoperate, 134
  evaluation of patients, 132
    neurological, orthopaedic, and psychiatric, 133
  refusion
    anterior, 136
    posterior, 134, 135
    posterolateral, 135
    problems, 134
  selection of patients, 141
Multiple myeloma in differential diagnosis of low back pain, 72

N

Neurological deficit and low back pain, 65
Nucleus pulposus, 2, 97

O

Ober's syndrome, 87
Odontoid process, fracture of, 23
Osteoporosis
  areas involved, 168
  causes, 168
  characteristics, 168, 170
  compression fractures, 168, 170
  dietary regimen, 171, 173
  in differential diagnosis of low back pain, 69
  of disuse, 169
  gross pathology, 170
  illustrative cases, 173 et seq.
  treatment
    ambulation, 170
    bed rest, 170
    exercises, 170
    fluoride, 171
    hormonal therapy, 170
    prophylactic, 179
Osteotomy of fused scoliotic spine, 265
  case reports, 268
  operative procedure, 266
  postoperative correction, 267

P

Pancreatitis in differential diagnosis of low back pain, 71
Pars interarticularis defects, 146 et seq.
  cause of low back pain, 63
Pathomechanics, 1; *see also* Biomechanics
Peptic ulcer in differential diagnosis of low back pain, 71
Piriformis syndrome, 86
Plantar flexion of foot test for malingering, 74
Plastic failure of substructures, 5
Postural foot deformities and low back pain, 65
Prostatic cancer in differential diagnosis of low back pain, 71
Pseudoarthritis repairs by fusion, 134, 135
Psychogenic disease in differential diagnosis of low back pain, 73

R

Rachischisis, 143
Restricted motion of spine and low back pain, 64
Retroperitoneal fibrosis in differential diagnosis of low back pain, 71

S

Sacralization and low back pain, 59
Sacroiliac joint disease in differential diagnosis of low back pain, 73
Sciatic scoliosis, 85
Sciatic tension tests and low back pain, 65
Sciatica; *see also* Low back pain
  age at onset, 55
  age at peak incidence, 55
  causes, 67
  defined, 54
  differential diagnosis, 84
  past observations, 84 et seq.
  as stage of low back pain, 55
  surgery for elderly, 82
  traction versus bed rest, 81
Scoliosis
  idiopathic; *see* Idiopathic scoliosis
  nonoperative treatment
    correlation of deformities, 190
    fusion following, 194
    historical review, 188
    Milwaukee brace and exercises, 188, 189, 193, 194
    of round back, 192
  osteotomy; *see* Osteotomy
  pulmonary function in
    abnormalities in lung, 180, 181
    alveolar ventilation, 184, 185
    cor pulmonale, 185
    increased vascular resistance, 185
    management of postoperative secretions, 187
    obstructive lesions, 180
    partial pressures, 183
    residual volume compared to total lung capacity, 180
    shunting of blood, 183
    ventilation/perfusion relationship (V/Q ratio), 181, 183

Scoliosis—cont'd
  pulmonary function in—cont'd
    ventilatory changes, 186
  review of surgery, 265
  thoracolumbar, and low back pain, 63
Shoe lifts for low back pain, 80
Spinal fusion; *see* Fusion
Spondylolisthesis
  of axis, traumatic, 26
  cause of low back pain, 63
  causes, 143
  in cervical vertebrae, 166
  classification, 144
    congenital, 145
    degenerative, 145
    isthmic, 144
    pathological, 145
    pedicular, 145
  conversion of spondylolysis to, 143
  derivation of term, 143
  etiology
    of congenital, 161
    of degenerative, 162
    of isthmic, 146, 157, 158, 161
      determining factors, 146 et seq.
    of pathological, 163
    of pedicular, 163
  reverse (retrograde), 164
  with scoliosis, 234
  surgical treatment, 115, 123
  terminology, 143
Spondylolysis
  cause of low back pain, 63
  conversion to spondylolisthesis, 143
  isthmic, 143
Spondyloschisis, 143
Stress-strain curves from tissue loading, 2
Substructures
  mechanical properties, 4
  relative motion between, 5
  types of failure, 5

T

Thoracic spine in low back pain
  kyphosis, 64
  ruptured disc, 64
  scoliosis, 63
Tissues
  elasticity, 4
  enumerated, 2
  hydrostatic pressure effect, 4
  loading studies, 2; *see also* Loading
  mechanical properties, 2
  specialized, 2
  stress-strain curves, 2
Traction versus bed rest for sciatica, 81
Turnbuckle cast for correction of scoliosis, 241
  application technique, 243
  selection of patients, 244

V

Vacuum phenomenon as evidence of disc degeneration, 60
Valleix's spots on sciatic nerve, 84
Vertebral artery syndrome, 13

W

Whiplash injuries
  associated injuries, 10
  experimental acceleration, 12
    muscle injuries and lesions, 12, 13, 15
  iatrogenic neurosis, 15
    avoidance, 15 et seq.
  litigation neurosis, 10-12
  symptoms, 10
  vertebral artery syndrome, 13
"Whiplash syndrome," 10
Williams' exercises for low back pain, 78